Pediatric **Success**

A Course Review Applying Critical Thinking to Test Taking

Pediatric **Success**

A Course Review Applying Critical Thinking to Test Taking

Beth Richardson, DNS, RN, CPNP, FAANP
Associate Professor
Coordinator of Pediatric Nurse Practitioner Program
Indiana University
Indianapolis, Indiana

F.A. Davis Company • Philadelphia

F. A. Davis Company
1915 Arch Street
Philadelphia, PA 19103
www.fadavis.com

Printed in the United States of America

Last digit indicates print number: 10 9 8 7 6 5 4 3 2

Publisher, Nursing: Robert G. Martone
Director of Content Development: Darlene D. Pedersen
Senior Project Editor: Padraic J. Maroney
Art and Illustration Manager: Carolyn O' Brien

As new scientific information becomes available through basic and clinical research, recommended treatments and drug therapies undergo changes. The author(s) and publisher have done everything possible to make this book accurate, up to date, and in accord with accepted standards at the time of publication. The author(s), editors, and publisher are not responsible for errors or omissions or for consequences from application of the book, and make no warranty, expressed or implied, in regard to the contents of the book. Any practice described in this book should be applied by the reader in accordance with professional standards of care used in regard to the unique circumstances that may apply in each situation. The reader is advised always to check product information (package inserts) for changes and new information regarding dose and contraindications before administering any drug. Caution is especially urged when using new or infrequently ordered drugs.

Contributors

Sherrilyn Coffman, DNS, RN, CPN
Professor and Assistant Dean
Nevada State College
Henderson, Nevada

Dawn Marie Daniels, DNS, RN,
PHCNS-BC
Clinical Nurse Specialist
Riley Hospital for Children
Indianapolis, Indiana

Mary Jo Eoff, RN, MSN, CPNP
Clinical Instructor
Indiana University
Indianapolis, Indiana

Joyce Foresman-Capuzzi, BSN, RN,
CEN, CPN, CCRN, CTRN, CPEN,
SANE-A, EMT-P
Clinical Nurse Educator/Emergency
Department
Lankenau Hospital
Wynnewood, Pennsylvania

Paige Johnson, RN, MSN, MPH,
CRNP
Pediatric Nurse Practitioner
Children's Mercy Hospital
Department of Hematology/Oncology
Kansas City, Missouri

Dominique Leveque, MSN, RN,
CPNP, FNP-C
Workplace Health Services
Clarian Health Partners
Indianapolis, Indiana

Christina Bittles McCarthy, MSN, RN,
CPNP
Pediatric Nurse Practitioner
Indiana University Dept. of Orthopedic
Surgery
Indianapolis, Indiana

Patricia A. Normandin, RN, MSN,
CEN, CPN, CPEN, DNP(c)
Pediatric Nursing Instructor
University of Massachusetts, Lowell
Lowell, Massachusetts

Julie A. Poore, RN, MSN
Visiting Lecturer
Indiana University
Indianapolis, Indiana

Susan P. Wade, MSN, RN, CPN,
CCRN
Clinical Nurse Specialist for Pediatrics and
PICU
Parkview Hospital
Fort Wayne, Indiana

Cele Walter, BSN, RN, CPN, NCSN
High School Nurse
Paul VI High School
Haddonfield, New Jersey

Candace F. Zickler, CPNP, RN, MSN
Supervisor, Health Services
Metropolitan School District of Perry
Township
Indianapolis, Indiana

Reviewers

Jacoline Sommer Albert, AND, RN, BScN, DI
Senior Instructor
The Aga Khan University
Karachi, Pakistan

Monique Alston-Davis, MSN, Ed, CPN
Assistant Professor
Montgomery College
Silver Spring, Maryland

Cathryn J. Baack, PhD, RN, CPNP
Assistant Professor
MedCentral College of Nursing
Mansfield, Ohio

Vicky H. Becherer, MSN, RN
Assistant Teaching Professor
University of Missouri, St. Louis
St. Louis, Missouri

Stacee Bertolla, RN, MSN, CPNP
Instructor
University of South Alabama
Mobile, Alabama

Kathleen Borge, MS, RNC
Faculty Chair, Women and Children's Health
Samaritan Hospital
Troy, New York

Pam Bowden, RN, MS, PNP
Faculty
North Hennepin Community College
Brooklyn Park, Minnesota

Twila J. Brown, PhD, RN
Assistant Professor
Southeast Missouri State University
Cape Girardeau, Missouri

Katherine Bydalek, MSN, FNP-BC, PhD
Assistant Professor
University of South Alabama
Mobile, Alabama

Dena Christianson, MSN, PNP
Adjunct Faculty
Nova Southeastern University
Fort Lauderdale, Florida

Karen Clancy, MS, RN, CNP
Clinical Instructor
Ohio State University
Neonatal Nurse Practitioner
Columbus Children's Hospital
Columbus, Ohio

Myra L. Clark, MS, FNP-C
Assistant Professor
North Georgia College and State University
Dahlonega, Georgia

Lori Clay, MSN, RN
Assistant Professor
Arkansas State University
Jonesboro, Arkansas

Jennifer Bell Frank, MSN, APRN, BC
Instructor
Jacksonville State University
Jacksonville, Alabama

Marianne Fraser, MSN, RN, BC
Assistant Professor
University of Utah
Salt Lake City, Utah

Susan Golden, MSN, RN
Nursing Faculty
Eastern New Mexico University, Roswell
Roswell, New Mexico

Kathy L. Ham, RN, EdD
Assistant Professor
Southeast Missouri State University
Cape Girardeau, Missouri

Brenda J. Walters Holloway, APRN, FNP, DNSc
Clinical Assistant Professor
University of South Alabama
Spanish Fort, Alabama

Mary C. Kishman, PhD, RN
Associate Professor
College of Mount St. Joseph
Cincinnati, Ohio

Katherine R. Kniest, RN, MSN, CNE
Professor
William Rainey Harper College
Palatine, Illinois

Robyn Leo, MSN
Associate Professor
Worcester State College
Worcester, Massachusetts

Barbara J. MacDougall, MSN, ARNP
Nova Southeastern University
Ft. Lauderdale, Florida

Kathleen T. Mohn, RN, MSEd, CLNC
Instructor
College of Southern Nevada
Las Vegas, Nevada

Jennifer Morton, MS, MPH, RN
Assistant Professor
University of New England
Portland, Maine

Irene Owens, MSN, APRN
Instructor
Lake Sumter Community College
Leesburg, Florida

Brenda Pavill, RN, FNP, PhD, IBCLC
Professor
Misericordia University
Dallas, Pennsylvania

Delia Pittman, PhD
Nursing Professor
MidAmerica Nazarene University
Olathe, Kansas

Deborah A. Roberts, RN, BSN, MSN, EdD
Assistant Professor
Humboldt State University
Arcata, California

Rebecca L. Shabo, RN, PNP-BC, PhD
Associate Professor
Kennesaw State University
Kennesaw, Georgia

Cynthia A. Shartle, RN, MSN, APRN, BC-FNP
ADN Faculty
South Texas College
McAllen, Texas

Patsy M. Spratling, RN, MSN
Nursing Instructor
Holmes Community College
Ridgeland, Mississippi

Bev Valkenier, BScN, RN, MSN
Lecturer
University of British Columbia
Vancouver, British Columbia, Canada

Elizabeth M. Wertz, RN, BSN, MPM, EMT-P, PHRN, FACMPE
Chief Executive Officer
Pediatric Alliance, PC
Carnegie, Pennsylvania

Sarah Whitaker, DNS, RN
Nursing Program Director
Dona Ana Community College
Las Cruces, New Mexico

Barbara White, RN, MSN, CCRN
Nursing Instructor
Southwestern Michigan College
Dowagiac, Michigan

Acknowledgments

I would like to thank my children, Jason and Sarah; my grandchildren, Caroline and Darren; and my friends, especially David, for all their love and support.

To students, graduates, and colleagues: thank you for all you do in caring for children and their families.

Contents

Fundamentals of Critical Thinking Related to Test Taking: The RACE Model

1

Pediatric Success: A Course Review Applying Critical Thinking to Test Taking is designed to help you, the student, complete your nursing program as well succeed on the NCLEX–RN examination.

This book applies critical thinking skills primarily to multiple choice questions as well as to some alternate test items. It provides practice test questions and test-taking hints to help you analyze each item and choose the correct response.

Another book in the Success series, *Fundamentals Success* by Nugent and Vitale, explains critical thinking and the RACE Model, which are used in each book in the series. This information will help you answer questions on tests in your nursing courses and on the NCLEX-RN examination. The key to successful studying is knowing the material that will be covered on the examinations. Course notes should be studied every night and corresponding readings done before class. This will help you learn the material and retain it longer. Once you know the material, it is important for you to be able to answer primarily multiple choice questions correctly. The RACE Model will help you succeed with answering questions.

HOW TO USE THIS REVIEW BOOK

The book contains 14 chapters, a final comprehensive examination, and practice questions on CD-ROM. Test-taking hints are included with each question.

This introductory chapter provides guidelines for course test preparation and includes an example of how to use the RACE Model. The RACE Model is an excellent strategy to help you analyze the stem and determine the correct response. The more you use it, the more comfortable you will feel, and then you will use it to answer all your multiple choice questions.

Chapter 2 focuses on growth and development of children from infancy through adolescence. Chapter 3 covers material on issues related to pediatric health. Chapters 4 through 12 follow problems through each of the body systems. Each chapter will have practice questions, answers, and rationales for the correct answer, including test-taking hints, keywords, and abbreviations.

Chapter 13, Leadership and Management, relates to pediatric nursing. Chapter 14, Pharmacology, has been included because of the expressed need of students for extra testing in this area. In the NCLEX-RN test plan (www.ncsbn.org), pharmacology and management of care have a large number of test items. Graduates need to have a working knowledge of issues in these areas. This chapter will include questions centered on what the student nurse caring for children of all ages needs to know about administering medications, actions, dosages, expected effects, adverse effects, and teaching families.

A final 100-question comprehensive examination is included. Two 75-question exit examinations on CD-ROM accompany the book. Students can take the CD-ROM tests prior to the final exam. Questions in this book are written primarily at the application and analysis level and are either multiple choice, with four response choices, or alternate item format. Nursing faculty members write tests in these formats to familiarize students with the NCLEX-RN examination style.

Test Preparation

One of the most important strategies for you is to study thoroughly and know the assigned material for the examination. It is best to study daily so you really learn the material and not wait and try to learn it all at one time. The more time you spend studying the topic, the better you will retain the material.

After you feel confident that you know the material, choose the chapter(s) in this book that correspond(s) with the assigned test material. Take the practice questions to determine your level of knowledge about the topic. Carefully review the questions you miss, making sure you read and understand the rationale for choosing the wrong distracter and why the correct response *is* correct. The rationales provide a great deal of information about the correct and incorrect options, which helps you understand the content better. The test-taking hints are strategies to help you logically determine the correct response. If you still feel uncomfortable with the content area, review that chapter in your textbook for better understanding. This method of preparing for an examination will help you identify your strengths and areas to focus on as you continue to study.

You may want to start with the last chapter, Pharmacology, because you will be administering medications to children throughout your pediatric nursing course. This chapter will help you focus on teaching strategies for families of children receiving medications, differences in delivering drugs to children, and calculating dosages.

RACE Model

The RACE Model is a critical thinking strategy to be used when answering multiple choice questions. The model will help you choose the correct response as you examine test questions critically. For more detailed information about the RACE Model, see *Test Success: Test Taking Techniques for Beginning Nursing Students* by Nugent and Vitale.

The RACE Model comprises:

R—Recognize the keywords in the stem.
A—Ask what the question is asking the nurse to do.
C—Critically analyze each option in relation to the information in the stem.
E—Eliminate as many options as possible to narrow your choice to the correct response.

Some students believe they know the material but have difficulty choosing the correct response when answering multiple choice questions. Using the RACE model will greatly increase your chances of choosing the correct response. In order to use it effectively during timed tests, you need to practice. Using the RACE Model as you prepare yourself with the chapter tests will help you. Following is a sample question:

1. A 6-month-old is being seen in the clinic for a well-child checkup. The parents want to know about starting solid foods. How should the nurse counsel them?
   a. "Since you started rice cereal from a spoon 2 months ago, you can add a new strained vegetable each week."
   b. "Introduce some mashed fruits first. After the infant is eating that well, start vegetables and rice cereal."
   c. "Infants do best eating solids if you spoon-feed a new strained vegetable every other day to see what their preferences are."
   d. "Add rice cereal to each bottle. Next you can add fruits and vegetables fed by spoon."

Using the RACE Model:

R—The client in the stem is the parent.
A—The parents want to know how to add solid foods to their infant's diet.
C—Infants start rice cereal between 4 and 6 months. This is fed to the infant by spoon unless there is an indication to place it in the bottle. That is not stated in the stem of this question. Either strained fruits or vegetables are added to the infant's diet about 6 months of age. The infant stays on that choice for several days to determine if the infant is allergic.
E—Now you can eliminate choices b., c., and d. because they do not contain choices that you know are correct. The remaining choice is a., the correct response.

Growth

KEYWORDS

Anemia
Auscultate
Autonomy
Dehydration
Detachment
Gynecomastia

Hepatitis B
Industry
Inguinal hernia
Initiative
Palpate

ABBREVIATIONS

Atrial septal defect (ASD)
Emergency room (ER)
Face, legs, action, consolability, crying
 (FLACC)
Failure to thrive (FTT)

Intramuscular (IM)
Intravenous (IV)
Nothing by mouth (NPO)
Pound (lb)

QUESTIONS

1. A 3-year-old female is hospitalized for a femur fracture. As her nurse, what nursing action would help foster the child's sense of autonomy?
   1. Allow the child to choose what time to take her oral antibiotics.
   2. Allow the child to have a doll for medical play.
   3. Allow the child to administer her own dose of Keflex (cephalexin) via oral syringe.
   4. Allow the child to watch age-appropriate videos.

2. A 16-year-old male is hospitalized for cystic fibrosis. He will be an inpatient for 2 weeks while he receives IV antibiotics. As the nurse caring for this patient, what action can you take that will most enhance his psychosocial development?
   1. Fax the teen's teacher, and have her send in his homework.
   2. Encourage the teen's friends to visit him in the hospital.
   3. Encourage the teen's grandparents to visit frequently.
   4. Tell the teen he is free to use his phone to call friends.

3. A 6-month-old male is at his well-child checkup. The nurse weighs him, and his mother asks if his weight is normal for his age. The nurse's best response is:
   1. "At 6 months his weight should be approximately three times his birth weight."
   2. "Each child gains weight at his or her own pace."
   3. "At 6 months his weight should be approximately twice his birth weight."
   4. "At 6 months a child should weigh about 10 lb more than his or her birth weight."

4. The nurse caring for a 4-year-old female in the ER is about to start a peripheral IV. The nurse's best method for explaining the procedure to the child is to:
   1. Show the child a pamphlet with pictures showing the IV placement procedure.
   2. Have the 5-year-old patient next door tell the 4-year-old about her experience with her IV placement.
   3. Show the child the IV placement equipment, and demonstrate the procedure on a doll.
   4. Tell the child that if she remains still, the procedure will be over quickly.

5. A 17-year-old male is being seen in the ER. In order to obtain the adolescent's health information, his nurse should:
   1. Interview the adolescent using direct questions.
   2. Gather information during a casual conversation.
   3. Interview the adolescent only in the presence of his parents.
   4. Gather information only from the parents.

6. A 7-year-old female is being admitted to the hospital for a diagnosis of acute lymphocytic leukemia. The nurse wants to gather information from the child regarding her feelings about her diagnosis. Which nursing action is most appropriate to gain information about how the child is feeling?
   1. The nurse should actively attempt to make friends with the child before asking her about her feelings.
   2. The nurse should ask the child's parents what feelings she has expressed in regard to her diagnosis.
   3. The nurse should provide the child with some paper to draw a picture of how she is feeling.
   4. The nurse should ask the child direct questions about how she is feeling.

7. How can the nurse best facilitate the trust relationship between infant and parent while the infant is hospitalized?
   1. The nurse should encourage the parents to remain at their child's bedside as much as possible.
   2. The nurse should keep parents informed about all aspects of their child's condition.
   3. The nurse should encourage the parents to hold their child as much as possible.
   4. The nurse should encourage the parents to participate actively in their child's care.

8. The nurse is caring for a 7-year-old female on the school-age unit. Her mother is concerned that she may have some developmental delays. Which of the following statements would indicate to the nurse that the child is not developmentally on track for her age:
   1. The child is able to follow a four-to-five-step command.
   2. The child started wetting the bed on this admission to the hospital.
   3. The child has an imaginary friend named Kelly.
   4. The child enjoys playing board games with her sister.

9. The nurse is caring for a 6-month-old in the ER. The physician orders the nurse to give the child a dose of Rocephin IM. The 1.5-mL dose arrives from the pharmacy. The nurse must do which of the following?
   1. Administer the injection in the deltoid muscle.
   2. Split the dose into two injections.
   3. Administer the injection in the dorsogluteal muscle.
   4. Administer the dose as a single injection to the vastus lateralis muscle.

10. A 3-year-old female is hospitalized for an ASD repair. Her parents have decided to go home for a few hours to spend time with her siblings. The child asks when her mommy and daddy will be back. The nurse's best response is:
    1. "Your mommy and daddy will be back after your nap."
    2. "Your mommy and daddy will be back at 6 p.m."
    3. "Your mommy and daddy will be back later this evening."
    4. "Your mommy and daddy will be back in 3 hours."

11. A male infant is visiting the pediatrician for his 6-month well-child checkup. His mother tells the nurse she wants to advance the infant's diet. Which statement by the infant's mother leads the nurse to believe that she needs further education about the nutritional needs of a 6-month-old?
    1. "I will continue to breastfeed my son and will give him rice cereal three times a day."
    2. "I will start my son on fruits and gradually introduce vegetables."
    3. "I will start my son on carrots and will introduce one new vegetable every few days."
    4. "I will not give my son any more than 8 ounces of baby juice per day."

12. An ER nurse is assessing a 12-month-old female. Which statement accurately describes the best method for assessing this child?
    1. The nurse should assess the child on the examining table.
    2. The nurse should assess the child in a head-to-toe sequence.
    3. The nurse should have the child's mother assist in holding her down.
    4. The nurse should assess the child while she is in her mother's lap.

13. An 11-year-old male is being evaluated in the ER for an inguinal hernia. Which statement accurately describes how the nurse should approach him for his physical assessment?
    1. The nurse should ask the child's parents to remain in the room during the physical exam.
    2. The nurse should auscultate the child's heart, lungs, and abdomen first.
    3. The nurse should explain to the child that the physical exam will not hurt.
    4. The nurse should explain to the child what the nurse will be doing in basic understandable terms.

14. The school nurse is planning an educational program centered on abstinence for adolescents. Which of the following methods does the nurse recognize as the most effective way to present this program?
    1. Use peer-led programs that emphasize the consequences of unprotected sexual contact.
    2. Teach students methods to resist peer pressure.
    3. Offer students the opportunity to care for a simulator infant for 1 week.
    4. Offer statistics, pamphlets, and films discussing the consequences of unprotected sexual contact.

15. The nurse is instructing a new breastfeeding mother in the need to provide her premature infant with an adequate source of iron in her diet. Which one of the following statements reflects a need for further education of the new mother?
    1. "I will use only breast milk or an iron-fortified formula as a source of milk for my baby until she is at least 12 months old."
    2. "My baby will need to have iron supplements introduced when she is 4 months old."
    3. "I will need to add iron supplements to my baby's diet when she is 9 months old."
    4. "When my baby begins to eat solid foods, I should introduce iron-fortified cereals to her diet."

16. A first-time mother brings in her 5-day-old baby for a well-child visit. The nurse weighs the infant and reports a weight of 7 lb 5 oz to the mother. The mother looks concerned and tells the nurse that her baby weighed 7 lb 10 oz when she was discharged 4 days ago. The nurse's best response to the mother is:
    1. "I will let the doctor know, and he will talk with you about possible causes of your infant's weight loss."
    2. "An initial weight loss of a few ounces is common among newborns, especially for breastfeeding mothers."
    3. "I can tell you are a first-time mother. Don't worry; we will find out why she is losing weight."
    4. "Maybe she isn't getting enough milk. How often are you breastfeeding her?"

17. The nurse is caring for a 12-month-old girl. The child's mother asks if the unit has any toys that her daughter can play with. The nurse goes to the toy area in search of a toy for the child. Which toy is the best choice for this child?
    1. A doll.
    2. A musical rattle.
    3. A board book.
    4. Colorful beads.

18. Which statement by the mother of an 18-month-old would lead the nurse to believe that the child should be referred for further evaluation for developmental delay?
    1. "My child is able to stand but is not yet taking steps independently."
    2. "My child has a vocabulary of approximately 15 words."
    3. "My child is still thumb sucking."
    4. "My child seems to be quite wary of strangers."

19. The mother of a child 2 years 6 months has arranged a play date with the neighbor and her 3-year-old daughter. During the play date the two mothers should expect that the children will do which of the following?
    1. The children will share and trade their toys while playing.
    2. The children will play with one another with little or no conflict.
    3. The children will play alongside one another but not actively with one another.
    4. The children will play with one or two items, ignoring most of the other toys.

20. A 2-year-old boy has been admitted to the hospital for anemia. His mother asks the nurse what foods to include in his diet to improve his nutritional status. Which of the following should the nurse recommend?
    1. Increase the child's intake of whole cow's milk to 32 ounces a day.
    2. Increase the child's intake of meats, eggs, and green vegetables.
    3. Increase the child's intake of fruits, whole grains, and rice.
    4. Increase the number of snacks the child eats during the day.

21. The parents of a 2-year-old boy are concerned about his behavior. Since the child's admission to the hospital 2 days ago he has been crying much more than usual and is inconsolable much of the time. The nurse's best response to the child's parents is:
    1. The child is in the detachment phase of separation anxiety, which is normal for children during hospitalization.
    2. The child is in the despair stage of separation anxiety, which is normal for children during hospitalization.
    3. The child is in the bargaining stage of separation anxiety, which is normal for children during hospitalization.
    4. The child is in the protest stage of separation anxiety, which is normal for children during hospitalization.

22. In order to prevent separation anxiety in a hospitalized toddler, which of the following should the nurse do?
    1. Assume the parental role when parents are not able to be at the bedside.
    2. Encourage the parents to remain at the bedside always.
    3. Establish a routine that is similar to that of the child's home.
    4. Rotate nursing staff so the child becomes comfortable with a variety of nurses.

23. A 5-year-old girl has been brought to the ER for suspected child abuse. What approach should the nurse use to gather information from the child?
    1. The nurse should promise the child that her parents will not know what she tells the nurse.
    2. The nurse should promise the child that she will not have to see the suspected abuser again.
    3. The nurse should use correct anatomical terms to discuss body parts.
    4. The nurse should tell the child that the abuse is not her fault and that she is a good person.

24. A 5-year-old is at the pediatrician's office for his well-child checkup. The nurse will be administering three immunizations to the child. The nurse should expect which reaction from the child when she gives his immunizations?
    1. The child will likely remain silent and still.
    2. The child will likely cry and tell the nurse that it hurts.
    3. The child will likely try to stall the nurse.
    4. The child will likely remain still while telling the nurse that she is hurting him.

25. An 8-year-old is NPO while he awaits surgery for central line placement later in the afternoon. The nurse is trying to engage the child in some form of activity to distract him from thinking about his upcoming surgery. Which is the best method of distraction for a child of this age in this situation?
    1. Encourage the child to use the telephone to call friends.
    2. Encourage the child to watch television.
    3. Encourage the child to play a board game.
    4. Encourage the child to read the central line pamphlet he was given.

26. According to developmental theories, which important event does the nurse understand is essential to the development of the toddler?
    1. The child learns to feed self.
    2. The child develops friendships.
    3. The child learns to walk.
    4. The child participates in being potty-trained.

27. The nurse caring for an 8-year-old boy is trying to encourage developmental growth. What activity can the nurse provide for the child to encourage his sense of industry?
    1. Allow the child to choose what time to take his medication.
    2. Provide the child with the homework his teacher has sent in.
    3. Allow the child to assist with his bath.
    4. Allow the child to help with his dressing change.

28. A female nurse caring for a 5-year-old boy is trying to encourage developmental growth. What can the nurse do to reinforce the child's intellectual initiative when he asks the nurse about his upcoming surgery?
    1. Answer the child's questions about his upcoming surgery in simple terms.
    2. Provide the child with a book that has vivid illustrations about his surgery.
    3. Tell the child he should wait and ask the doctor his questions.
    4. Tell the child that she will answer his questions at a later time.

29. The mother of 11-year-old fraternal twins tells the nurse at their well-child checkup that she is concerned because her daughter has gained more weight and height than her twin brother. The mother is concerned that there is something wrong with her son. The nurse's best response is:
    1. "I understand your concern. I will talk with the physician, and we can draw some lab work."
    2. "I understand your concern. Has your son been ill lately?"
    3. "It is normal for girls to grow a little taller and gain more weight than boys at this age."
    4. "It is normal for you to be concerned, but I am sure your son will catch up with your daughter eventually."

30. A 9-year-old girl builds a clubhouse in her backyard. She hangs a sign outside her clubhouse that says "No boys allowed." The child's parents are concerned that she is excluding their neighbor's son, and they are upset. What should the school nurse tell the child's parents?
    1. Her behavior is cause for concern and should be addressed.
    2. Her behavior is common among school-age children.
    3. Her feelings about boys will subside within the next year.
    4. They should have their daughter speak with the school counselor.

31. The school nurse is preparing a discussion on nutrition with the fourth-grade class. Based on the childrens' developmental level, what information should she include in her presentation?
    1. A review of the number of calories that a fourth-grade child should consume in a day.
    2. A review of a list of high-calorie foods that all fourth-graders should avoid.
    3. A review of how to read food labels so children know which foods are good for them.
    4. A review of nutritious foods with basic scientific information about how they affect the body organs and systems.

32. An 18-year-old boy comes to the ER complaining of a rash and itching in the groin area. He is concerned that he has contracted a sexually transmitted disease and worries that his parents will find out. The nurse's best response is:
    1. "We will need to contact your parents to let them know you are in the ER."
    2. "We will not contact your parents regarding this visit."
    3. "Who would you like us to contact about your visit here today?"
    4. "We cannot promise that the hospital will not contact your parents."

33. A 2-day-old girl is being discharged home. The nurse is working on discharge teaching with her parents. They are asking the nurse about how to use the infant car seat and where it should be placed in their vehicle. Which of the following should the nurse do?
    1. Give the parents a pamphlet explaining how to install the car seat.
    2. Accompany the parents to the car, and show them how to install the car seat.
    3. Contact the hospital's car-seat safety officer, and ask the officer to accompany the parents to the car for car-seat installation.
    4. Show the parents a video on car-seat installation and safety, and ask if they are comfortable with the information.

34. A 3-year-old girl is attending her grandfather's funeral. Her parents have told her that her grandfather is in heaven with God. The child is taken up to the open casket with her parents. Which statement by the child describes a 3-year-old child's understanding of spirituality?
    1. "Grandpa's body is here with us on Earth, and his spirit is in heaven."
    2. "Grandpa is in heaven. Is this heaven?"
    3. "Grandpa's spirit is no longer in his body."
    4. "Grandpa won't need his body in heaven."

35. A 13-year-old boy is hospitalized for a femur fracture. He was hit by a car while he and his friends were racing bikes near a major intersection. The child's parents are concerned about his judgment. What should the nurse understand?
    1. The child's behavior is typical of young teens.
    2. The child's behavior is related to hormonal surges during adolescence.
    3. This was an isolated incident and will not likely happen again.
    4. The child's behavior is related to teen rebellion.

36. A 2-day-old girl is being discharged from the hospital. Her mother asks the nurse when she will receive her first hepatitis B immunization. Which is the nurse's best response?
    1. "Babies receive the hepatitis B vaccine only if their mother is hepatitis B–positive."
    2. "She will receive her first dose of the hepatitis B vaccine prior to discharge today."
    3. "She will receive her first hepatitis B vaccine when she is 1 year of age."
    4. "She will receive her first hepatitis B vaccine at 6 months of age."

37. The nurse is performing a physical assessment on a 6-month-old baby. Which finding should the nurse understand as abnormal for this child?
    1. The child's posterior fontanel is open.
    2. The child's anterior fontanel is open.
    3. The child has the beginning signs of tooth eruption.
    4. The child is able to track and follow objects.

38. A 16-year-old girl is having a discussion with her nurse about her recent diagnosis of lupus. The nurse understands how to best answer the young woman's questions about her prognosis because she understands that cognitively:
    1. Adolescents are preoccupied with thoughts of the here and now.
    2. Adolescents are able to understand and imagine possibilities for the future.
    3. Adolescents are capable of thinking only in concrete terms.
    4. Adolescents are overly concerned with past events and relationships.

39. The mother of a 13-year-old girl tells the nurse that she is concerned because her daughter has gained 10 lb since she began puberty. The child's mother asks the nurse for advice about what to do about her daughter's weight gain. Which of the following should the nurse do?
    1. Provide the child's mother with some pamphlets on nutrition and healthy eating.
    2. Provide the child's mother with information about a new exercise program for teens.
    3. Inform the child's mother that it is common for teen girls to gain weight during puberty.
    4. Inform the child's mother that her daughter will likely gain another 5 to 10 lb in the next year.

40. A 13-year-old boy is visiting the pediatrician's office for his well-child checkup. The child tells the nurse that he is worried because his breasts are growing and they hurt. He tells the nurse he is afraid to take his shirt off in front of the other boys during gym class. What should the nurse tell him?
    1. "The pediatrician will draw some blood to find out why your breasts are growing."
    2. "It is just a slight hormonal imbalance that can be easily corrected with medication."
    3." This is a normal condition of puberty that will resolve within a year or two."
    4. "This is a rare finding that occurs in about 5% of boys during puberty."

41. An 8-year-old girl is at the pediatrician's office for a well-child checkup. Her mother tells the nurse that she has been having some difficulty getting her daughter to complete her chores. The child's mother asks the nurse for techniques for gaining the child's cooperation with chores. Which of the following should the nurse suggest the mother do?
    1. Use "grounding" as a technique.
    2. Use "time-out" as a technique.
    3. Use a reward system as a technique.
    4. Use spanking as a technique.

42. A 5-year-old boy has always been one of the shortest children in class since pre-school. His mother tells the school nurse that her husband is 6' and she is 5'7". She is concerned about her son's height. Based on her knowledge of a child's physical growth during the school-age years, what should the nurse tell the child's mother?
    1. She should expect him to grow about 3 inches every year from ages 6 to 9 years.
    2. She should expect him to grow about 2 inches every year from ages 6 to 9 years.
    3. She should have him seen by an endocrinologist for growth hormone injections.
    4. Be sure to have her son's growth reevaluated when he is 7 years old.

43. A 2-year-old girl has just become a big sister. Her mother has been a stay-at-home mother. Based on the developmental level of a 2-year-old, which comment should the child's mother expect from her toddler about her new baby brother?
    1. "Mommy, when my baby brother takes a nap, will you play with me?"
    2. "Mommy, can I play with my baby brother?"
    3. "Mommy, he is so cute. I love him."
    4. "Mommy, it is time to put him away so we can play."

44. A mother requests that her child receive the varicella vaccine at her 9-month well-child checkup. The nurse tells the mother that:
    1. Children who are vaccinated will likely develop a mild case of the disease from the vaccine.
    2. The nurse cannot give the vaccine.
    3. The nurse will administer the vaccine after the physician examines the child.
    4. The child will need a booster vaccination at 18 months of age.

45. A 16-year-old boy has a diagnosis of new onset diabetes. The child is meeting with the nurse educator regarding changes that will need to be made in his diet. What would most influence a teenager's food choices?
    1. Parents and their dietary choices.
    2. Cultural background.
    3. Peers and their dietary choices.
    4. Television and other forms of media influence.

46. The parents of a 7-month-old girl are attending a class on child safety. Following the class, what should the child's parents understand as one of the most common causes of injury and death for a 7-month-old child?
    1. Poisoning.
    2. Child abuse.
    3. Aspiration.
    4. Dog bites.

47. A 3-year-old boy has been hospitalized because he fell down the stairs. His mother is crying and states, "This is all my fault." Which is the nurse's best response to the child's mother?
    1. "Accidents happen. You shouldn't blame yourself."
    2. "Falls are one of the most common injuries for toddlers."
    3. "It may be a good idea to put a baby gate on the stairs."
    4. "Your son should be proficient at walking down the stairs by now."

48. A 9-year-old boy has been hospitalized following a bicycle injury. What should the nurse recommend to the child's parents to prevent future injury?
    1. Their son should wear safety equipment while riding bicycles.
    2. Their son should read educational material on bicycle safety.
    3. Their son should watch a video on bicycle safety.
    4. Their son should ride his bike in the presence of adults.

49. An 8-day old female was admitted to the hospital with vomiting and dehydration. The nurse has just obtained vital signs. The child's heart rate is 185, her respiratory rate is 44, her blood pressure is 85/52, and her temperature is 99°F (37.2° C). The child's parents ask the nurse if her vital signs are within normal limits. What is the nurse's best response to the parents?
    1. "Your daughter's blood pressure is elevated, but the other vital signs are within normal limits."
    2. "Your daughter's temperature is elevated, but the other vital signs are within normal limits."
    3. "Your daughter's respiratory rate is elevated, but the other vital signs are within normal limits."
    4. "Your daughter's heart rate is elevated, but the other vital signs are within normal limits."

50. An 11-month-old girl has a diagnosis of iron-deficiency anemia. The child's mother tells the nurse that her daughter is currently taking iron and a multivitamin. Which statement made by the mother should be of concern to the nurse?
    1. "I give my daughter her iron and multivitamin at the same time each morning."
    2. "I give my daughter her iron and her multivitamin in her morning 6-oz bottle."
    3. "I give my daughter her iron and multivitamin in a nipple before I feed her the morning bottle."
    4. "I give my daughter her iron and multivitamin in oral syringes toward the back of her cheek."

51. The mother of a 15-year-old boy is frustrated because he spends much of his weekend time sleeping. She informs the nurse, "My son sleeps longer now than he did when he was in kindergarten." What is the nurse's best response to the child's mother's frustration?
    1. "Your son may be trying to catch up on the sleep he misses during the week while he is studying."
    2. "Developmental theorists believe that teens require more sleep as they begin to integrate new roles into their lives."
    3. "Teens require more sleep due to the rapid physical growth that is occurring during adolescence."
    4. "Teens require more sleep due to the increase in their social obligations."

52. A 5-year-old boy is being screened for developmental delays using the Denver Developmental Screening Test. The child's mother is explaining to the nurse her understanding of the screening test. The nurse realizes that the child's mother needs further education about the test when she states which of the following?
    1. "It screens my son's gross motor skills."
    2. "It screens my son's fine motor skills."
    3. "It screens my son's intelligence level."
    4. "It screens my son's language development."

53. The mother has brought her 16-year-old daughter to the ER because she is concerned her daughter is anorexic. During the child's initial physical assessment, the nurse notes the daughter has signs and symptoms of nutritional deficit. Which assessment item led the nurse to this initial conclusion?
    1. The child has a protein level within normal limits.
    2. The child's blood pressure is 110/66.
    3. The child's hair and nails are brittle and dry.
    4. The child's teeth appear to be eroded.

54. A 3-year-old was admitted to the hospital with croup. His nurse just obtained vital signs. The child's heart rate is 90, his respiratory rate is 44, his blood pressure is 100/52, and his temperature is 98.8°F (37.1° C). The parents ask the nurse if his vital signs are appropriate for a child his age. The nurse's best response to the parents is:
    1. "Your son's blood pressure is elevated, but the other vital signs are within normal limits."
    2. "Your son's temperature is elevated, but the other vital signs are within normal limits."
    3. "Your son's respiratory rate is elevated, but the other vital signs are within normal limits."
    4. "Your son's heart rate is elevated, but the ogther vital signs are within normal limits."

55. The nurse caring for a 9-month-old is using the FLACC scale to rate her pain level. The child's parents ask the nurse what the FLACC scale is. Which is the nurse's best response?
    1. "It estimates a child's level of pain utilizing vital sign information."
    2. "It estimates a child's level of pain based on parents' perception."
    3. "It estimates a child's level of pain utilizing behavioral and physical responses."
    4. "It estimates a child's level of pain utilizing a numeric scale from 0 to 5."

56. A 12-month-old boy weighed 8 lb 2 oz at birth. Understanding developmental milestones, what should the nurse caring for the child calculate his current weight as?
    1. Approximately 16 lb 4 oz.
    2. Approximately 20 lb 5 oz.
    3. Approximately 24 lb 6 oz.
    4. Approximately 32 lb 8 oz.

57. An 8-week-old male has just had surgery for pyloric stenosis. His nurse is assessing his level of pain. The child's mother asks the nurse what vital sign changes she should expect to see in a child who is experiencing pain. The nurse's best response is:
    1. "We expect to see a child's heart rate decrease and respiratory rate increase."
    2. "We expect to see a child's heart rate and blood pressure decrease."
    3. "We expect to see a child's heart rate and blood pressure increase."
    4. "We expect to see a child's heart rate increase and blood pressure decrease."

58. A 17-year-old male has had some recent behavioral changes. His mother calls the nurse at the pediatrician's office and tells her that her son has been coming home from school every day, closing his door, and refraining from interaction with his parents. The child's mother does not know what she should do about her son's unsociable behavior. The nurse's best response to the child's mother is:
    1. "You should go speak with your son and ask him directly what is wrong with him."
    2. "You should set limits with your son and tell him that this is unacceptable behavior."
    3. "Your son's behavior is abnormal, and he is going to need a psychiatric referral."
    4. "Your son's behavior is normal. You should listen to him without being judgmental."

59. A 4-year-old is visiting the pediatrician's office for his well-child checkup. The nurse needs to take his blood pressure. Which action by the nurse is a developmentally appropriate method for eliciting the child's cooperation?
    1. Have the child's parents help put on the blood pressure cuff.
    2. Tell the child that if he sits still, the blood pressure machine will go quickly.
    3. Ask the child if he feels a squeezing of his arm.
    4. Tell the child that blood pressures do not hurt.

60. A 4-year-old has been hospitalized with FTT. The child has orders for daily weights, strict input and output, and calorie counts as a means of measuring her nutritional status. Which action by the nurse would be a concern?
    1. The nurse weighs the child every morning before the child eats breakfast.
    2. The nurse weighs the child with no clothing except for undergarments.
    3. The nurse sits with the child when the child eats her meals.
    4. The nurse weighs the child using the same scale every morning.

61. Which of the following are stressors common to hospitalized toddlers? Select all that apply.
    1. Social isolation.
    2. Interrupted routine.
    3. Sleep disturbances.
    4. Self-concept disturbances.
    5. Fear of being hurt.

1. 1. Medication administration times must be adhered to. A 3-year-old should not be allowed to choose administration times.
   2. A doll for medical play is an excellent method for teaching children about medical procedures, but it will not enhance her sense of autonomy.
   3. **Allowing toddlers to participate in actions of which they are capable is an excellent way to enhance their autonomy.**
   4. Age-appropriate videos are a good way to occupy the child while she is hospitalized, but they will not enhance her autonomy.

   TEST-TAKING HINT: The test taker must understand the meaning of the word "autonomy" in order to answer this question. The question also requires knowledge of Erickson's stages. The test taker also needs to consider safe nursing care. Answer 1 could be detrimental to the welfare of the child.

2. 1. The teen may want to continue his schoolwork while in the hospital, but it is not the best means of enhancing his psychosocial development.
   2. **Teens are most concerned about being like their peers. Having the teen's friends visit will help him feel he is still part of the school and social environment.**
   3. The teen may want to see his grandparents, but they are not the primary focus in his life.
   4. Calling friends is a good means of remaining in contact with peers. However, having direct contact with friends is a better means of maintaining social contact.

   TEST-TAKING HINT: The age of the child is essential to answering this question. The test taker must understand that peers are central to an adolescent's life.

3. 1. At 6 months his weight should be approximately two times his birth weight.
   2. Children gain weight at their own pace but should double the birth weight by 4 to 6 months.
   3. **Children should double their birth weight by 4 to 6 months of age.**
   4. By 6 months an infant should have doubled the birth weight; 10 lb is a lot of weight to gain in 4 to 6 months.

   TEST-TAKING HINT: This is a specific physical developmental milestone that should be memorized.

4. 1. The child is too young to understand the procedure using pamphlets.
   2. Children 4 years old are egocentric and will not relate the other child's experience to their own.
   3. **A 4-year-old child understands things in very concrete and simple terms. Therefore, medical play is an excellent method for helping her understand the procedure.**
   4. The nurse has no idea how long the procedure will take and should not give the child information that may not be reliable.

   TEST-TAKING HINT: The age of the child is essential to answering this question. The test taker must understand the developmental level of the child in order to choose the appropriate intervention. Most 4-year-old patients are unable to read, so choice 1 can be eliminated.

5. 1. Teens may not speak as freely when asked direct questions.
   2. **Frequently adolescents will share more information when it is gathered during a casual conversation.**
   3. Teens may share more information when they are not in the presence of their parents. It is important to interview the child first. Parent information can be obtained following the interview with the child.
   4. It is important to gather information from both the teen and the parent.

   TEST-TAKING HINT: The age of the child is essential to answering this question. Answers 3 and 4 contain the word "only." There are rare instances in nursing when the word "only" would apply. These answers can usually be eliminated.

6. 1. The nurse should not attempt to make friends with the child too quickly. The child should be given the opportunity to observe the nurse working in order to increase her comfort level with the nurse.
   2. The child's parents are a good source of information, but the child may not have expressed all of her feelings to her parents.
   3. **Often children will include much more detail of their feelings in drawings. They will often express things in pictures they are unable to verbalize.**
   4. School-age children do not often share all of their feelings verbally, especially to people with whom they are not familiar.

TEST-TAKING HINT: The age of the child is essential to answering this question. The test taker must also have knowledge of psychosocial development of the school-age child.

7. 1. Having parents close to the child is important, but infants are most secure when they are being held, patted, and talked to.
2. It is important that the nurse keep the parents informed about their child's condition, but it does not have any impact on the child's trust versus mistrust relationship with the parents.
3. **Having parents hold their child while in the hospital is an excellent means of building the trust relationship. Infants are most secure when they are being held, patted, and spoken to.**
4. Parents should be encouraged to learn their child's care, but it is not the best means of enhancing the trust relationship.

TEST-TAKING HINT: The test taker must understand Erickson's stages, including the individual tasks that are met during each stage.

8. 1. School-age children should be able to follow a four- to five-step command, so this does not indicate that the child has a developmental delay.
2. The child was potty-trained before entering the hospital, and it is important to inform her mother that bedwetting is a common form of regression seen in hospitalized children. The child will likely return to her normal toileting habits when she returns home.
3. **Most school-age children do not have imaginary friends. This is much more common for children of 3 and 4 years of age.**
4. Most school-age children do enjoy playing board games.

TEST-TAKING HINT: The test taker must also understand the stressors that affect children who are hospitalized and how they will react to those stressors based on their developmental level.

9. 1. The deltoid of a 6-month-old is not developed enough and should not be used for IM injections.
2. **A nurse should not deliver more than 1 mL per IM injection to a child of 6 months.**
3. The dorsogluteal muscle should not be used in children until they have been walking for at least 2 years.

4. The vastus lateralis is the site of choice for an IM injection for a child 6 months old. However, the injection should not be more than 1 mL for a single injection.

TEST-TAKING HINT: The test taker must have knowledge of IM injections sites and acceptable volumes for children of varying ages.

10. 1. **Preschoolers understand time in relation to events.**
2. Preschoolers cannot tell time.
3. Preschoolers want concrete information, and the words "this evening" are not meaningful to them.
4. Preschoolers have no concept how long an hour is.

TEST-TAKING HINT: The age of the child is essential to answering this question. The test taker must have knowledge of a child's understanding of the concept of time. Answers 2, 3, and 4 can be eliminated because they provide choices for time measurement that would only be understandable to children school-age or older.

11. 1. Breastfeeding is the ideal nutrition for the first year of life. Cereal can be introduced between 4 and 6 months of age.
2. **Infants should be started on vegetables prior to fruits. The sweetness of the fruits may inhibit them from taking vegetables.**
3. It is essential to introduce new foods one at a time to determine if a child has any allergies.
4. Infants can be given fruit juice by 6 months of age, but it is recommended not to exceed 4 to 6 ounces per day.

TEST-TAKING HINT: The test taker must have knowledge of the recommended nutrition for an infant.

12. 1. Children 12 months old are best assessed in proximity to their parents.
2. The appropriate sequence for assessment with an infant is to auscultate first, palpate next, and assess ears, eyes, and mouth last. Least invasive procedures are recommended first.
3. Infants do not like to be held down. This will likely cause the child distress. If the child needs to be held down, it is best to enlist the aid of another staff member.
4. **Infants are most secure when in proximity to the parent. The parent's lap is an excellent place to assess the child.**

TEST-TAKING HINT: Health-care professionals must use developmentally appropriate methods to approach children. The test taker must have knowledge of a child's psychosocial development. Answers 1 and 2 can be eliminated because these methods of assessment would be used on an older child.

13. 1. Privacy is very important to school-age children. The child should be given the choice whether his parents are present for the exam.
    2. School-age children can be assessed in a head-to-toe sequence.
    3. The nurse should not promise that the exam will not hurt. Palpation of the area of the hernia may hurt the child, and that may jeopardize the trust relationship between the nurse and the child.
    4. **School-age children are capable of understanding basic functions of the body and should be taught about their diagnosis in simple, basic terms.**

TEST-TAKING HINT: Health-care professionals must approach children using developmentally appropriate methods. The test taker must have knowledge of a child's psychosocial development. Answers 1 and 2 can be eliminated because they are methods of assessment used for younger children.

14. 1. **Adolescents are most concerned with what their peers think and feel. They are most receptive to information that comes from another adolescent.**
    2. It is very difficult for teens to resist peer pressure even with the appropriate tools of resistance.
    3. Infant simulators are useful, but they are very expensive and often difficult to obtain.
    4. Pamphlets are helpful aids in relaying information to teens, but hearing the information firsthand from a peer is the most effective method of education.

TEST-TAKING HINT: The test taker must understand the psychosocial development of an adolescent in order to choose the appropriate intervention. Adolescents focus on their relationships with peers and are much more influenced by peers than by multimedia information or by information provided by an adult.

15. 1. Breast milk or an iron-fortified formula is recommended as the primary source of nutrition for the first year of life.
    2. Premature infants have iron stores from the mother that last approximately 2 months, so it is important to introduce an iron supplement by 2 months.
    3. **Premature infants have iron stores from the mother that last approximately 2 months, so it is important to introduce an iron supplement by 2 months. Full-term infants have iron stores that last approximately 4 to 6 months.**
    4. Iron-fortified cereals are a good source of iron once a child is old enough to consume solid foods.

TEST-TAKING HINT: The test taker must have knowledge of the recommended nutrition for an infant.

16. 1. The nurse should inform the physician how many ounces the infant lost. However, a loss of a few ounces during the first few days of life is normal. There will be reason for concern if the infant does not gain weight within the next week.
    2. **Newborns can lose up to 10% of their birth weight without concern but should regain their birth weight by 2 weeks of age.**
    3. The nurse should not make this comment. The mother will likely feel belittled, and she may be afraid to ask questions in the future.
    4. A loss of a few ounces during the first few days of life is normal. Many times infants of breastfeeding mothers lose weight initially because the mother's milk has not come in yet.

TEST-TAKING HINT: The test taker can eliminate 3. This is a non-therapeutic response. Remembering that newborns can lose up to 10% of their birth weight will help you choose the right response.

17. 1. The child can play with a small doll, but she will likely just put the doll in her mouth. She is not old enough to play appropriately with this toy.
    2. **A musical rattle is the perfect toy for this child. Infants have short attention spans and enjoy auditory and visual stimulation.**
    3. Reading to children is essential throughout childhood. However, the child will

likely just chew on the book, so it is not the ideal choice.

4. Beads are not appropriate for infants due to the risk of choking.

TEST-TAKING HINT: The test taker must understand the developmental level of the child in order to choose the appropriate toy. The test taker must also understand safety issues for a child this age.

18. 1. **The child should be walking independently by 15 to 18 months. Because this toddler is 18 months and not walking, a referral should be made for a developmental consult.**

2. The vocabulary of an 18-month-old should be 10 words or more.

3. Thumb sucking is still common for 18-month-olds and may actually be at its peak at that age.

4. It is very common for a child of 18 months to exhibit stranger anxiety.

TEST-TAKING HINT: The age of the child is essential to answering this question. The test taker must understand basic developmental milestones in order to choose the appropriate intervention.

19. 1. Toddlers do not share their possessions well. One of their favorite words is "mine."

2. Because toddlers do not share well, they are often in conflict with one another during play.

3. **Toddlers engage in parallel play. They often play alongside another child but they rarely engage in activities with the other child.**

4. Toddlers have very short attention spans and commonly play with various items for short periods.

TEST-TAKING HINT: The age of the child is essential to answering this question. The test taker must understand the developmental level of the child in order to choose the appropriate form of play.

20. 1. One of the primary reasons toddlers develop anemia is because they are consuming too much milk, which is limiting their intake of iron-rich foods. Milk is a poor source of iron and should be limited to 24 ounces per day for a child with anemia.

2. **Meat, eggs, and green vegetables are excellent sources of iron.**

3. Iron-enriched cereals are a good choice for children, but this list of foods is not the choice of the most iron-rich foods.

4. Increasing the number of snacks the child consumes is not the focus. Instead, the focus is on providing the child with the most iron-rich foods.

TEST-TAKING HINT: The test taker must have knowledge of the recommended nutrition for children. The test taker must also have knowledge of foods that are high in iron.

21. 1. During the detachment phase of separation anxiety, children are usually fairly cheerful, and they often lack a preference for their parents.

2. During the despair stage of separation anxiety, children usually have a loss of appetite, altered sleep patterns, and a lack of much interest in play.

3. The bargaining stage is not a stage of separation anxiety; it is one of the stages of grief.

4. **During the protest stage of separation anxiety, children are often inconsolable, and they often cry more than they do when they are at home. These children also frequently ask to go home.**

TEST-TAKING HINT: The test taker must have knowledge of the stages of separation anxiety.

22. 1. The nurse should try to comfort the child and be friendly, but she should not try to replace the parent.

2. Parents should be encouraged to be with their child as much as possible. However, parents may feel guilty if they leave knowing the staff believes the parents should always be at the bedside.

3. **It is very important to try to maintain a child's home routine both when parents are present and when they have to leave the hospital. This will increase the child's sense of security and decrease anxiety.**

4. Providing consistent nursing care is important, not rotating staff. The child needs consistent care to decrease anxiety.

TEST-TAKING HINT: The test taker must have knowledge of the stages of separation anxiety. Answer 1 can be ruled out because the nurse should never assume a parental role with a child. Answer 4 can be eliminated because it is essential that children be provided with continuity of care.

23. 1. The nurse should not promise not to tell. The nurse should always be honest with the child in order to develop a level of trust.
2. The nurse should not make a promise that cannot be kept. Once again, the trust relationship could be jeopardized if the child feels the nurse lied to her.
3. The nurse should discuss body parts in relation to the child's vocabulary.
4. **Many young children believe abuse or illness is their fault, and they should be reminded they are not to blame. Many children of this age believe they have acquired a disease or have been abused because they are bad people.**

TEST-TAKING HINT: Children of this age often believe an injury or abuse is their fault. They sometimes feel they are being punished for being bad. The safety and security of the child is paramount in this situation. The child needs to know she is now safe and she did not cause the abuse. Answers 1 and 2 can be eliminated because of the word "promise." The nurse needs to build a trusting relationship with the child and should never make a promise that cannot be kept.

24. 1. Teens are more likely to be stoic and remain still and silent during injections.
2. **The common response of a 5-year-old is to cry and protest during an immunization.**
3. School-age children are most likely to try to stall the nurse.
4. Teens usually remain still, and they may calmly tell the nurse that they are feeling pain during the injection.

TEST-TAKING HINT: The age of the child is essential to answering this question. The test taker must understand the child's psychosocial development in order to choose the appropriate response.

25. 1. Talking to friends may distract the child for some time. However, the conversation could revert to a discussion about the upcoming surgery.
2. Watching television may distract the child for some time, but he may still be thinking about his surgery.
3. **A board game is the optimal choice because school-age children enjoy being engaged in an activity with others that will require some skill and challenge.**
4. Reading material about the surgery will only increase his thoughts about the surgery.

TEST-TAKING HINT: The age of the child is essential to answering this question. The test taker must understand the cognitive developmental level of the child in order to choose the appropriate method of distraction.

26. 1. Toddlers are in a stage of life where they like to do for themselves. However, developmental theorists like Erickson and Freud believe that toilet training is the essential event that must be mastered by the toddler.
2. Toddlers engage in more parallel play. Building friendships is not common until school age and adolescence.
3. Walking should be mastered by 18 months of age.
4. **Developmental theorists like Erickson and Freud believe that toilet training is the essential event that must be mastered by the toddler.**

TEST-TAKING HINT: The test taker must have knowledge of Freud and Erickson's developmental theories.

27. 1. Giving the child choices while in the hospital is important. However, medications should be kept on schedule. It is essential to give them at the prescribed time.
2. **The school-age child is focused on academic performance; therefore the child can achieve a sense of industry by completing his homework and staying on track with his classmates.**
3. The child should have already mastered bathing. It is not likely to give him a sense of accomplishment.
4. The child may enjoy assisting with his dressing change, but it is not the best example of industry.

TEST-TAKING HINT: The test taker must have knowledge of Erickson's stages of development. Answer 1 can be eliminated because it could be detrimental to children to allow them to choose medication times. Answers 3 and 4 can be eliminated because they are not activities that help the child achieve a sense of industry.

28. 1. **The child is taking the initiative to ask questions, as all toddlers do, and the nurse should always answer those questions as appropriately and accurately as possible.**
2. A book illustrating what will happen to the child may help him, but it will not encourage his intellectual initiative.

3. By not answering the child's questions, the nurse may actually be stifling his sense of initiative.

4. By not answering the child's questions, the nurse may actually be stifling his sense of initiative.

TEST-TAKING HINT: The age of the child is essential to answering this question. The test taker must understand the cognitive level of the child in order to choose the appropriate intervention. Answers 3 and 4 can be eliminated because the nurse is avoiding the child's questions.

29. 1. This is not an appropriate response. The nurse should be aware that it is normal for girls to grow taller and gain more weight than boys near the end of middle childhood.

2. This is not an appropriate response. The nurse should be aware that it is normal for girls to grow taller and gain more weight than boys near the end of middle childhood.

3. **This is the appropriate response. The nurse understands that it is normal for girls to grow taller and gain more weight than boys near the end of middle childhood.**

4. This is not the best response. The boy will likely surpass his sister when he reaches adolescence.

TEST-TAKING HINT: This is a specific physical developmental milestone that should be memorized.

30. 1. The child's behavior is normal. Girls of 9 and 10 generally prefer to have friends who are of the same gender.

2. **This is common behavior. Girls of 9 and 10 generally prefer to have friends who are of the same gender.**

3. Girls of 9 and 10 generally prefer to have friends who are of the same gender. The child will likely have the same feelings next year.

4. There is no need for the child to see the counselor. Girls of 9 and 10 generally prefer to have friends who are of the same gender.

TEST-TAKING HINT: The age of the child is essential to answering this question. The test taker must understand the psychosocial development of the child in order to choose the appropriate behavior. Answer 3 can be eliminated because it is too absolute. There is no way to determine

exactly how long the child will have these feelings about boys.

31. 1. School-age children do not engage in calorie counting. This is an adult activity.

2. Children may not want to hear this information, as most of them enjoy consuming high-calorie foods that taste good.

3. School-age children do not engage in calorie counting. This is an adult activity.

4. **Reviewing nutritious choices keeps the lesson on a positive note, and school-age children are very interested in how food affects their bodies. They are capable of understanding basic medical terminology.**

TEST-TAKING HINT: The test taker must have knowledge of the school-age children's cognitive level and their ability to process and understand information.

32. 1. An 18-year-old has a right to privacy; if he does not want his parents contacted, as long as no harm has come to him they do not need to be contacted.

2. **An adolescent has every right to privacy as long as the situation is not life-threatening.**

3. The nurse can ask if the patient would like the nurse to contact someone; again, if the teen says no, that is his or her right.

4. An adolescent has every right to privacy as long as the situation is not life-threatening. Therefore, the hospital can promise not to contact the parents.

TEST-TAKING HINT: The test taker must have knowledge of the psychosocial development of an adolescent and what the state law says about privacy.

33. 1. Pamphlets may be a useful tool to reinforce teaching. However, a hands-on approach is best in this situation.

2. The nurse could accompany the parents if she is proficient in car-seat safety and installation.

3. **The car-seat safety officer is the best choice, as that individual would have the needed information and certification to help the family.**

4. A video may be a useful tool to reinforce teaching. However, a hands-on approach is best in this situation.

TEST-TAKING HINT: The question requires knowledge of the safety concerns involving improper car-seat installation. The question also requires the test taker to

implement teaching and learning strategies for educating parents. Most people learn best with demonstration and return demonstration. Therefore the test taker can eliminate answers 1 and 4.

34. 1. Children 3 years old do not understand the difference between body and spirit. Their understanding of spirituality is literal in nature.
    2. **Children 3 years old are literal thinkers. The child's parents told her that Grandpa was in heaven. She sees his body, so she thinks they are all in heaven.**
    3. Children 3 years old do not understand the difference between body and spirit. Their understanding of spirituality is literal in nature.
    4. Children 3 years old think of spirituality in literal terms and do not understand the concept of heaven.

    TEST-TAKING HINT: The age of the child is essential to answering this question. The test taker must understand the cognitive development of the child in order to choose the appropriate response. Answers 1, 3, and 4 can be eliminated because they demonstrate the understanding of an older school-age child.

35. 1. **The brains of young teens are not completely developed, which often leads to poor judgment and low impulse control.**
    2. Hormonal changes in teens play a primary role in the development of secondary sex characteristics.
    3. The child may be prone to other lapses in judgment. The brains of young teens are not completely developed, which often leads to poor judgment and low impulse control.
    4. The child's behavior had nothing to do with rebellion.

    TEST-TAKING HINT: The age of the child is essential to answering this question. The test taker must understand the psychosocial and cognitive development of the adolescent in order to choose the appropriate intervention.

36. 1. Babies born to mothers positive for hepatitis B receive the first dose of hepatitis B vaccine within 12 hours of delivery.
    2. **The first dose of hepatitis B vaccine is recommended between birth and 2 months. Most hospitals give the vaccine prior to discharge home.**

3. The first dose of hepatitis B vaccine is recommended between birth and 2 months. Most hospitals give the vaccine prior to discharge home.
4. The first dose of hepatitis B vaccine is recommended between birth and 2 months. Most hospitals give the vaccine prior to discharge home.

TEST-TAKING HINT: The test taker must have knowledge of vaccination schedules for children of varying ages.

37. 1. **The posterior fontanel should close between 6 and 8 weeks of age.**
    2. The anterior fontanel usually closes between 12 and 18 months.
    3. The infant usually has a first tooth by 6 months.
    4. The infant should be able to track objects.

    TEST-TAKING HINT: This is a specific physical developmental milestone that should be memorized.

38. 1. Adolescents are becoming abstract thinkers and are able to imagine possibilities for the future.
    2. **Adolescents are becoming abstract thinkers and are able to imagine possibilities for the future.**
    3. Preschool and school-age children think in concrete terms. Adolescents are beginning to think in abstract terms.
    4. Adolescents are becoming abstract thinkers and are able to imagine possibilities for the future. They are not preoccupied with past events.

    TEST-TAKING HINT: The test taker must understand the cognitive level of an adolescent in order to choose the appropriate answer.

39. 1. The child's mother may be interested in information relating to proper nutrition and exercise. However, the most important thing is for the nurse to let the child's mother know that this is a normal finding in teenage girls as they enter puberty.
    2. The child's mother may be interested in information relating to proper nutrition and exercise. However, the most important thing is for the nurse to let the mother know that this is a normal finding in teenage girls as they enter puberty.
    3. **The nurse should tell the child's mother that this is a normal finding in teenage girls as they enter puberty.**
    4. The nurse knows that it is normal for girls to gain weight during puberty but has no

idea how much weight the child will gain or if she will gain any more.

TEST-TAKING HINT: The test taker must have knowledge of the physical development of adolescent girls.

40. 1. Gynecomastia and breast tenderness are common for about a third of boys during middle puberty. Gynecomastia usually resolves in 2 years.
2. Gynecomastia and breast tenderness are common for about a third of boys during middle puberty. Gynecomastia usually resolves in 2 years.
3. **Gynecomastia and breast tenderness are common for about a third of boys during middle puberty. Gynecomastia usually resolves in 2 years.**
4. Gynecomastia and breast tenderness are common for about a third of boys during middle puberty. Gynecomastia usually resolves in 2 years.

TEST-TAKING HINT: The test taker must have knowledge about the physical development of adolescent boys.

41. 1. Grounding is a technique that generally works well with adolescents.
2. Time-out is a technique that is primarily used for toddler and preschool children.
3. **School-age children usually respond very well to a reward system and often enjoy the rewards so much that they will continue chores without continual reminders.**
4. Spanking is never a suggestion that should be given to families.

TEST-TAKING HINT: The age of the child is essential to answering this question. The test taker must understand the psychosocial development of the child in order to choose the appropriate intervention. Answer 4 can be eliminated because physical punishment should never be suggested. Answer 1 can be eliminated because it is a technique that works best with adolescents. Answer 2 can be eliminated because it is a technique that works best with toddlers and preschool children.

42. 1. During the school-age years, a child grows approximately 2 inches per year.
2. **During the school-age years, a child grows approximately 2 inches per year.**
3. This is not the appropriate time to have the child evaluated. His mother needs to reserve her concerns until he is older. He will likely begin to catch up with his peers within the next year.

4. The child should continue to see his pediatrician for annual visits, but there is no need for a special visit to reevaluate his growth at this time.

TEST-TAKING HINT: This is a specific physical developmental milestone that should be memorized.

43. 1. Toddlers are egocentric and are not yet capable of delayed gratification. It is unlikely that the child will wait to play with her mother until the baby sleeps.
2. Toddlers do not usually engage in play with others. They are generally involved in parallel play.
3. Toddlers usually initially resent the presence of new siblings because they take away some of the parents' time and attention.
4. **This is a typical statement that would be made by a toddler. Toddlers are very egocentric and do not consider the needs of the other child.**

TEST-TAKING HINT: The age of the child is essential to answering this question. The test taker must understand the psychosocial development of the toddler in order to choose the appropriate statement.

44. 1. It is possible for children to develop a mild rash after receiving the varicella vaccine. However, the varicella vaccine is not usually administered prior to 1 year of age.
2. **The nurse should not give the vaccine. The varicella vaccine is not usually administered prior to 1 year of age.**
3. The varicella vaccine is not usually administered prior to 1 year of age.
4. The recommendation is that a second dose be administered at 4 to 6 years of age.

TEST-TAKING HINT: The test taker must understand basic immunization schedules to answer the question.

45. 1. The child's family does have some influence on his dietary choices, but teens are more focused on being like their peers.
2. The child's culture does affect his food choices. However, teens are more likely to choose "junk foods" and foods that their peers are eating.
3. **As a teen, the child is most influenced by his peers. Teens long to be like others around them.**
4. Television does affect personal food choices, but the peer group still has the most prevalent impact in a teen's life.

TEST-TAKING HINT: The age of the child is essential to answering this question. The test taker must understand that peers are central to an adolescent's life.

46. 1. Poisoning is more common among toddlers and preschoolers who are ambulating.
2. Child abuse is not one of the leading causes of injury and death in children. Accidents are the most common cause of injury and death.
3. **Aspiration is a common cause of injury and death among children of this age. These children often find small objects lying on the floor and place them in their mouths. Older siblings are often responsible for leaving small objects around.**
4. Dog bites are not a leading cause of injury or death in children.

TEST-TAKING HINT: The test taker must have knowledge of the primary safety concerns of infants. Answer 1 can be eliminated as poisoning is more common among preschoolers. Child abuse and dog bites, answers 2 and 4, are not common causes of injury and death in infants.

47. 1. This comment will not make the mother feel any better. The mother is going to blame herself regardless of where the blame lies. The nurse would do better to just listen than to make this sort of comment.
2. **Falls are one of the most common injuries, and it may make the parent feel better to know that this is common among all toddlers.**
3. It may be a good idea to put up a baby gate, but in this situation the nurse's comment may be interpreted as judgmental.
4. Toddlers are still working on maintaining stability while walking, climbing stairs, and running. The toddler should not be expected to be proficient at this time.

TEST-TAKING HINT: The test taker must understand the psychological state of the parent. Most parents blame themselves whenever their children are injured, so answer 1 can be eliminated. Answer 3 implies that the injury is the parent's fault, so it too can be eliminated.

48. 1. **Safety equipment is essential for bicycling, skateboarding, and participating in contact sports. Most injuries occur during the school-age years, when** children are more active and participate in contact sports.
2. Educational material is a good way to reinforce the use of safety equipment, but the parents must insist that the child use his safety equipment.
3. Video material is a good way to reinforce the use of safety equipment, but the parents must insist that the child use his safety equipment.
4. The child's parents may not always be present when he rides his bike, so the use of safety equipment is the primary concern.

TEST-TAKING HINT: This is a question focusing on safety. The test taker must understand that educational material may reinforce a child's knowledge of safety. However, in order to avoid injury, the best thing a parent can do is insist on the use of safety equipment.

49. 1. A normal systolic blood pressure for a child from birth to 1 month is 50 to 101. A normal diastolic blood pressure for a child from birth to 1 month is 42 to 64.
2. A normal temperature is 96.6°F to 100°F (35.8° C to 37.7° C).
3. A normal respiratory rate for a child from birth to 1 month is 30 to 60.
4. **A normal heart rate for a child from birth to 1 month is 90 to 160.**

TEST-TAKING HINT: Normal vital signs for each age group should be memorized in order to understand abnormalities that occur with different disease processes.

50. 1. It is always a good idea for parents to administer medications at the same time each day.
2. **Medications should never be mixed in a large amount of food or formula because the parent cannot be sure that the child will take the entire feeding. Formula decreases the absorption of iron.**
3. Giving medications in a nipple is an acceptable method of administering liquid oral medications to infants.
4. An oral syringe is a good method of administering oral medications. The syringe should be placed in the back side of the cheek. Small amounts of the medication should be given at a time.

TEST-TAKING HINT: The test taker must have knowledge of medication administration. Answers 1, 3, and 4 can be eliminated as they are all appropriate methods for administering medications to infants.

51. 1. Teens require more sleep due to the rapid physical growth that occurs during adolescence.
    2. Teens are trying to integrate new roles into their lives. However, that has no impact on their need for increased sleep.
    3. **Teens require more sleep due to the rapid physical growth that occurs during adolescence.**
    4. Teens are generally more social and may be staying out late. However, their increased requirement for sleep is related to their rapid growth during adolescence.

    TEST-TAKING HINT: The test taker must have knowledge of the physical growth and development of adolescents.

52. 1. The Denver Developmental Test, which evaluates children from 1 month to 6 years, is used to screen gross motor skills, fine motor skills, language development, and personal/social development.
    2. The Denver Developmental Test, which evaluates children from 1 month to 6 years, is used to screen gross motor skills, fine motor skills, language development, and personal/social development
    3. **The Denver Developmental Test does not test a child's level of intelligence.**
    4. The Denver Developmental Test, which evaluates children from 1 month to 6 years, is used to screen gross motor skills, fine motor skills, language development, and personal/social development.

    TEST-TAKING HINT: The test taker must have knowledge of the Denver Developmental Test and what it screens for.

53. 1. A low protein level could indicate a nutritional deficit. However, this would not be an indication that the nurse sees on an initial assessment. Lab work would be required to have this information.
    2. This is a normal blood pressure for a teen.
    3. **Dry and brittle hair and nails are common among people who have a nutritional deficit.**
    4. Eroded teeth are more common of people who have frequent vomiting. The acidic nature of the vomitus causes the enamel of the teeth to deteriorate causing erosion. This practice is most common among teens with bulimia.

    TEST-TAKING HINT: The test taker must have knowledge of the nutritional needs of an adolescent. Answer 1 can be eliminated because it states that the value is normal. Answer 2 can be eliminated
because it is a normal blood pressure. Answer 4 can be eliminated because it relates more to bulimia than anorexia.

54. 1. A normal systolic blood pressure for a child from 3 to 6 years is 78 to 111. A normal diastolic blood pressure for a child from 3 to 6 years is 42 to 70.
    2. A normal temperature is 96.6°F to 100°F (35.8° C to 37.7° C).
    3. **A normal respiratory rate for a child from 3 to 6 years is 20 to 30 breaths per minute.**
    4. A normal heart rate for a child from 3 to 6 years is 75 to 120.

    TEST-TAKING HINT: Normal vital signs for each age group should be memorized in order to understand abnormalities that occur with different disease processes.

55. 1. Vital signs are not considered when measuring pain using the FLACC scale.
    2. The parents' perception of their child's pain level is not considered when using the FLACC scale.
    3. **The FLACC scale utilizes behavioral and physical responses of the child to measure the child's level of pain. The scale utilizes facial expression, leg position, activity, intensity of cry, and level of consolability.**
    4. The FLACC scale assigns a numeric value to a child's pain level, which is from 0 to 10.

    TEST-TAKING HINT: The test taker must have knowledge of pain rating scales used to measure the pain of nonverbal children.

56. 1. Children should double their birth weight by 6 months of age.
    2. Children should triple their birth weight by 12 months of age.
    3. **Children should triple their birth weight by 12 months of age.**
    4. Children should triple their birth weight by 12 months of age.

    TEST-TAKING HINT: This is a specific physical developmental milestone that should be memorized.

57. 1. When a child is experiencing pain, the normal physiological response is for the heart rate and respiratory rate to increase.
    2. When a child is experiencing pain, the normal physiological response is for the heart rate and blood pressure to increase.
    3. **When a child is experiencing pain, the normal physiological response is for the heart rate, respiratory rate, and blood pressure to increase.**

4. When a child is experiencing pain, the normal physiological response is for the heart rate, respiratory rate, and blood pressure to increase.

TEST-TAKING HINT: The test taker must have knowledge of vital sign changes that occur when a child is in pain.

58. 1. If the child's parents confront him, he may feel like they are being judgmental, and he will likely not want to communicate with them. When parents begin a dialogue with their child early on in life, they are more capable of approaching the child when they do notice behavioral changes.
    2. Setting limits is always a good thing to do with children. However, the child's parents are not addressing the reason for his behavioral changes.
    3. The child's behavior is typical of a teen's response to developmental and psychosocial changes of adolescence. He does not need a psychological referral at this time.
    4. **The child's behavior is typical of a teen's response to developmental and psychosocial changes of adolescence.**

TEST-TAKING HINT: The age of the child is essential to answering this question. The test taker must understand the psychosocial development of an adolescent in order to choose the appropriate answer. Adolescents focus on their relationships with peers and are much more influenced by peers than parents. Adolescents also want privacy, so the best thing parents can do is listen to their teens.

59. 1. The child is preschool age. Preschool children like to do things for themselves and will not likely behave any better for the parents than the nurse.
    2. The nurse should not promise the child that the procedure will go quickly. The nurse needs to develop a trusting relationship with the child so only promises than can be kept should be made.
    3. **Preschool children enjoy games, and it is a good way to elicit their assistance and cooperation during a procedure.**
    4. The nurse should not promise the child that the procedure will not hurt. Each child's perception of pain is individual in nature. The nurse needs to develop a trusting relationship with the child so only promises that can be kept should be made.

TEST-TAKING HINT: The age of the child is essential to answering this question. The

test taker must understand the psychosocial and cognitive development of a preschooler in order to choose the appropriate intervention. Answers 2 and 4 can be eliminated because nurses should never make promises to children that they may not be able to keep. It is difficult to build a trusting relationship with children unless the nurse is completely honest.**

60. 1. **The child should be weighed every day before she eats. Her weight will not be an accurate reflection if she is fed prior to being weighed.**
    2. The child should be weighed only in undergarments. The weight of clothing must not be included.
    3. The nurse should remain in the room while the child eats in order to accurately record a calorie count.
    4. The child should be weighed on the same scale every time. All scales are not equally accurate, so it is important to use the same scale in order to obtain an accurate trend.

TEST-TAKING HINT: The test taker must have knowledge of a child's nutrition and how to obtain an accurate weight.

61. 2, 3, 5.
    1. Social isolation is a stressor of the hospitalized teen.
    2. **Common stressors of the hospitalized toddler include interrupted routine, sleep pattern disturbances, and fear of being hurt.**
    3. **Common stressors of the hospitalized toddler include interrupted routine, sleep pattern disturbances, and fear of being hurt.**
    4. Self-concept disturbance is a stressor of the hospitalized teen.
    5. **Common stressors of the hospitalized toddler include interrupted routine, sleep pattern disturbances, and fear of being hurt. The stressors of social isolation and self-concept disturbances are stressors of the hospitalized teen.**

TEST-TAKING HINT: The age of the child is essential to answering this question. The test taker must understand the developmental level of the child in order to choose the appropriate intervention. The test taker must also have knowledge of common stressors that affect children during hospitalization.

Issues Related to Pediatric Health

KEYWORDS

100% Oxygen via non-rebreather mask
Activated charcoal
Alcohol poisoning
Airway
Anticipatory guidance
Assessment
Bacterial meningitis
Breathing
Carbon monoxide poisoning
Cervical spine precautions
Child abuse
Childproofing measures
Chronically ill child
Circulation
Concussion
Congenital hypothyroidism
Contact precautions
Cystic fibrosis
Death of a child
Digoxin
Droplet (airborne) precautions
Early intervention services
Epinephrine 1:1000 subcutaneous injection
Erythema infectiosum (fifth disease)
Exanthema subitum (roseola)
Eye trauma
Galactosemia
Genetic counseling
Grief reaction
Hepatitis B antigen
Hepatitis B immune globulin
Hepatitis B vaccine

Home care nursing
Immunizations
Initial neurological assessment
Injury prevention
Jaw thrust maneuver
Kawasaki disease
Lead poisoning
Low phenylalanine diet
Maple syrup urine disease
Miscarriages
Munchausen syndrome by proxy
Near-drowning
Newborn assessment
Normal growth and development
Nursing intervention
Pediatric trauma
Poisonings
Renal diet
Respiratory precautions
Rheumatic fever
Rotovirus vaccine
Serial neurological assessments
Sexual abuse
Shaken baby syndrome
Spinal cord injuries
Tay-Sachs disease
Terminally ill child
Therapeutic open communication
Tuberculosis
Vaccine information statement
Varicella (chickenpox)
Varicella vaccine

ABBREVIATIONS

Diphtheria, tetanus toxoid, and acellular pertussis (DTaP)

Haemophilus influenza type B (Hib)

Human immunodeficiency virus (HIV)

Inactivated polio vaccine (IPV)

Phenylketonuria (PKU)

QUESTIONS

1. The mother of a 21-day-old male tells the nurse she is residing in a homeless shelter and is concerned about his mild cough, poor appetite, low-grade fever, weight loss, and irritability over the last 2 weeks. Which nursing intervention would be the nurse's highest priority?
   1. Weigh the baby to have an accurate weight using standard precautions.
   2. Reassure the mother that the baby may only have a cold, which can last a few weeks.
   3. Immediately initiate droplet face-mask precautions, and isolate the infant.
   4. Take a rectal temperature while completing the assessment using standard precautions.

2. The nurse received a report on a new admission: a 3-year-old with Kawasaki disease. Understanding the etiology and major complications of Kawasaki disease, the priority nursing intervention would be:
   1. Continuous cardiovascular and oxygen saturation monitoring.
   2. Vital signs every 4 hours until stable.
   3. Strict intake and output monitoring hourly.
   4. Begin aspirin therapy after fever has resolved.

3. The nurse is assessing a 3-week-old with suspected bacterial meningitis. Isolation and respiratory precautions have already been initiated. Which clinical assessment by the nurse would warrant immediate intervention?
   1. The neonate is irritable.
   2. The neonate has a rectal temperature of 100.6° F (38.1°C).
   3. The neonate is quieter than usual.
   4. The neonate's respiratory rate is 24 breaths per minute.

4. The mother of an 18-month-old is discharged from the hospital after the child has a febrile seizure secondary to exanthem subitum (roseola). On discharge, the mother asks the nurse if her 6-year-old twins will get sick. Which teaching about the transmission of roseola would be most accurate?
   1. The child should be isolated in the home until the vesicles have dried.
   2. The child does not need to be isolated from the older siblings.
   3. Administer acetaminophen to the older siblings to prevent seizures.
   4. Monitor older children for seizure development.

5. A child is diagnosed with erythema infectiosum (fifth disease). You observe the mother crying, and she says, "I am afraid. Will my unborn baby die? I have a planned cesarian section next week." Which statement would be the most therapeutic response?
   1. "Let me get the physician to come and talk with you."
   2. "I understand. I would be afraid, too."
   3. "Would you like me to call your obstetrician to have you seen as soon as possible?"
   4. "I understand you are afraid. Can we can talk about your concerns?"

6. Which of the following would be the priority intervention the nurse should initiate for a child suspected of having varicella (chickenpox)?
   1. Contact precautions.
   2. Contact and droplet respiratory precautions.
   3. Droplet respiratory precautions.
   4. Universal precautions and standard precautions.

7. Which of the following would be the priority teaching to the parent of a child diagnosed with chickenpox (varicella) who was prescribed diphenhydramine (Benadryl) for itching?
   1. Give a warm bath with mild soap before lotion application.
   2. Avoid Caladryl lotion while taking diphenhydramine (Benadryl).
   3. Apply Caladryl lotion generously to decrease itching.
   4. Give a cool shower with mild soap to decrease itching.

8. Which signs and symptoms would the nurse expect to assess in a child with rheumatic fever?
   1. Joint pain in ankles and knees.
   2. Negative group A beta streptococcal culture.
   3. Large red "bulls eye"–appearing rash.
   4. Stiff neck with photophobia.

9. The parents of a 12-month-old male with HIV are concerned about his receiving routine immunizations. What will the nurse tell them about immunizations?
   1. "Your child will not receive routine immunizations today."
   2. "Your child will receive the recommended vaccines today; regular immunizations help prevent childhood illnesses."
   3. "Your child is not severely immunocompromised, but I would still be concerned about his receiving them. Let's not give them today."
   4. "Your child may develop infections if he gets his routine immunizations. Your child will not be immunized today."

10. After airway, breathing, and circulation have been assessed and stabilized, which intervention should the nurse implement for a child diagnosed with encephalitis?
    1. Assist with a lumbar puncture, and give reassurance.
    2. Obtain a throat culture, then begin antibiotics.
    3. Perform initial and serial neurological assessments.
    4. Administer antibiotics and antipyretics.

11. Expected nursing assessments of a newborn with suspected cystic fibrosis would include:
    1. Observe frequency and nature of stools.
    2. Provide chest physical therapy.
    3. Observe for weight gain.
    4. Assess parent's compliance with fluid restrictions.

12. Which treatment would the nurse anticipate for a 2-week-old boy diagnosed with PKU?
    1. There is no treatment or special diet.
    2. A high phenylalanine diet.
    3. A low phenylalanine diet.
    4. The mother would be advised not to breastfeed the infant.

13. Which teaching would be important to discuss with the family of a child born with PKU?
    1. Studies have shown that children with PKU outgrow the disease.
    2. Consumption of decreased amounts of protein and dairy products is advised.
    3. High-protein and high-dairy products consumption must be maintained.
    4. Exclusive breastfeeding is encouraged for maximal nutrition for the child.

14. Which teaching is most important for a child with PKU during a well-child visit?
    1. The child is able to eat a quarter-pound hamburger and drink a milkshake daily.
    2. If the child wants soda, diet soda is preferred over milk or dairy products.
    3. The child may have ice cream in an unlimited quantity once a week.
    4. Diet soda or anything with the sweetener aspartame should be avoided.

15. Which intervention should the nurse implement for a newborn diagnosed with galactosemia?
    1. Eliminate all milk and lactose-containing foods.
    2. Encourage breastfeeding as long as possible.
    3. Encourage lactose-containing formulas.
    4. Avoid feeding soy-protein formula to the newborn.

16. Which statement by the parent of a newborn male diagnosed with galactosemia demonstrates successful teaching?
    1. "This is a rare disorder that usually does not affect future children."
    2. "Our newborn looks normal; he may not have galactosemia."
    3. "Our newborn may need to take penicillin and other medications to prevent infection."
    4. "Penicillin and other drugs that contain lactose as fillers need to be avoided."

17. Which signs and symptoms would the nurse expect to assess in a newborn with congenital hypothyroidism?
    1. Preterm, diarrhea, and tachycardia.
    2. Post-term, constipation, and bradycardia.
    3. High-pitched cry, colicky, and jittery.
    4. Lethargy, diarrhea, and tachycardia.

18. Which of the following families would be appropriate to refer for genetic counseling?
    1. Parents with macrosomic infant.
    2. Parents with neonatal abstinence syndrome infant.
    3. Couple with a history of planned abortions.
    4. Couple with a history of multiple miscarriages.

19. Which statement from parents of a newborn male diagnosed with Tay-Sachs disease indicates successful understanding of his long-term prognosis?
    1. "If we give our baby a proper diet, early intervention, and physical therapy, he can live to adulthood."
    2. "He will have normal development for about 6 months before progressive developmental delays develop."
    3. "With intense physical therapy and early intervention, we can prevent developmental delays."
    4. "If we give our baby a lactose-free diet for life, we can minimize developmental delays and learning disabilities."

20. Which intervention might the nurse anticipate in a 2-day-old infant diagnosed with maple syrup urine disease?
    1. High-protein, high-amino-acid diet.
    2. Low-protein, limited amino-acid diet.
    3. Low-protein, low-sodium diet.
    4. Phenylalanine-restricted diet.

21. What would be the priority nursing action on finding the varicella vaccine at room temperature on the shelf in the medication room?
    1. Ensure the varicella vaccine's integrity is intact; if intact, follow the five rights of medication administration.
    2. Do not administer this batch of vaccine.
    3. Ensure the varicella vaccine's integrity is intact; if intact, give the vaccine after verifying proper physician orders.
    4. Ask the mother if the child has had any prior reactions to varicella.

22. What would the most therapeutic response if the mother of a 6-month-old female tells the nurse she does not want her infant to have the DTaP vaccine because the infant had localized redness the last time she received the vaccine?
    1. "I will let the physician know, and we will not administer the DTaP vaccination today."
    2. "Every child has that allergic reaction, and your child will still get the DTaP today."
    3. "I will let the physician know that you refuse further immunizations for your daughter."
    4. "Would you mind if we discussed your concerns?"

23. Which nursing intervention should take place prior to all vaccination administrations?
    1. Document the vaccination to be administered on the immunization record and medical record.
    2. Provide the vaccine information statement handout, and answer all questions.
    3. Administer the most painful vaccination first, and then alternate injection sites.
    4. Refer to the vaccination as "baby shots" so the parent understands the baby will be receiving an injection.

24. Which would be the nurse's best response if a mother asks if her baby still needs the Hib vaccine because he already had Hib?
    1. "Yes, it is recommended that the baby still get the Hib vaccine."
    2. "No, if he has had Hib, he will not need to receive the vaccine."
    3. "Let me take a nasal swab first; if it is negative, he will receive the Hib vaccine."
    4. "The physician will order a blood test, and depending on results, your child may need the vaccine."

25. What would be the nurse's best response if the foster mother of a 15-month-old with an unknown immunization history comes to the clinic requesting immunizations?
    1. "Your foster child will not receive any immunizations today."
    2. "Your foster child will receive the measles, mumps, rubella (MMR); and Hib; IPV; and hepatitis B vaccines."
    3. "Your foster child could have harmful effects if we revaccinate with prior vaccines."
    4. "Your foster child will receive only the Hib and DTaP vaccines today."

26. Which medication is most important to have available in all clinics and offices if immunizations are administered?
    1. Benadryl (diphenhydramine) injection.
    2. Epinephrine 1:10,000 injection.
    3. Epinephrine 1:1000 injection.
    4. Benadryl (diphenhydramine) liquid.

27. Which is the nurse's best response when the mother of a 2-month-old who is going to get the IPV tells the nurse the older brother is immunocompromised?
    1. "Your baby should not be immunized because your immunocompromised son could develop polio."
    2. "Your baby should receive the oral poliovirus vaccine instead so your immunocompromised son does not get sick."
    3. "You should separate your 2-month-old child from the immunocompromised son for 7 to 14 days after the IPV."
    4. "Your baby can be immunized with the IPV; he will not be contagious."

28. Which of the following would be the priority intervention for the newborn of a mother positive for hepatitis antigen?
    1. The newborn should be given the first dose of hepatitis B vaccine by 2 months of age.
    2. The newborn should receive the hepatitis B vaccine and hepatitis B immune globulin within 12 hours of birth.
    3. The newborn should receive the hepatitis B vaccine and hepatitis B immune globulin within 24 hours of birth.
    4. The newborn should receive hepatitis B immune globulin only within 12 hours of birth.

29. Which instruction would be of highest priority for the mother of an infant receiving his first oral rotavirus vaccine?
    1. "Call the physician if he develops fever or cough."
    2. "Call the physician if he develops fever, redness, or swelling at the injection site."
    3. "Call the physician if he develops a bloody stool or diarrhea."
    4. "Call the physician if he develops constipation and irritability."

30. What would be the best plan of care for a newborn whose mother's hepatitis B antigen status is unknown?
    1. Give the infant the hepatitis B vaccine within 12 hours of birth.
    2. Give the infant the hepatitis B vaccine and hepatitis B immune globulin within 12 hours of birth.
    3. Give the infant the hepatitis B vaccine within 24 hours of birth.
    4. Give the infant the hepatitis B vaccine and hepatitis B immune globulin within 24 hours of birth.

31. When discharging a newborn, which injury prevention instruction would be of highest priority to tell the parents?
    1. "Place safety locks on all medicine cabinets and household cleaning supplies."
    2. "Transport the infant in the front seat when driving alone so you can see the baby."
    3. "Never leave the baby unattended on a raised, unguarded area."
    4. "Place safety guards in front of any heating appliance, stove, fireplace, or radiator."

32. A 10-month-old female is carried into the emergency department by her parents after she fell down 15 stairs in her walker. Which would be your highest priority nursing intervention?
    1. Assess airway while simultaneously maintaining cervical spine precautions.
    2. Assess airway, breathing, and circulation simultaneously.
    3. Prepare for diagnostic radiological testing to check for any injuries.
    4. Obtain venous access and draw blood for testing.

33. Which would be the most appropriate discharge instructions for a child with a right wrist sprain 3 hours ago?
    1. "You should rest, elevate the wrist above the heart, apply heat wrapped in a towel, and use the sling when walking."
    2. "You can use the wrist, but stop if it hurts; elevate the wrist when not in use, and use the sling when walking."
    3. "You should rest, apply ice wrapped in a towel, elevate the wrist above the heart, and use the sling when walking."
    4. "You do not have to take any special precautions; do not use any movements that cause pain, and apply alternate heat and ice, each wrapped in a towel.

34. A child with a newly applied left leg cast initially feels fine, then starts to cry and tells his mother his leg hurts. Which assessment would be the nurse's first priority?
    1. Cast integrity.
    2. Neurovascular integrity.
    3. Musculoskeletal integrity.
    4. Soft-tissue integrity.

35. An adolescent male comes in for his yearly physical. Which would be the most appropriate injury prevention/safety teaching for him?
    1. Inquire which are his favorite sports and discuss his knowledge and application of appropriate safety principles.
    2. Tell him to be careful performing sports activities because every sport has the potential for injury.
    3. Tell him not to let his friends encourage him to drink or smoke or take any drugs.
    4. Ask his mother what sports he plays and if he wears a helmet with contact sports.

36. Which assessment is most important after any injury in a child?
    1. History of loss of consciousness and length of time unconscious.
    2. Serial assessments of level of consciousness.
    3. Initial neurological assessment.
    4. Initial vital signs and oxygen saturation level.

37. Which would be the most appropriate nursing intervention when caring for a child newly admitted with a mild head concussion and no cervical spine injury?
    1. Keep head of bed flat, side rails up, and safety measures in place.
    2. Elevate head of bed, side rails up, and safety measures in place.
    3. Observe for drainage from any orifice and notify physician immediately.
    4. Continually stimulate the child to keep awake to check neurological status.

38. Which would be the most appropriate teaching to the parents of a female child in the emergency department who is awake, alert, and has no respiratory distress after a near-drowning experience?
    1. "She will most likely be discharged, and you should watch for any cough or trouble breathing."
    2. "She will need to have a preventive tube for breathing and ventilation to ensure her lungs are clear."
    3. "She will be fine but sometimes antibiotics are started as a preventive."
    4. "She will most likely be admitted for at least 24 hours and observed for respiratory distress or any swelling of the brain."

39. What would be the most appropriate advice to give to the parent of a boy with slight visual blurring after being hit in the face with a basketball?
    1. "Apply ice, observe for any further eye complaints, and bring him back if he has increased pain."
    2. "Take him to the emergency department to ensure that he does not have any internal eye damage."
    3. "Call your pediatrician if he starts vomiting, is hard to wake up, or has worsening of eye blurring."
    4. "Observe for any further eye complaints, headaches, dizziness, or vomiting, and if worsening occurs, take him to your pediatrician."

40. Which would be the best response to the mother of a 13-year-old boy who continues to ask to ride his 16-year-old cousin's all-terrain vehicle?
    1. Emphasize that if he wears safety apparel and has adult supervision, it is fine.
    2. Explain to the mother that he is developing increased physical skills and, if he wears safety apparel and shows maturity, it should be fine.
    3. Discuss that all-terrain vehicles are not recommended for those younger than 16 years of age.
    4. Discuss with the mother that this is a stage where the child is seeking independence and should be allowed to participate in new physical activities.

41. Which response about safety measures is the most appropriate advice to the 2-year-old girl's mother who had her older home remodeled to reduce the lead level?
    1. "Wash and dry the child's hands and face before eating."
    2. "Remodeling the home to remove the lead is all you need to do."
    3. "It is best to use hot water to prepare the child's food to decrease the lead."
    4. "Diet does not matter in reducing lead levels in the child."

42. Which intervention would be most appropriate for a 3-year-old boy who had just ingested dish detergent?
    1. Discuss childproofing measures in the home in a nonthreatening manner.
    2. Inquire about the circumstances of the ingestion.
    3. Discuss having ipecac and the Poison Control phone number in the home.
    4. Tell the mother you will be giving the boy medicine to make him throw up.

43. Which would be the most appropriate intervention for a 4 year-old boy brought to the emergency department after ingesting a small watch battery?
    1. No treatment would be needed; assess and monitor airway, breathing, circulation, and abdominal pain.
    2. Ask the mother the time of the ingestion; if it was more than 2 hours ago, it will probably pass in his bowel movement.
    3. Assess and monitor airway, breathing, circulation, and abdominal pain; anticipate admission and prepare for surgical intervention.
    4. Discuss childproofing measures needed in the home with a 4-year-old child; provide anticipatory guidance concerning other possible poisonous ingestions.

44. Which nursing intervention would be of highest priority for a 2-year-old suspected of ingestion of his grandmother's digoxin?
    1. Provide supplemental oxygen.
    2. Establish intravenous access.
    3. Draw blood for a STAT digoxin level.
    4. Provide continuous cardiac monitoring.

45. Which would be the priority nursing intervention for a child with carbon monoxide poisoning?
    1. Provide supplemental 100% oxygen.
    2. Provide continuous oxygen saturation monitoring.
    3. Establish intravenous access.
    4. Draw blood for a STAT carbon monoxide level.

46. Which of the following would be appropriate anticipatory guidance for a well-care visit of a 17-year-old?
    1. Discuss alcohol use and potential for alcohol poisoning.
    2. Discuss secondary sex characteristics that will develop.
    3. Teach about anger management and safe sex.
    4. Teach about peer pressure and desire for independence.

47. Which would be the best response to a 10-year-old girl who asks if she can take acetaminophen daily if she gets aches and pains?
    1. Tell her it is better not to take medication if she gets aches and pains; she should check with her mother before taking any medication.
    2. Teach her that nonprescription drugs like acetaminophen can be a poisoning hazard if too many are taken; it is best for her to check with her mother.
    3. Encourage her to keep a log of when she takes acetaminophen to try to establish what is causing her aches and pains.
    4. Sometimes it is okay to take acetaminophen daily, but it depends on why she has aches and pains.

48. What would be the nurse's best advice to a mother who says her 3-year-old son ingested his father's Visine eye solution?
    1. "Initiate vomiting immediately."
    2. "Call the Poison Control Center."
    3. "Call the pediatrician right away."
    4. "Dilute with milk 1:1 volume of suspected ingestion."

49. What would be the best response if a mother tells the nurse that the only way she can get her 2-year-old daughter to take medicine is to call it candy?
    1. Tell her that is fine as long as the child takes all of the medicine.
    2. Discuss the importance of not calling medicine candy to prevent accidental drug ingestion.
    3. Discuss with the mother that the child does not have to take the medicine if she does not want it.
    4. Tell the mother her child will have to go to "time out" if she does not take her medicine.

50. Which nursing plan would be most successful if the nurse has to administer activated charcoal to a 5-year-old boy?
    1. Have his parents tell him he has to drink it while providing a movie to distract him.
    2. Tell him it is candy, it tastes good, do not let him look at it, and tell him he will get a toy after he takes it all down.
    3. Mix it with a sweetening flavoring, provide a straw, give in an opaque cup with a cover.
    4. Have his mother take some first to show the boy it does not taste too bad, and then administer it to him quickly.

51. Which statement most accurately describes child abuse?
    1. Intentional physical abuse and neglect.
    2. Intentional and unintentional physical and emotional abuse and neglect.
    3. Sexual abuse of children, usually by an adult.
    4. Intentional physical, emotional, and sexual abuse and neglect.

52. What is the most likely cause of a child's illness if it is unexplained, prolonged, recurrent, extremely rare, and usually occurs when the mother is present?
    1. Genetic disorder.
    2. Munchausen syndrome by proxy.
    3. Duchenne muscular dystrophy.
    4. Syndrome of inappropriate antidiuretic hormone.

53. Which statement would be most therapeutic to a child the nurse suspects has been abused?
    1. "Who did this to you? This is not right."
    2. "This is wrong that your mother did not protect you."
    3. "This is not your fault; you are not to blame for this."
    4. "I will not tell anyone."

54. The mother of a 6-month-old states that since yesterday, the child cries when anyone touches her arm. Which would be the priority assessment after the airway, breathing, and circulation had been assessed and found stable?
    1. Ask the mother if she knows what happened.
    2. Assess child for other signs of potential physical abuse.
    3. Prepare for radiological diagnostic studies.
    4. Establish intravenous access, and draw blood for diagnostic testing.

55. Which assessment of a 2-year-old with burns on his feet would cause suspicion of child abuse?
    1. Splash marks on his right lower leg.
    2. Burns noted on right arm.
    3. Symmetrical burns on both feet.
    4. Burns mainly noted on right foot.

56. Which would be the nurse's priority intervention if a 7-year-old girl's mother tells the nurse she has noticed excessive masturbation?
    1. Tell her it is normal development for children of her age.
    2. Ask the mother if anyone is abusing the daughter that she knows about.
    3. Talk with the child and find out why she is touching herself down there.
    4. Investigate thoroughly the circumstances in which she masturbates.

57. Which statement by the mother would lead the nurse to suspect sexual abuse in a 4-year-old girl?
    1. Masturbation.
    2. Increased temper tantrums.
    3. She is not grateful.
    4. She does not demonstrate loyalty.

58. What would be the priority intervention when a 10-year-old girl comes to the nurse's office because of a headache, and the nurse notices various stages of bruising on her inner upper arms?
    1. Call her mother and ask her if acetaminophen can be given for the headache.
    2. Ask the girl what happened to her arms, and have her describe the headache.
    3. Inquire about her headache and the bruising on her arms; file mandatory reporting forms.
    4. Call her mother to pick her up from school, and complete required school nurse visit forms.

59. Which statement is true of abused children?
    1. They will tell the truth if asked about their injuries.
    2. They will repeat the same story as their parents.
    3. They usually are not noted to have any changes in behavior.
    4. They will have outgoing personalities and be active in school activities.

60. Which statement is true of shaken baby syndrome?
    1. There may be absence of external signs of injury.
    2. Shaken babies usually do not have retinal hemorrhage.
    3. Shaken babies usually do not have signs of a subdural hematoma.
    4. Shaken babies have signs of external head injury.

61. What would be the best response if the mother of a 10-year-old boy on kidney dialysis tells the nurse he has no appetite and only eats bananas?
    1. "Right now his stomach is upset, and as long as he is eating something to give him strength, it is fine."
    2. "Let's talk about your son and his diet."
    3. "Bananas are good to eat; they are rich in needed nutrients."
    4. "Did you try asking him what else he may want to eat?"

1. 1. Weighing the child would be important but not the priority when concerned about an infectious cause. Initiating droplet precautions to prevent infecting others would be a priority, then weighing the infant.
   2. The symptoms are not suggestive of a cold but something more serious. Infants do not usually lose weight, nor are they irritable with a simple cold.
   3. **Children with tuberculosis may have a history of living in a crowded home or could be homeless. Other symptoms may include a cough, cold symptoms, low-grade fever, irritability, poor appetite, and exposure to a person with tuberculosis. Initiation of droplet precautions and isolation of the infant would be warranted in this situation.**
   4. Taking the infant's temperature is important, but initiating droplet precautions would be the priority.

   TEST-TAKING HINT: The test taker should be highly suspicious of tuberculosis given the family and patient history. Health-care personnel need to be vigilant to contain and prevent further spread of communicable diseases. This child could have meningitis, which would also require isolation and respiratory precautions.

2. 1. **Cardiovascular manifestations of Kawasaki disease are the major complications in pediatric patients. Continuous cardiac monitoring is required to alert the nurse of any cardiovascular complications. Decreased oxygen saturation and respiratory changes have been shown to be early indicators of potential complications.**
   2. Vital signs would be taken every 1 to 2 hours until stable on a new admission with Kawasaki disease.
   3. Strict intake and output is very important, but because the major complications with Kawasaki disease are cardiovascular, continuous cardiac monitoring is the priority.
   4. High-dose aspirin therapy is begun and continued until the child has been afebrile for 48 to 72 hours; then the child is placed on low-dose therapy.

   TEST-TAKING HINT: The test taker should understand that cardiovascular manifestations of Kawasaki disease are the major complications in pediatric patients.

3. 1. With the diagnosis of suspected bacterial meningitis, the neonate is expected to be irritable, which frequently accompanies increased intracranial pressure.
   2. A rectal temperature of 38.1°C or 100.6°F indicates a low-grade fever and is not as concerning as the slower-than-normal respiratory rate of 24.
   3. The fact the infant is quieter than normal is in response to the slow respiratory rate and sepsis the neonate is experiencing.
   4. **A normal neonate's respiratory rate is 30 to 60 breaths per minute. Neonates' respiratory systems are immature, and the rate may initially double in response to illness. If no immediate interventions are begun when there is respiratory distress, a neonate's respiratory rate will slow down, develop worsening respiratory distress and, eventually, respiratory arrest. Neonates with slower or faster respiratory rates are true emergencies cases; they require identification of cause of distress.**

   TEST-TAKING HINT: The test taker needs to know the normal range of vital signs and when to be concerned.

4. 1. **The rash is pink and maculopapular, not vesicular. The period of communicability is unknown, and the incubation period is 5 to 15 days and more commonly seen in children 6 months to 3 years of age. Isolating the siblings is not necessary.**
   2. Roseola transmission is unknown and more commonly seen in children 6 months to 3 years of age, so siblings do not need to be isolated.
   3. Because the siblings have no history of seizures, it is not necessary to administer acetaminophen to prevent seizures.
   4. Febrile seizures are not usually seen in children older than 6 years, and because they have no history of seizures, it is not necessary to monitor them for seizure development.

   TEST-TAKING HINT: The test taker should understand that exanthema subitum (roseola) transmission is unknown, usually limited to children 6 months to 3 years of age, and isolation is not necessary.

5. 1. Having the physician come back and talk with the pregnant mother of a 2-year-old with fifth disease is appropriate, but these are certainly concerns the nurse can address by using therapeutic communication.
   2. Acknowledging the mother's fear is therapeutic, and it is appropriate to intervene.
   3. Informing the obstetrician would be appropriate after dealing therapeutically with the mother's concerns.
   4. **There is less risk of fetal death in the second half of the pregnancy. It is more therapeutic to acknowledge a client's fears. After acknowledging her fears, the appropriate response would be to discuss concerns and clarify any misconceptions.**

   TEST-TAKING HINT: The test taker should understand there is a 10% risk of death if a mother is exposed to erythema infectiosum (fifth disease) during the first half of her pregnancy.

6. 1. The primary source of transmission is secretions of the respiratory tract (droplet) of infected persons (airborne). Transmission occurs by direct contact, skin lesions to a lesser extent, and contaminated objects.
   2. **Varicella (chickenpox) is highly contagious. Contact and droplet respiratory precautions should be started immediately because the primary source of transmission is secretions of the respiratory tract (droplet) and also by contaminated objects.**
   3. Droplet precaution is very important because that is the primary source of transmission. Transmission also occurs by direct contact and contaminated objects.
   4. Standard precautions (formerly universal precautions) should always be maintained; the term refers to protecting oneself from patient's blood or body fluids.

   TEST-TAKING HINT: The test taker should understand that the primary source of transmission of varicella (chickenpox) is secretions of the respiratory tract of infected persons (airborne). Transmission occurs by direct contact, skin lesions to a lesser extent, and contaminated objects.

7. 1. To help decrease itching, a cool bath is a better option. Soap and warm water can cause more itching.
   2. **Caladryl lotion contains diphenhydramine (Benadryl), and the child would be at risk for toxicity if the Caladryl is applied to open lesions.**

3. Caladryl lotion is applied in an amount to cover the lesions.
4. A cool shower can be soothing and decrease itching. Mild soap is drying to the lesions and can cause more itching.

TEST-TAKING HINT: The test taker should understand that Caladryl lotion contains Benadryl.

8. 1. **Joint pain or arthritis is the most common symptom of acute rheumatic fever (60% to 80% of first attacks). The joint pain usually occurs in two or more large joints (ankle, knee, wrist, or elbow).**
   2. Rheumatic fever usually follows group A streptcococcal infection, and the culture is usually positive.
   3. Large red "bulls-eye" lesions are more characteristic of Lyme disease. The rash associated with rheumatic fever is erythematous with a demarcated border.
   4. A stiff neck with photophobia is more indicative of meningitis.

   TEST-TAKING HINT: The test taker should remember the major and minor criteria of rheumatic fever to answer this question.

9. 1. **It is the nurses' function to acknowledge a client's fears and then discuss concerns to clarify any misconceptions. Immunizations and influenza vaccine are recommended to prevent infection. Immunocompromised HIV-infected children should not receive the varicella and MMR live vaccines.**
   2. Recommended immunizations for a 12-month-old include varicella and MMR (live vaccines), which are not administered to an immunocompromised child.
   3. Recommended vaccines will be administered because the child is not immunocompromised.
   4. The recommendation is for the child to receive routine immunizations unless the child is immunocompromised.

   TEST-TAKING HINT: The test taker should know that families and patients who are HIV-positive should be taught ways to prevent infections, including the administration of immunizations.

10. 1. Airway, breathing, and circulation are part of the primary patient assessment. Neurological assessment is the next assessment to perform.
    2. The child has been diagnosed with encephalitis. Unless there is a concern about

the child's having strep throat, a throat culture would not be obtained.

3. **In a child with a neurological problem, initial and serial neurological assessments would be a priority nursing intervention to monitor for changes in neurological status.**

4. Encephalitis is usually caused by a virus; therefore, antibiotics are not ordered. Antipyretics may be used to help control fevers.

TEST-TAKING HINT: The test taker should understand that the primary assessment includes ensuring patent airway, breathing, circulation, and intact neurological status. In a child with a neurological problem, continue monitoring for changes in neurological status.

11. 1. **Cystic fibrosis is inherited as an autosomal-recessive trait, causing exocrine gland dysfunction. About 7% to 10% of newborns with cystic fibrosis present with meconium ileus, so assessing stool frequency and consistency is important.**

2. Chest physical therapy would not be initiated in a newborn without a definitive diagnosis.

3. Assessing weight is important in newborns because they can lose up to 10% of their birth weight, and it can take up to 2 weeks for them to regain their birth weight.

4. The newborn would not be placed on fluid restriction even if diagnosed with cystic fibrosis.

TEST-TAKING HINT: The test taker should understand that cystic fibrosis is inherited as an autosomal-recessive trait that causes exocrine gland dysfunction and affects several body systems, including respiratory, gastrointestinal, and reproductive.

12. 1. PKU is inherited as an autosomal-recessive trait. The enzyme phenylalanine hydroxylase controlling the conversion of phenylalanine to tyrosine is missing. A low-phenylalanine diet is the treatment to prevent brain damage.

2. PKU is inherited as an autosomal-recessive trait. The enzyme phenylalanine hydroxylase controlling the conversion of phenylalanine to tyrosine is missing. A low-phenylalanine diet is the treatment to prevent brain damage.

3. **PKU is inherited as an autosomal-recessive trait. The enzyme phenylalanine hydroxylase controlling the**

conversion of phenylalanine to tyrosine is missing. A low-phenylalanine diet is the treatment to prevent brain damage.

4. Breast milk has low amounts of phenylalanine so the mother can breastfeed with monitoring of phenylalanine levels in the infant.

TEST-TAKING HINT: The test taker should understand that PKU is a genetic inherited autosomal-recessive trait caused by a missing enzyme. This enzyme is needed to metabolize the essential amino acid phenylalanine.

13. 1. PKU is a genetic autosomal-recessive inherited trait. Phenylalanine is an essential amino acid, which makes it impossible to remove totally from the diet. Treatment is a low-phenylalanine diet, which includes some vegetables, fruits, juice, bread and starches.

2. **Many high-protein foods such as meats and dairy products are restricted or eliminated from the diet due to the high phenylalanine content.**

3. High-protein foods such as meat and dairy products are restricted to small amounts or eliminated because of their high phenylalanine content.

4. Breast milk contains PKU and, if the mother wanted to breast feed, the infant would need careful monitoring of PKU levels.

TEST-TAKING HINT: The test taker should understand that PKU is a genetic autosomal-recessive inherited trait. Strict, lifelong dietary restrictions and monitoring are required. Diet management includes meeting the child's nutritional and growth needs while maintaining phenylalanine levels within a safe range.

14. 1. High-protein foods like meats and dairy products are restricted because of their high phenylalanine content.

2. The sweetener aspartame (NutraSweet, Equal) should be avoided because it is converted to phenylalanine in the body.

3. Because of their high-protein content, dairy products are limited or eliminated from the diet.

4. **Artificial sweeteners such as aspartame are converted to phenylalanine in the body and should be avoided.**

TEST-TAKING HINT: The test taker should understand how PKU is treated to successfully answer this question.

15. 1. **Galactosemia is a rare autosomal-recessive disorder involving an inborn error of carbohydrate metabolism. The hepatic enzyme galactose-1-phosphate uridyl transferase is absent, causing the failure of galactose to be converted into glucose. Glucose builds up in the bloodstream, which can result in liver failure, cataracts, and renal tubular problems. Treatment of galactosemia involves eliminating all milk and lactose-containing foods, including breast milk.**
    2. Galactosemia is a rare autosomal-recessive disorder involving an inborn error of carbohydrate metabolism so that all milk and lactose-containing foods including breast milk are eliminated.
    3. Galactosemia is a rare autosomal-recessive disorder involving an inborn error of carbohydrate metabolism so that all milk and lactose-containing foods including breast milk are eliminated.
    4. Galactosemia is a rare autosomal-recessive disorder involving an inborn error of carbohydrate metabolism so that all milk and lactose-containing foods including breast milk are eliminated. Soy protein is the preferred formula.

    TEST-TAKING HINT: The test taker should understand that galactosemia is a rare autosomal-recessive disorder involving an inborn error of carbohydrate metabolism.

16. 1. Galactosemia is a rare genetic autosomal-recessive disorder involving an inborn error of carbohydrate metabolism that may affect future children.
    2. Infants usually appear normal at birth, but within a few days of ingesting milk begin to vomit and lose weight.
    3. Many drugs, such as penicillin, contain unlabeled lactose as filler and need to be avoided.
    4. **Many drugs, such as penicillin, contain unlabeled lactose as filler and need to be avoided.**

    TEST-TAKING HINT: The test taker should understand that galactosemia is a rare genetic autosomal-recessive disorder involving an inborn error of carbohydrate metabolism that may affect future children.

17. 1. Congenital hypothyroidism clinical manifestations may include bradycardia, constipation, poor feeding, lethargy, galactose-1-phosphate uridyl transferase, jaundice prolonged for more than than 2 weeks, cyanosis, respiratory difficulties, hoarse cry, large anterior/posterior fontanels, post-term, birth weight greater than 4000 g.
    2. **Congenital hypothyroidism clinical manifestations may include bradycardia, constipation, poor feeding, lethargy, jaundice prolonged for more than 2 weeks, cyanosis, respiratory difficulties, hoarse cry, large anterior/posterior fontanels, post-term, and birth weight greater than 4000 g.**
    3. High-pitched cry and being colicky and jittery usually indicate drug withdrawal or a neurological problem.
    4. Congenital hypothyroidism clinical manifestations may include bradycardia, constipation, poor feeding, lethargy, jaundice prolonged for more than 2 weeks, cyanosis, respiratory difficulties, hoarse cry, large anterior/posterior fontanels, post-term, and birth weight greater than 4000 g.

    TEST-TAKING HINT: The test taker needs to know clinical manifestations of hypothyroidism to answer this question.

18. 1. Macrosomia (large for gestational age) does not require genetic counseling.
    2. Neonatal abstinence syndrome is a term used to describe a set of symptoms displayed by infants exposed to chemicals in utero.
    3. Couples with planned abortions would not need genetic counseling unless there were genetic problems with children and/or adults in their families.
    4. **Couples with a history of multiple miscarriages, stillbirths, or infertility should be referred for genetic counseling to try to determine the cause of their problems with maintaining a pregnancy.**

    TEST-TAKING HINT: The test taker should understand that couples with multiple miscarriages, stillbirths, or infertility should be referred to genetic counseling to assist in a successful pregnancy.

19. 1. Tay-Sachs disease is a genetic disorder in which the infant has normal development for the first 6 months. After 6 months, developmental delays and neurological worsening occur. Dietary restriction or providing physical therapy does not change the outcome.

2. Tay-Sachs disease is a genetic disorder in which the infant has normal development for the first 6 months. After 6 months, developmental delays and neurological worsening occur. Dietary restriction or providing physical therapy does not change the outcome.

3. Tay-Sachs disease is a genetic disorder in which the infant has normal development for the first 6 months. After 6 months, developmental delays and neurological worsening occur. Dietary restriction or providing physical therapy does not change the outcome.

4. Tay-Sachs disease is a genetic disorder in which the infant has normal development for the first 6 months. After 6 months, developmental delays and neurological worsening occur. Dietary restriction or providing physical therapy does not change the outcome.

TEST-TAKING HINT: The test taker should understand that Tay-Sachs disease is a genetic disorder in which the infant dies in childhood.

20. 1. Maple syrup urine disease is a genetic inborn error of metabolism. It is a deficiency of decarboxylase, which is needed to degrade some amino acids. If left untreated, altered tone, seizures, and death can occur.

2. **A child with maple syrup urine disease will be on a low-protein, limited amino-acid diet for life. Patients need a diet high in thiamine.**

3. A child with maple syrup urine disease will be on a low-protein, limited amino-acid diet for life. Patients need a diet high in thiamine.

4. A child with maple syrup urine disease will be on a low-protein, limited amino-acid diet for life. Patients need a diet high in thiamine.

TEST-TAKING HINT: Maple syrup urine disease is a genetic disorder with restricted branched-chain amino acids; for example, valine, leucine, and isoleucine.

21. 1. Varicella vaccine should be kept frozen in the lyophilized form. After reconstitution, the varicella vaccine should be given within 30 minutes to ensure viral potency. The 5 rights of patient medication should always be followed prior to administration.

2. **The varicella vaccine integrity cannot be ensured if the vaccine is at room temperature, so do not administer.**

3. Varicella vaccine should be kept frozen in the lyophilized form. After reconstitution, the varicella vaccine should be given within 30 minutes to ensure viral potency. If the vaccine is not frozen, do not administer.

4. This is an important question to ask the mother but does not address the questions of the nurse finding the varicella vaccine at room temperature.

TEST-TAKING HINT: Varicella vaccine should be kept frozen in the lyophilized form. The vaccine diluents can be kept at room temperature.

22. 1. A common reaction to the DTaP vaccine is local swelling and redness at the injection site, which disappears in a few days. The nurse should not speak for the physician.

2. This local reaction is not considered an allergic reaction or an indication the child should not receive this immunization again.

3. The nurse is interpreting what the mother is stating to include refusal of all vaccines.

4. **This is the therapeutic response, discussing the mother's concerns about the immunizations and local reactions.**

TEST-TAKING HINT: The test taker needs to know common local reactions to immunizations.

23. 1. Written information about the vaccine should always be given prior to any immunization administered as well as allowing time for questions. Accurate documentation should always occur after immunizations are given.

2. **Written information about the vaccine should always be given prior to any immunization administered as well as allowing time for questions.**

3. Administer the most painful immunization last.

4. The word "shots" has a negative connotation to parents and should be avoided.

TEST-TAKING HINT: The test taker should understand that the vaccine information statement must be given and discussed with the parent before administering the vaccine.

24. 1. **The infant needs the Hib vaccine to ensure protection against many serious infections caused by Hib, such as bacterial meningitis, bacterial pneumonia, epiglottitis, septic arthritis, and sepsis.**

2. The infant needs the Hib vaccine to ensure protection against many serious infections caused by Hib, such as bacterial

meningitis, bacterial pneumonia,
epiglottitis, septic arthritis, and sepsis.
3. A nasal swab is used to diagnose a respiratory syncytial virus infection, which is unrelated to an Hib infection.
4. A blood test does not diagnose previous Hib infection in a healthy child.

TEST-TAKING HINT: The test taker should understand that the Hib vaccine protects against serious infections.

25. 1. The option is to try to determine immunization status by contacting previous health-care providers for a record of vaccines received. If previous providers are unknown, then the child will receive recommended immunizations for the age.
2. MMR, Hib, IPV, or hepatitis B vaccines would not routinely be due at this visit.
3. There are usually no harmful effects to a child with unknown immunization status if revaccinated.
4. **Vaccines routinely due at 15 months include Hib and DTaP. To catch up missed immunizations the nurse would need the child's immunization record to verify what he has received.**

TEST-TAKING HINT: The test taker would need to know what to do when the child's immunization status is unknown.

26. 1. Epinephrine 1:10,000 injection should be given intravenously only. Most children in a clinic or office setting receive immunizations during their well-child visit and do not have intravenous catheters in place for immediate access.
2. Epinephrine 1:10,000 injection should be given intravenously only. Most children in a clinic or office setting receive immunizations during their well-child visit and do not have intravenous catheters in place for immediate access.
3. **Epinephrine 1:1000 injection would be the drug of choice for subcutaneous injection if a severe allergic reaction occurs in an office or clinic setting.**
4. Epinephrine 1:10,000 injection should be given intravenously only. Most children in a clinic or office setting receive immunizations during their well-child visit and do not have intravenous catheters in place for immediate access.

TEST-TAKING HINT: The test taker should understand that in all offices and clinics offering immunizations, epinephrine is

the most important medication to have on hand in the event of an allergic reaction. Epinephrine's usual dose is 0.01 mg/kg of 1:1000 subcutaneous solution.

27. 1. IPV does not contain live poliovirus, so the virus cannot be transmitted to the immunocompromised sibling.
2. The oral polio vaccine contains weakened poliovirus; rarely, the virus can be transmitted to someone immunocompromised. The virus is shed in the stool.
3. There is no need to isolate the sibling from the child receiving the inactive poliovirus vaccine because the virus cannot be transmitted.
4. **The infant sibling can and should be immunized as recommended. The infant will not shed the poliovirus.**

TEST-TAKING HINT: The test taker should understand that household contacts and siblings of immunocompromised children are able to receive the IPV. They should not receive the oral poliovirus vaccine because there is a rare risk of vaccine-associated polio paralysis.

28. 1. Immunizing the neonate with hepatitis B immune globulin within 12 hours of birth provides prophylaxis against hepatitis B infection
2. The newborn should receive both hepatitis B vaccine and hepatitis B immune globulin within 12 hours of birth to prevent hepatitis B infection.
3. **The newborn should receive both hepatitis B vaccine and hepatitis B immune globulin within 12 hours of birth to prevent hepatitis B infection.**
4. The newborn should receive both hepatitis B vaccine and hepatitis B immune globulin within 12 hours of birth to prevent hepatitis B infection.

TEST-TAKING HINT: The test taker should understand that infants born to mothers positive for hepatitis B antigen should receive hepatitis B vaccine and hepatitis B immune globulin within 12 hours of birth to prevent infection.

29. 1. There is a very small incidence of infants developing intussusception–bloody stool or diarrhea after receiving oral rotovirus vaccine. Cough is not associated with this vaccine.
2. This is an oral vaccine, not an injectable vaccine.

3. There is a very small incidence of infants developing intussusception–bloody stool or diarrhea after receiving oral rotavirus vaccine.
4. There is a very small incidence of infants developing intussusception–bloody stool or diarrhea after receiving oral rotavirus vaccine.

TEST-TAKING HINT: The test taker should know potential adverse effects from the oral rotavirus vaccine.

30. 1. Infants born to mothers of unknown hepatitis B antigen status should be given the hepatitis B immune globulin and hepatitis B vaccine within 12 hours of birth. If the mother is positive for hepatitis B antigen, then the baby should receive the hepatitis B immune globulin as soon as possible within 12 hours of birth. Timely administration of the hepatitis B vaccine is important to prevent passive acquisition of hepatitis B from the mother.
2. **Infants born to mothers of unknown hepatitis B antigen status should be given the hepatitis B immune globulin and hepatitis B vaccine within 12 hours of birth. If the mother is positive for hepatitis B antigen, then the baby should receive the hepatitis B immune globulin as soon as possible within 12 hours of birth. Timely administration of the hepatitis B vaccine is important to prevent passive acquisition of hepatitis B from the mother.**
3. Infants born to mothers of unknown hepatitis B antigen status should be given the hepatitis B immune globulin and hepatitis B vaccine within 12 hours of birth. If the mother is positive for hepatitis B antigen, then the baby should receive the hepatitis B immune globulin as soon as possible within 12 hours of birth. Timely administration of the hepatitis B vaccine is important to prevent passive acquisition of hepatitis B from the mother.
4. Infants born to mothers of unknown hepatitis B antigen status should be given the hepatitis B immune globulin and hepatitis B vaccine within 12 hours of birth. If the mother is positive for hepatitis B antigen, then the baby should receive the hepatitis B immune globulin as soon as possible within 12 hours of birth. Timely administration of the hepatitis B vaccine is important to prevent passive acquisition of hepatitis B from the mother.

TEST-TAKING HINT: The test taker should understand that infants born to mothers with unknown hepatitis B antigen status should be given the hepatitis B vaccine within 12 hours of birth.

31. 1. The priority is to prevent the infant from rolling off a raised surface. Placing safety locks is done when the infant is a few months old.
2. The infant should be transported in the middle of the back seat of the vehicle, which is considered the safest place.
3. **The highest priority in newborn injury prevention is to never leave the baby unattended on a raised, unguarded surface. Involuntary reflexes may cause the infant to move and fall.**
4. Placing safety guards is the priority when the infant is a few months old and mobile.

TEST-TAKING HINT: The test taker needs to know developmentally appropriate injury prevention and then discuss it with the parent.

32. 1. **Priority nursing intervention with pediatric trauma patients is airway assessment while maintaining cervical spine precautions. If the airway is compromised, immediate corrective action should be taken prior to assessment of breathing.**
2. Assessing airway, breathing, and circulation will be done in that order, not simultaneously.
3. Diagnostic radiological testing is done after the child is stabilized.
4. Venous access and blood draws are done after airway, breathing, and circulation have been assessed.

TEST-TAKING HINT: The test taker should understand pediatric trauma patients can also have spinal cord injuries and what the priorities are in those situations.

33. 1. For the first 24 hours, rest, ice, compression, and elevation are recommended for acute injury. This is best remembered by the acronym RICE (rest, ice, compression, and elevation).
2. The wrist should be kept immobile and elevated.
3. **For the first 24 hours, rest, ice, compression, and elevation are recommended for acute injury. This is best remembered by the acronym RICE (rest, ice, compression, and elevation).**

4. For the first 24 hours, rest, ice, compression, and elevation are recommended for acute injury. This is best remembered by the acronyms RICE (rest, ice, compression, and elevation) and ICES (ice, compression, elevation, and support).

TEST-TAKING HINT: The test taker should remember the acronym RICE (rest, ice, compression, and elevation).

34. 1. Neurovascular integrity should be assessed first and frequently because neurovascular compromise may cause serious consequences. Neurovascular integrity should be assessed for pain: increased Pain out of proportion with injury, Pallor of extremity, Paresthesia, Pulselessness at distal part of extremity, and Paralysis post cast application (5 Ps). Cast integrity would be assessed, but neurovascular integrity is the highest priority.
    2. **Neurovascular integrity should be assessed first and frequently because neurovascular compromise may cause serious consequences. Neurovascular integrity should be assessed for pain: increased Pain out of proportion with injury, Pallor of extremity, Paresthesia, Pulselessness at distal part of extremity, and Paralysis post cast application (5 Ps). Cast integrity would be assessed, but neurovascular integrity is the highest priority.**
    3. Neurovascular integrity should be assessed first and frequently because neurovascular compromise may cause serious consequences. Neurovascular integrity should be assessed for pain: increased Pain out of proportion with injury, Pallor of extremity, Paresthesia, Pulselessness at distal part of extremity, and Paralysis post cast application (5 Ps). Musculoskeletal integrity would be assessed after neurovascular integrity.
    4. Neurovascular integrity should be assessed first and frequently because neurovascular compromise may cause serious consequences. Neurovascular integrity should be assessed for pain: increased Pain out of proportion with injury, Pallor of extremity, Paresthesia, Pulselessness at distal part of extremity, and Paralysis post cast application (5 Ps). Cast integrity would be assessed, but neurovascular integrity is the highest priority. Soft-tissue integrity is assessed last.

TEST-TAKING HINT: The test taker should understand that neurovascular integrity should be assessed first.

35. 1. **Adolescence is a time of need for independence and learning to make appropriate decisions. Safety is always a concern, and tying a safety discussion to the teen's interest in sports will help keep him safe. The nurse needs to inquire and build on the teen's interests and knowledge.**
    2. Lecturing to an adolescent would not be appropriate; the nurse needs to determine what the teen knows about safety measures for that sport and then build on that information.
    3. Determining whether the teen drinks, smokes, or uses drugs and what he thinks about those activities is the first step. Lecturing is never appropriate.
    4. The teen should be addressed directly.

TEST-TAKING HINT: The test taker should understand that age and developmentally appropriate injury prevention teachings are most effective.

36. 1. Serial assessments of level of consciousness are the most important observations of a child after any injury. History of loss of consciousness and length of time unconscious is important information, but serial assessments give current information.
    2. **Serial assessments of level of consciousness are the most important observations of a child after any injury. That information tells you if the child's condition is changing.**
    3. Initial neurological assessments are important but only provide a baseline.
    4. Initial vital signs and oxygen saturation level give a baseline and help when looking at serial assessments.

TEST-TAKING HINT: The test taker should understand that serial observations of the child's level of consciousness are the most important nursing observations.

37. 1. The head of the bed should be elevated to decrease intracranial pressure. Side rails should be up to help ensure the child stays in bed, and age-appropriate safety measures should be instituted.
    2. **The head of the bed should be elevated to decrease intracranial pressure. Side rails should be up to help ensure the child stays in bed, and age-appropriate safety measures should be instituted.**

3. Drainage from the nose or ear would indicate more severe head injury and would be reported to the physician. The priority would be elevating the head of the bed to decrease intracranial pressure.

4. The child may sleep, but frequent assessments will be made, and the child will be awakened often.

TEST-TAKING HINT: The test taker should understand that the appropriate nursing intervention would be to elevate the head of the bed to decrease intracranial pressure.

38. 1. Any child who has had a near-drowning experience should be admitted for observation. Even if a child does not appear to have any injury from the event, complications can occur within 24 hours. Respiratory compromise and cerebral edema can be delayed complications.

2. A ventilation tube would not be inserted unless she needs it as determined by her blood gases, x-rays, and clinical picture.

3. Any child who has had a near-drowning experience should be admitted for observation. Even if a child does not appear to have any injury from the event, complications can occur within 24 hours. Respiratory compromise and cerebral edema can be delayed complications.

4. **Any child who has had a near-drowning experience should be admitted for observation. Even if a child does not appear to have any injury from the event, complications can occur within 24 hours after the event. Respiratory compromise and cerebral edema can be delayed complications.**

TEST-TAKING HINT: The test taker should understand that respiratory compromise and cerebral edema may occur 24 hours after near-drowning. This means that children with a near-drowning event should be admitted.

39. 1. Trauma to the eyes and surrounding structures is the leading cause of blindness in children. This incident would be considered blunt trauma to the eyes, and the child should receive immediate medical attention.

2. **This type of eye injury is considered blunt force trauma to the eyes, and the child should be evaluated medically for assessment and prevention of eye damage. Slight blurring could indicate eye**

injuries, such as detached retina and hyphema, which need immediate medical intervention.

3. This type of eye injury is considered blunt force trauma to the eyes, and the child should be evaluated medically for assessment and prevention of eye damage. Slight blurring could indicate eye injuries, such as detached retina and hyphema, which need immediate medical intervention.

4. This type of eye injury is considered blunt force trauma to the eyes, and the child should be evaluated medically for assessment and prevention of eye damage. Slight blurring could indicate eye injuries, such as detached retina and hyphema, which need immediate medical intervention.

TEST-TAKING HINT: The test taker should understand that trauma to the eyes and supporting structures are the leading cause of blindness in children.

40. 1. He may be at the developmental stage of seeking independence, but adolescents do not yet have the emotional or physical development to operate all-terrain vehicles. The American Academy of Pediatrics states that those younger than 16 years should not operate all-terrain vehicles. Wearing safety apparel is important in all sports.

2. He may be at the developmental stage of seeking independence, but adolescents do not yet have the emotional or physical development to operate all-terrain vehicles. The American Academy of Pediatrics states that those younger than 16 years should not operate all-terrain vehicles.

3. **He may be at the developmental stage of seeking independence, but adolescents do not yet have the emotional or physical development to operate all-terrain vehicles. The American Academy of Pediatrics states that those younger than 16 years should not operate all-terrain vehicles.**

4. He may be at the developmental stage of seeking independence, but adolescents do not yet have the emotional or physical development to operate all-terrain vehicles. The American Academy of Pediatrics states that those younger than 16 years should not operate all-terrain vehicles.

TEST-TAKING HINT: The test taker should understand that school-age children do not have the physical or emotional development to handle all-terrain vehicles.

41. 1. **Washing and drying hands and face, especially before eating, decrease lead ingestion.**
2. Other measures can be taken to decrease ingestion of lead, such as washing hands and face before eating.
3. Hot water absorbs lead more readily than cold water.
4. Diet does matter; regular meals, adequate iron, calcium, and less fat help the child absorb little lead.

TEST-TAKING HINT: The test taker should understand lead poisoning usually occurs with hand-to-mouth activity in toddlers.

42. 1. This is not the time to teach about child-proofing the home. The parent will feel guilty, and anxiety would prevent the parent from remembering the advice.
2. **The most therapeutic approach is to inquire about the circumstances of the ingestion in a nonjudgmental manner.**
3. Ipecac is no longer recommended to be kept in the home because of the increasing number of medications where its use is contraindicated. All households should have the Poison Control number by a telephone.
4. This is not the time to teach about child-proofing the home. The parent will feel guilty, and anxiety would prevent the parent from remembering the advice.

TEST-TAKING HINT: The test taker needs knowledge of therapeutic communication to answer this question.

43. 1. A battery is considered a corrosive poison, and medical attention should be sought.
2. Determining the time of ingestion is important, but treatment should be started when a battery is ingested.
3. **Batteries are considered corrosives; the child will be admitted, and surgery may be necessary for removal.**
4. This is not the time to discuss child-proofing measures. The parent would be anxious and feel guilty about the ingestion.

TEST-TAKING HINT: The test taker should understand that a battery is considered a poison and to seek medical attention.

44. 1. Continuous cardiac monitoring would be the priority because of the bradycardia and dysrhythmias that can occur with digoxin toxicity. Oxygen may be needed if there is enough bradycardia causing a decrease in oxygen saturation.

2. The priority is to establish continuous cardiac monitoring. If it is determined that venous access is necessary, then that can be established.
3. The digoxin level would be good to know, but that is not the priority.
4. **Bradycardia and cardiac dysrhythmias are common signs of digoxin toxicity in children. Continuous cardiac monitoring is the highest priority to detect dysrhythmias before they became lethal.**

TEST-TAKING HINT: The test taker should understand that bradycardia and cardiac dysrhythmia are common signs of digoxin toxicity in children.

45. 1. **100% oxygen via non-rebreather mask is given as quickly as possible if carbon monoxide poisoning is suspected because the signs and symptoms of carbon monoxide poisoning are related to tissue hypoxia.**
2. When carbon monoxide enters the blood, it readily combines with hemoglobin to form carboxyhemoglobin. Tissue hypoxia reaches dangerous levels because carbon monoxide does not release easily. Oxygen saturation obtained by oximetry will be normal because oxygen saturation monitoring does not measure dysfunctional hemoglobin.
3. The priority is to provide supplemental oxygen, then establish intravenous access.
4. Although a carbon monoxide level may be ordered, the highest priority nursing intervention is to administer oxygen.

TEST-TAKING HINT: The test taker should understand that 100% oxygen via non-rebreather mask is given as quickly as possible if carbon monoxide poisoning is suspected.

46. 1. **Age- and developmentally appropriate anticipatory guidance teachings for a 17-year-old are to discuss alcohol use and potential for alcohol poisoning.**
2. The development of secondary sex characteristics would be discussed with a younger adolescent.
3. Discussing their thoughts about anger management and safe sex would be initiated with younger teens.
4. Discussions about peer pressure would be done with younger teens when it is more prominent.

TEST-TAKING HINT: The test taker should understand that alcohol poisoning can

occur with binge drinking and should be discussed during older adolescent well visits.

47. 1. Tell the child occasional use of acetaminophen for aches and pains is recommended. Daily use can cause rebound so that when she stops taking the medication, her aches and pains will be worse. At this age, her parents should be involved in her over-the-counter drug use.
   2. Too much acetaminophen can cause liver damage; she should check with her mother before taking it.
   3. Keeping a log can be helpful in determining what triggers her aches and pains. The priority would be to recommend that she not take pain medication daily.
   4. **If she needs pain medication daily, a cause needs to be determined.**

   TEST-TAKING HINT: The test taker needs to know what would be considered therapeutic management of the child's pain.

48. 1. Vomiting is contraindicated with this medication, the best advice is to call Poison Control first. Visine (topical sympathomimetic) can cause serious or fatal consequences if even a little is ingested.
   2. **Calling Poison Control is the first step for ingestion of any known or unknown substance. Visine (topical sympathomimetic) can cause serious or fatal consequences if even a little is ingested.**
   3. The parents of any child who has had an unintentional ingestion should be counseled to call Poison Control to determine treatment. Visine (topical sympathomimetic) can cause serious or fatal consequences if even a little is ingested.
   4. Overdoses are not treated with diluted milk unless indicated.

   TEST-TAKING HINT: The test taker should understand that in cases of drug poisonings, Poison Control should be called immediately.

49. 1. Medications should never be called candy so as to prevent accidental ingestion of medication by children thinking it is candy.
   2. **Medications should never be called candy so as to prevent accidental ingestion of medication by children thinking it is candy.**
   3. This is one of those instances when the toddler has to do something he may not want to do.

4. The medication has to be taken, and the toddler is not given an option. Going to "time out" delays the administration of the medication.

   TEST-TAKING HINT: The test taker should understand that medication should never be called candy to prevent accidental ingestion.

50. 1. Charcoal is odorless and tasteless, but the black color should be masked. Providing a movie is a good distraction but is not the best answer.
   2. Never tell a child that medicine is candy in order to prevent accidental overdose.
   3. **Mixing charcoal with a sweetening agent may help the child ingest it. Children usually like sweeter drinks. Hiding the black color in an opaque container with a lid may also make it more palatable.**
   4. A parent can help by tasting the charcoal first, but getting the child to drink it quickly probably will not happen.

   TEST-TAKING HINT: The test taker should understand that masking the taste and black color will make the activated charcoal more tolerable.

51. 1. Child abuse is intentional physical, emotional, and/or sexual abuse and/or neglect.
   2. Child abuse is intentional physical, emotional, and/or sexual abuse and/or neglect.
   3. Child abuse is intentional physical, emotional, and/or sexual abuse and/or neglect.
   4. **Child abuse is intentional physical, emotional, and/or sexual abuse and/or neglect.**

   TEST-TAKING HINT: The test taker needs to know the definition.

52. 1. Genetic disorders can usually be explained by specific testing. Munchausen syndrome by proxy may be the cause of unexplained, prolonged, rare, recurrent illnesses. It usually occurs when the caregiver is present.
   2. **Munchausen syndrome by proxy may be the cause of unexplained, prolonged, rare, recurrent illnesses. It usually occurs when the caregiver is present.**
   3. Duchenne muscular dystrophy is a genetic disorder characterized by muscle weakness usually appearing in the third year of life.

4. Syndrome of inappropriate antidiuretic hormone results from hypothalamic dysfunction and is not unexplained.

TEST-TAKING HINT: The test taker needs to know the definition of Munchausen syndrome by proxy or else eliminate other options and make an educated guess.

53. 1. Immediately asking who did this is not therapeutic.
2. Blaming the mother for not protecting the child is inappropriate.
3. **When communicating with a child you think may have been abused, it is the most therapeutic to tell the child it is not the child's fault.**
4. Someone has to be told, so lying to the child is not appropriate or therapeutic.

TEST-TAKING HINT: The test taker should understand that if someone verbalizes abuse, therapeutic communication is extremely important to use.

54. 1. **The health-care provider's highest priority should be to try to get history information from the parent.**
2. Assess the child for other signs of potential physical abuse after you have determined the child is stable. Children who are physically abused may have other injuries in various stages of healing.
3. Radiological studies will be ordered, but more information as to what may have caused the injury is important information to obtain.
4. Intravenous access and blood tests may not be indicated.

TEST-TAKING HINT: The test taker should understand that history information is very important in trying to determine the cause of the arm pain.

55. 1. Burns on both feet are more indicative of a child being held in hot water, thus indicating abuse.
2. Burns on the arm may or may not indicate abuse. History information is important to determine that.
3. **Physical abuse has certain characteristics. Symmetrical burns on both feet indicate abuse.**
4. Burns mainly on the right foot might indicate the child got into a tub of hot water and then got out without putting the other foot in, which would not indicate abuse.

TEST-TAKING HINT: The test taker should understand that physical signs suggestive

of abuse are symmetrical burns with absence of splash marks.

56. 1. Masturbation is most common in 4-year-olds and during adolescence.
2. **Masturbation may indicate sexual abuse. It is imperative that the nurses do a thorough investigation if a parent is concerned about a child's masturbation.**
3. Talking with the child to find out why she is masturbating would be one component of a thorough investigation. Children do not have insight into their behaviors, however, so she may not be able to state why.
4. Masturbation may indicate sexual abuse. It is imperative that the nurse do a thorough investigation if a parent is concerned about a child's masturbation.

TEST-TAKING HINT: The test taker should understand that masturbation may indicate sexual abuse.

57. 1. Sexual exploration may be more prominent during this stage.
2. **Increased temper tantrums, increased sleep disorders, and depression may indicate sexual abuse.**
3. The child's being grateful has nothing to do with suspecting sexual abuse.
4. Children at 4 years of age are loyal to their parents. They may get angry at them, but they still love them, seek their approval, and do not talk badly about them to others. These behaviors could be normal development for a 4-year-old.

TEST-TAKING HINT: The test taker should understand that increased temper tantrums, increased sleep disorders, and depression may indicate sexual abuse.

58. 1. The priority at this time is to ensure her safety. Coming to the school nurse may be a cry for help.
2. **Her safety should be ensured first, then discuss physical complaints. School nurses are mandatory reporters of any suspected child abuse.**
3. Ensuring the child's safety is the highest priority when a health professional suspects child abuse.
4. Ensuring the child's safety is the highest priority when a health professional suspects child abuse.

TEST-TAKING HINT: Accurate assessment, description, and documentation should be recorded by the nurse. Child protective personnel should be notified.

59. 1. Abused children frequently lie about their injuries from fear about what will happen to them.
    2. **Abused children frequently repeat the same story as their parents.**
    3. Changes in behavior may suggest abuse.
    4. Children who are abused may become withdrawn and not participate in school activities.

TEST-TAKING HINT: The test taker should understand that abused children commonly repeat the same story as their parents to avoid being punished.

60. 1. **There may be absence of external signs of injury in shaken baby syndrome because the injury can cause retinal hemorrhage and subdural hematoma.**
    2. Retinal hemorrhage is indicative of shaken baby syndrome in an infant without external signs of injury.
    3. Subdural hematoma is indicative of shaken baby syndrome in an infant without external signs of injury.
    4. Infants with shaken baby syndrome do not usually have signs of external head injury.

TEST-TAKING HINT: The test taker should understand that there may be an absence of external signs of injury in shaken baby syndrome.

61. 1. It would be most therapeutic to discuss with the mother and child the best foods to eat and to avoid on a renal diet. Bananas should be limited because of their high potassium content. Potassium is excreted in the urine.
    2. **It would be most therapeutic to discuss with the mother and child the best foods to eat and to avoid on a renal diet. Bananas should be limited because of their high potassium content.**
    3. Bananas are high in potassium, so the number needs to be limited.
    4. It would be most therapeutic to discuss with the mother and child the best foods to eat and to avoid on a renal diet. Bananas should be limited because of their high potassium content.

TEST-TAKING HINT: The test taker should know dietary restrictions for a child with chronic kidney disease.

Respiratory Disorders 4

QUESTIONS

1. The nurse caring for a female pediatric client with CF sends a stool for analysis. The results show an excessive amount of azotorrhea and steatorrhea. What does the nurse realize about the laboratory values?
   1. They reflect that the patient is not compliant with taking her vitamins.
   2. They reflect that the patient is not compliant with taking her enzymes.
   3. They reflect that the patient is eating too many foods high in fat.
   4. They reflect that the patient is eating too many foods high in fiber.

2. Which of the following statements about the inheritance of CF is most accurate?
   1. CF is an autosomal-dominant trait that is passed on from the child's mother.
   2. CF is an autosomal-dominant trait that is passed on from the child's father.
   3. The child of parents who are both carriers of the gene for CF has a 50% chance of acquiring CF.
   4. The child of a mother who has CF and a father who is a carrier of the gene for CF has a 50% chance of acquiring CF.

3. The parent of a 4-month-old with CF asks the nurse what time to begin the child's first CPT each day. Which is the nurse's best response?
   1. "You should do the first CPT 30 minutes before feeding the child breakfast."
   2. "You should do the first CPT after deep-suctioning the child each morning."
   3. "You should do the first CPT 30 minutes after feeding the child breakfast."
   4. "You should do the first CPT only when the child has congestion or coughing."

4. The parent of a 10-month-old with CF asks the nurse how to meet the child's increased nutritional needs. Which is the nurse's best suggestion?
   1. "You may need to increase the number of fresh fruits and vegetables you give your child each day."
   2. "You may need to advance your child's diet to whole cow's milk because it is higher in fat than formula."
   3. "You may need to change your child to a higher-calorie formula."
   4. "You may need to increase your child's carbohydrate intake each day."

5. The parent of an 18-year-old with CF is excited about the possibility of the child receiving a double lung transplant. What should the parent understand?
   1. The transplant will cure the child of CF and allow the child to lead a long and healthy life.
   2. The transplant will not cure the child of CF but will allow the child to have a longer life.
   3. The transplant will help to reverse the multisystem damage that has already been caused by CF.
   4. The transplant will be the child's only chance at surviving long enough to graduate college.

6. A 2-year-old has just been diagnosed with CF. The parents ask the nurse what early respiratory symptoms they should expect to see in their child. Which is the nurse's best response?
   1. "You can expect your child to develop a barrel-shaped chest."
   2. "You can expect your child to develop a chronic productive cough."
   3. "You can expect your child to develop bronchiectasis."
   4. "You can expect your child to develop wheezing respirations."

7. A female child with CF is hospitalized with constipation. The parent asks the nurse what will need to be done to relieve the child's constipation. Which is the nurse's best response?
   1. "Your child likely has an obstruction and will require surgery."
   2. "Your child will likely be given IV fluids to relieve her constipation."
   3. "Your child will likely be given GoLYTELY to relieve her constipation."
   4. "Your child will be placed on a clear liquid diet to relieve her constipation."

8. The parents of a 5-week-old have just been told that their child has CF. The mother had a sister who died of CF when she was 19 years of age. The parents are sad and ask the nurse several questions about CF and the current projected life expectancy. What is the nurse's best initial intervention?
   1. The nurse should tell the parents that the life expectancy for CF patients has improved significantly in recent years.
   2. The nurse should tell the parents that their child might not follow the same course that the mother's sister did.
   3. The nurse should listen to the parents and tell them that the physician will come to speak to them about treatment options.
   4. The nurse should listen to the parents and be available to them anytime during the day to answer their questions.

9. A 7-month-old is taken to the pediatrician's office with a low-grade fever, nasal congestion, and a mild cough. Which should the nursing care management of this child include?
   1. Maintaining strict bedrest.
   2. Avoiding contact with family members.
   3. Instilling saline nose drops and bulb suctioning.
   4. Keeping the head of the bed flat.

10. A school-age child has been diagnosed with nasopharyngitis. The parent is concerned because the child has had little or no appetite for the last 24 hours. The parent asks the nurse if this is a concern. Which is the nurse's best response?
   1. "Do not be concerned; it is common for children to have a decreased appetite for several days during a respiratory illness."
   2. "Be sure your child is taking an adequate amount of fluid. The appetite should return soon."
   3. "Try offering the child some favorite food. Maybe that will improve the appetite."
   4. "You need to force your child to eat whatever you can; adequate nutrition is essential."

11. A physician diagnoses a school-age child with strep throat and pharyngitis. The child's parent asks the nurse what treatment the child will need. Which is the nurse's best response?
   1. "Your child will be sent home on bedrest and should recover in a few days without any intervention."
   2. "Your child will need to have the tonsils removed to prevent future strep infections."
   3. "Your child will need oral penicillin for 10 days and should feel better in a few days."
   4. "Your child will need to be admitted to the hospital for 5 days of intravenous antibiotics."

12. A 5-year-old female is diagnosed with pharyngitis. The child is complaining of throat pain. Which of the following statements by the mother indicates that she needs more education regarding the care and treatment of her daughter's throat pain?
   1. "I will have my daughter gargle with warm saline three times a day."
   2. "I will offer my daughter ice chips several times a day."
   3. "I will give my daughter Tylenol every 4 to 6 hours as needed."
   4. "I will give my daughter her amoxicillin until all doses of the antibiotic are gone."

13. A school-age child has been diagnosed with strep throat. The parent asks the nurse when the child can return to school. Which is the nurse's best response?
    1. "48 hours after the first documented normal temperature."
    2. "24 hours after the first dose of antibiotics."
    3. "48 hours after the first dose of antibiotics."
    4. "24 hours after the first documented normal temperature."

14. A school-age child is admitted to the hospital for a tonsillectomy. The nurse caring for this patient is assessing the child 8 hours after surgery. During the nurse's assessment, the child's parent tells the nurse that the child is in pain. Which of the following observations should be of most concern to the nurse?
    1. The child's heart rate and blood pressure are elevated.
    2. The child complains of having a sore throat.
    3. The child is refusing to eat solid foods.
    4. The child is swallowing excessively.

15. A pediatric client had a tonsillectomy 24 hours ago. The nurse is reviewing discharge instructions with the parents. The parents tell the nurse that the child is a big eater, and they want to know what foods to give the child for the next 24 hours. What is the nurse's best response?
    1. "The child's diet should not be restricted at all."
    2. "The child's diet should be restricted to clear liquids."
    3. "The child's diet should be restricted to ice cream and cold liquids."
    4. "The child's diet should be restricted to soft foods."

16. A pediatric client is admitted to the ER with an acute asthma exacerbation. The nurse tells the parents that blood will have to be drawn for some diagnostic laboratory studies. Which laboratory result will provide the health-care team with the most important information regarding the child's respiratory status?
    1. A CBC.
    2. An ABG.
    3. A BUN.
    4. A PTT.

17. A pediatric client is admitted in status asthmaticus. The parent reports that the child is currently taking Singulair, albuterol, and Flovent. What is the most important piece of information that the nurse must ask the parent in order to best treat the patient?
    1. "What time did your child eat last?"
    2. "Has your child been exposed to any of the usual asthma triggers?"
    3. "When was your child last admitted to the hospital for asthma?"
    4. "When was your child's last dose of medication?"

18. A 2-year-old is diagnosed with asthma. The parents are big sports fans and want their child to play sports. The parents ask the nurse what impact asthma will have on the child's future in sports. Which is the nurse's best response?
    1. "As long as your child takes prescribed asthma medication, the child will be fine."
    2. "The earlier a child is diagnosed with asthma, the more significant the symptoms."
    3. "The earlier a child is diagnosed with asthma, the better the chance the child has of growing out of the disease."
    4. "Your child should avoid playing contact sports and sports that require a lot of running."

19. The parent of a pediatric client with asthma is talking to the nurse about administering the child's albuterol inhaler. Which statement by the parent leads the nurse to believe that the parent needs further education on how to administer the medication?
    1. "I should administer two quick puffs of the albuterol inhaler using a spacer."
    2. "I should always use a spacer when administering the albuterol inhaler."
    3. "I should be sure that my child is in an upright position when administering the inhaler."
    4. "I should always shake the inhaler before administering a dose."

20. A 7-year-old female with asthma is playing a soccer game in gym class. During the game the child begins to cough, wheeze, and have difficulty catching her breath. The school nurse is called to the soccer field. Which of the following should the nurse administer to provide quick relief?
    1. Prednisone.
    2. Singulair.
    3. Albuterol.
    4. Flovent.

21. There are several children in the ER waiting area who all have asthma. The nurse has only one room left in the ER. Based on the following information, which child should be seen first?
    1. A 5-year-old who is speaking in complete sentences, is pink in color, is wheezing bilaterally, and has an oxygen saturation of 93%.
    2. A 9-year-old who is quiet, is pale in color, and is wheezing bilaterally with an oxygen saturation of 92%.
    3. A 12-month-old who has a mild cry, is pale in color, has diminished breath sounds, and has an oxygen saturation of 93%.
    4. A 16-year-old who is speaking in short sentences, is wheezing, is sitting upright, and has an oxygen saturation of 93%.

22. A 3-year-old female is admitted to the hospital with asthma. The nurse is trying to work with the child on breathing exercises to increase her expiratory phase. What should the nurse have the child do?
    1. Use an incentive spirometer.
    2. Breathe into a paper bag.
    3. Blow a pinwheel.
    4. Take several deep breaths.

23. The parents of a 6-year-old who has a new diagnosis of asthma asks the nurse what to do to make their home a more allergy-free environment for the child. Which is the nurse's best response?
    1. "Use a humidifier in your child's room."
    2. "Have your carpet cleaned chemically once a month."
    3. "Wash household pets weekly."
    4. "Avoid purchasing upholstered furniture."

24. A pediatric client was seen at the pediatrician's office and was diagnosed with viral tonsillitis. The parent asks how to care for the child at home. Which is the nurse's best response?
    1. "You will need to give your child a prescribed antibiotic for 10 days."
    2. "You will need to schedule a follow-up appointment in 2 weeks."
    3. "You can give your child Tylenol every 4 to 6 hours as needed for pain."
    4. "You can place warm towels around your child's neck for comfort."

25. A 2-month-old is seen in the pediatrician's office for his 2-month well-child checkup. The nurse is assessing the patient and reports to the physician that the child is exhibiting early signs of respiratory distress. Which of the following would indicate an early sign of distress?
    1. The infant is breathing shallowly.
    2. The infant has tachypnea.
    3. The infant has tachycardia.
    4. The infant has bradycardia.

26. Nursing care management of the pediatric client with a diagnosis of mononucleosis should include which of the following?
    1. Limit the child's visitors to family only.
    2. Limit the child's activity to bedrest.
    3. Limit the child's diet to clear liquids.
    4. Limit the child's daily fluid intake.

27. The school nurse is planning to educate kindergarten children on how to stop the spread of influenza in the classroom. Which of the following should the nurse instruct the children?
    1. Stay home if they have a runny nose and cough.
    2. Wash their hands after using the restroom.
    3. Wash their hands after sneezing.
    4. Have a flu shot annually.

28. Which of the following is the highest priority for receiving the flu vaccine?
    1. An 18-year-old who is living in a college dormitory.
    2. A healthy 8-month-old who attends day care.
    3. A 7-year-old who attends public school.
    4. A 3-year-old who is undergoing chemotherapy.

29. The parent of a pediatric client with influenza is concerned about when the child will be able to return to school. The parent asks the nurse when the child is most infectious. Which is the nurse's best response?
    1. "24 hours before and after the onset of symptoms."
    2. "1 week after the onset of symptoms."
    3. "1 week before the onset of symptoms."
    4. "24 hours after the onset of symptoms."

30. A 6-week-old male is admitted to the hospital with influenza. The child is crying, and the father tells the nurse that his son is hungry. The nurse explains that the baby is taking nothing by mouth. The parent does not understand why the child cannot eat. Which is the nurse's best response to the parent?
    1. "We are giving your child intravenous fluids, so there is no need for anything by mouth."
    2. "The shorter and narrower airway of infants increases their chances of aspiration."
    3. "When your child eats, he burns too many calories; we want to conserve the child's energy."
    4. "Your child has too much nasal congestion; if we feed the child by mouth, the distress will likely increase."

31. The nurse is caring for a 22-month-old male who has had repeated bouts of otitis media. The nurse is educating the parents about otitis media. Which of the following statements from the parents indicates they need additional teaching?
    1. "If I quit smoking, my child may have less chance of getting an ear infection."
    2. "As my child gets older, he should have fewer ear infections, because his immune system will be more developed."
    3. "My child will have fewer ear infections if he has his tonsils removed."
    4. "My child may need a speech evaluation."

32. The parent of a 10-month-old male brings the child to the pediatrician's office with URI symptoms and a fever. The parent asks the nurse what can be done at home to improve the child's current condition. Which is the nurse's best response?
   1. "Give your child small amounts of fluid every hour to prevent dehydration."
   2. "Give your child Robitussin at night to reduce his cough and help him sleep."
   3. "Give your child a baby aspirin every 4 to 6 hours to help reduce the fever."
   4. "Give your child an over-the-counter cold medicine at night."

33. A physician prescribes 10 days of amoxicillin to treat a 6-year-old male with an ear infection. The nurse is reviewing discharge instructions with the parent. Which information should be included in the discharge instructions?
   1. "Administer the amoxicillin until the child's symptoms subside."
   2. "Administer an over-the-counter antihistamine with the antibiotic."
   3. "Administer the amoxicillin until all the medication is gone."
   4. "Allow your child to administer his own dose of amoxicillin."

34. The parent of a pediatric client who has had frequent ear infections asks the nurse if there is anything that can be done to help the child avoid future ear infections. Which is the nurse's best response?
   1. "Your child should be put on a daily dose of Singulair."
   2. "Your child should be kept away from tobacco smoke."
   3. "Your child should be kept away from other children with otitis."
   4. "Your child should always wear a hat when outside."

35. Which of the following children would benefit most from having ear tubes placed?
   1. A 2-month-old who has had one ear infection.
   2. A 2-year-old who has had five previous ear infections.
   3. A 7-year-old who has had two ear infections this year.
   4. A 3-year-old whose sibling has had four ear infections.

36. A 2-month-old is diagnosed with otitis. The parent asks the nurse if the otitis will have any long-term effects for the child. Understanding the complications that can occur with otitis, which is the nurse's best response?
   1. "The child could suffer hearing loss."
   2. "The child could suffer some speech delays."
   3. "The child could suffer recurrent ear infections."
   4. "The child could require ear tubes."

37. A 6-month-old is diagnosed with an ear infection. The parents report that the child is not sleeping well and is crying frequently. The child also has a moderate amount of yellow drainage coming from the infected ear. This is the parents' first baby. Which of the following nursing objectives is the priority for this family at this time?
   1. Educating the parents about signs and symptoms of an ear infection.
   2. Providing emotional support for the parents.
   3. Providing pain relief for the child.
   4. Promoting the flow of drainage from the ear.

38. A 2-year-old is admitted to the hospital in respiratory distress. The physician tells the parents that the child probably has RSV. The parents ask the nurse how they will determine if their child has RSV. Which is the nurse's best response?
   1. "We will need to do a simple blood test to determine whether your child has RSV."
   2. "There is no specific test for RSV. The diagnosis is made based on the child's symptoms."
   3. "We will swab your child's nose and send those secretions for testing."
   4. "We will have to send a viral culture to an outside lab for testing."

39. An 8-month-old male twin is in the hospital with RSV. The nurse educated the parent on how to prevent the healthy twin at home from contracting RSV. Which statement indicates the parent needs further teaching?
    1. "I should make sure that both my children receive Synagis injections for the remainder of this year."
    2. "I should be sure to keep my infected son away from his brother until he has recovered."
    3. "I should insist that all people who come in contact with my twins thoroughly wash their hands before playing with them."
    4. "I should insist that anyone with a respiratory illness avoid contact with my children until the children are well."

40. Which of the following patients is at highest risk for requiring hospitalization as a result of RSV?
    1. A 3-year-old with a congenital heart defect.
    2. A 2-month-old who is a former 32-week preemie.
    3. A 4-year-old who is a former 30-week preemie.
    4. A sixteen-month-old with a tracheostomy.

41. A 6-month-old is admitted to the hospital with RAD. The nurse is assessing the child. Which of the following physical findings should be of most concern?
    1. The baby has tachypnea.
    2. The baby has mild retractions.
    3. The baby is wheezing.
    4. The baby is grunting.

42. A 6-year-old presents to the ER with respiratory distress and stridor. The child is diagnosed with RSV. The parent asks the child's nurse how the child will be treated. Which is the nurse's best response?
    1. "We will treat your child with intravenous antibiotics."
    2. "We will treat your child with intravenous steroids."
    3. "We will treat your child with nebulized racemic epinephrine."
    4. "We will treat your child with alternating doses of Tylenol and Motrin."

43. The parent of a pediatric client calls the ER. The parent reports that the child has had a barky cough for the last 3 days and it always gets worse at night. The parent asks the nurse what to do. Which is the nurse's best response?
    1. "Take your child outside in the night air for 15 minutes."
    2. "Bring your child to the ER immediately."
    3. "Give your child an over-the-counter cough suppressant."
    4. "Give your child warm liquids to soothe the throat."

44. Which of the following children is in the greatest need of emergency medical treatment?
    1. A 6-year-old who has high fever, no spontaneous cough, and frog-like croaking.
    2. A 3-year-old who has a barky cough, is afebrile, and has mild intercostal retractions.
    3. A 7-year-old who has abrupt onset of moderate respiratory distress, a mild fever, and a barky cough.
    4. A 13-year-old who has a high fever, stridor, and purulent secretions.

45. A pediatric client is seen in the ER with a nonproductive cough, clear nasal drainage, and congestion. The child is diagnosed with nasopharyngitis. What information should the nurse include in the discharge instructions?
    1. Inform the parents to complete the entire prescription of antibiotics.
    2. Recommend that the parents avoid sending the child to day care.
    3. Educate the parents on comfort measures for the child.
    4. Instruct the parents to restrict the child to clear liquids for 24 hours.

46. A 15-month-old is brought to the ER. The parents tell the nurse that the child has not been eating well and has had an increased respiratory rate. Which of the following assessments is of greatest concern?
    1. The patient is lying down and has moderate retractions, low-grade fever, and nasal congestion.
    2. The patient is in the tripod position and has diminished breath sounds and a muffled cough.
    3. The patient is sitting up and has coarse breath sounds, coughing, and fussiness.
    4. The patient is restless, crying, has bilateral wheezes and poor feeding.

47. A 3-year-old female is admitted to the ER with drooling, difficulty swallowing, sore throat, and a fever of 39°C (102.2° F). The physician suspects epiglottitis. The parents ask the nurse how the physician will know for sure if their daughter has epiglottitis. Which is the nurse's best response?
    1. "A simple blood test will tell us if your daughter has epiglottitis."
    2. "We will swab your daughter's throat and send it for culture."
    3. "We will do a lateral neck x-ray of the soft tissue."
    4. "The diagnosis is made based on your daughter's signs and symptoms."

48. A 2-year-old child is brought to the ER with a high fever, dysphagia, drooling, rapid pulse, and tachypnea. What should the nurse's first action be?
    1. Prepare for immediate IV placement.
    2. Prepare for immediate respiratory treatment.
    3. Place the child on a stretcher for a thorough physical assessment.
    4. Allow the child to sit in the parent's lap while awaiting an x-ray.

49. A pediatric client is diagnosed with epiglottitis. The parents ask the nurse what treatment their child will receive. Which is the nurse's best response?
    1. "Your child will need to complete a course of intravenous antibiotics."
    2. "Your child will need to have surgery to remove her tonsils."
    3. "Your child will need 10 days of aerosolized ribavirin."
    4. "Your child will recover without any intervention in about 5 days."

50. A 3-year-old is admitted to the hospital with a diagnosis of epiglottitis. The child is in severe distress and needs to be intubated. The mother is crying and tells the nurse that she should have brought her son in yesterday when he said his throat was sore. Which is the nurse's best response?
    1. "Children this age rarely get epiglottitis; you should not blame yourself."
    2. "It is always better to have your child evaluated at the first sign of illness rather than wait until symptoms worsen."
    3. "Epiglottitis is slowly progressive, so early intervention may have decreased the extent of your son's symptoms."
    4. "Epiglottitis is rapidly progressive; you could not have predicted that his symptoms would worsen so quickly."

51. A 2-year-old is admitted to the hospital with croup. The parent tells the nurse that her 7-year-old just had croup and it cleared up in a couple of days without intervention. She asks the nurse why her 2-year-old is exhibiting worse symptoms and needs to be hospitalized. Which is the nurse's best response?
    1. "Some children just react differently to viruses. It is best to treat each child as an individual."
    2. "Younger children have wider airways that make it easier for bacteria to enter and colonize."
    3. "Younger children have short and wide eustachian tubes, making them more susceptible to respiratory infections."
    4. "Children younger than 3 years usually exhibit worse symptoms because their immune systems are not as developed."

52. A 5-year-old is brought to the ER with a temperature of 99.5° F (37.5°C), a barky cough, stridor, and hoarseness. Which of the following nursing interventions should the nurse prepare for?
1. Immediate IV placement.
2. Respiratory treatment of racemic epinephrine.
3. A tracheostomy set at the bedside.
4. Informing the child's parents about a tonsillectomy.

53. A 3-year-old is seen in the physician's office for a dry, hacking cough that is preventing the child from sleeping. The child is diagnosed with a URI. Which of the following interventions is most appropriate for this patient?
1. The child should be given cough suppressants at night.
2. The child should be given a cough expectorant every 4 hours.
3. The child should be given cold and flu medication every 8 hours.
4. The child should be given 1/2 teaspoon honey four to five times per day.

54. Which of the following statements about pneumonia is accurate?
1. Pneumonia is most frequently caused by bacterial agents.
2. Children with bacterial pneumonia are usually sicker than children with viral pneumonia.
3. Children with viral pneumonia are usually sicker than those with bacterial pneumonia.
4. Children with viral pneumonia must be treated with a complete course of antibiotics.

55. Which of the following children diagnosed with pneumonia would benefit most from hospitalization?
1. A 14-year-old with a fever of 38.6°C (101.5°F), rapid breathing, and a decreased appetite.
2. A 15-year-old who has been vomiting for 3 days and has a fever of 38.5°C (101.3°F).
3. A 13-year-old who is coughing, has coarse breath sounds, and is not sleeping well.
4. A 16-year-old who has a cough, chills, fever of 38.5°C (101.3°F), and wheezing.

56. A pediatric client is admitted to the hospital with left-sided pneumonia. The client is complaining of pain and wants to be repositioned in the bed. The nurse knows the patient may be most comfortable in which position?
1. Lying in the Trendelenburg position.
2. Lying on the left side.
3. Lying on the right side.
4. Lying in the supine position.

57. A pediatric client with severe cerebral palsy is admitted to the hospital with aspiration pneumonia. What is the most beneficial educational information that the nurse can provide to the parents?
1. The signs and symptoms of aspiration pneumonia.
2. The treatment plan for aspiration pneumonia.
3. The risks associated with recurrent aspiration pneumonia.
4. The prevention of aspiration pneumonia.

58. A 3-year-old is brought to the ER with coughing and gagging. The parent reports that the child was eating carrots when she began to gag. What diagnostic evaluation will be used to determine if the child has aspirated the carrot?
1. A chest x-ray will be taken.
2. A bronchoscopy will be performed.
3. A blood gas will be drawn.
4. A sputum culture will be done.

59. The parent of a 9-month-old calls the ER because his child is choking on a marble. The parent tells the nurse that he knows cardiopulmonary resuscitation. The parent asks how to help his child while waiting for Emergency Medical Services. Which is the nurse's best response?
1. "You should administer five abdominal thrusts followed by five back blows."
2. "You should try to retrieve the object by inserting your finger in your daughter's mouth."
3. "You should perform the Heimlich maneuver."
4. "You should administer five back blows followed by five chest thrusts."

60. The community health nurse is teaching a child-safety class to parents of toddlers. Which information will be most helpful in teaching the parents about the primary prevention of foreign body aspiration?
1. Knowledge of the signs and symptoms of foreign body aspiration.
2. Knowledge of the therapeutic management of foreign body aspiration patients.
3. Knowledge of the most common objects that toddlers aspirate.
4. Knowledge of the risks associated with foreign body aspiration.

61. What does the therapeutic management of CF patients include? Select all that apply.
1. Providing a high-protein, high-calorie diet.
2. Providing a high-fat, high-carbohydrate diet.
3. Encouraging exercise.
4. Minimizing pulmonary complication.
5. Encouraging medication compliance.

62. A sweat chloride test is used to diagnose CF. A chloride level greater than _____ is a positive diagnostic indicator of CF.

1. 1. The patient's compliance with vitamins would not be reflected in a lab result of azotorrhea and steatorrhea. If the patient were not taking her daily vitamin supplements, she might be deficient in those vitamins.
   2. **If the patient were not taking her enzymes, the result would be a large amount of undigested food, azotorrhea, and steatorrhea in the stool. CF patients must take digestive enzymes with all meals and snacks. Pancreatic ducts become clogged with thick mucus that blocks the flow of digestive enzymes from the pancreas to the duodenum. Therefore, patients must take digestive enzymes to aid in absorption of nutrients. Often, teens are noncompliant with their medication regimen because they want to be like their peers.**
   3. Steatorrhea is an increased amount of fat in the stool. However, in CF patients, it is not a result of eating too many fatty foods.
   4. Azotorrhea is an increased amount of protein in the stool. Steatorrhea is an increased amount of fat in the stool. This is not a result of eating too many foods high in fiber.

   TEST-TAKING HINT: The test taker needs to understand the pathophysiology of CF and the impact it has on the gastrointestinal system. The test taker also must be familiar with the conditions azotorrhea and steatorrhea.

2. 1. CF is not an autosomal-dominant trait. It is a recessive trait. Therefore, both parents must be carriers of the gene in order for their children to inherit the disease. If a child is born to parents who are both carriers of the gene for CF, the child has a 25% chance of acquiring the disease and a 50% chance of being a carrier of the disease. If the child is born to a mother with CF and a father who is a carrier, the child has a 50% chance of acquiring the disease and a 50% chance of being a carrier of the disease.
   2. CF is not an autosomal-dominant trait. It is a recessive trait. Therefore, both parents must be carriers of the gene in order for their children to inherit the gene. If a child is born to parents who are both carriers of the gene for CF, the child has a 25% chance of acquiring the disease and a 50% chance of being a carrier of the disease. If the child is born to a mother with CF and a father who is a carrier, the child has a 50% chance of acquiring the disease and a 50% chance of being a carrier of the disease.
   3. If a child is born to parents who are both carriers of the gene for CF, the child has a 25% chance of acquiring the disease and a 50% chance of being a carrier of the disease.
   4. **If the child is born to a mother with CF and a father who is a carrier, the child has a 50% chance of acquiring the disease and a 50% chance of being a carrier of the disease.**

   TEST-TAKING HINT: Answers 1 and 2 can be eliminated with knowledge of the genetic inheritance of CF. CF is not an autosomal-dominant trait.

3. 1. **CPT should be done in the morning prior to feeding to avoid the risk of the child vomiting.**
   2. Infants with CF are not routinely deep-suctioned. Occasionally if they have a weak cough reflex, infants may be suctioned following CPT to stimulate them to cough.
   3. If CPT is done following feeding, it increases the likelihood that the child may vomit.
   4. CPT should be done as a daily regimen with all CF patients. CPT helps to break up the secretions in the lungs and makes it easier for the patient to clear those secretions.

   TEST-TAKING HINT: Answer 4 can be eliminated because of the word "only." There are very few times in health care when an answer will be "only." Answer 3 can be eliminated when one considers the risk of vomiting and aspiration that may occur if percussion is performed following eating.

4. 1. Children with CF have difficulty absorbing nutrients because of the blockage of the pancreatic duct. Pancreatic enzymes cannot reach the duodenum to aid in digestion of food. These children often require up to 150% of the caloric intake of their peers. The nutritional recommendation for CF patients is high-calorie and high-protein.
   2. Whole cow's milk is a good source of fat but is not an increased source of protein that is recommended for CF patients. Another consideration here is that whole cow's milk is not recommended until 12 months of age.

3. Often infants with CF need to have a higher-calorie formula to meet their nutritional needs. Infants may also be placed on hydrolysate formulas that contain added medium-chain triglycerides.

4. An increase in carbohydrate intake is not usually necessary. The nutritional recommendation for CF patients is high-calorie and high-protein.

TEST-TAKING HINT: Answers 1, 2, and 4 can be eliminated with understanding of the nutritional needs of the child with CF. Answer 2 can also be eliminated because whole cow's milk is not recommended until 12 months of age.

5. 1. A lung transplant does not cure CF, but the transplanted lungs do not contain the CF genes. Although the new lungs do not contain CF, the sinuses, pancreas, intestines, sweat glands, and reproductive tract do. The new lungs are more susceptible to infection because of the immunosuppressive therapy that must be given post transplant. Immunosuppressive drugs make it difficult for the body to fight infection, which can lead to lung damage.

2. A lung transplant does not cure CF, but it does offer the patient an opportunity to live a longer life. The concerns are that, after the lung transplant, the child is at risk for rejection of the new organ and for development of secondary infections because of the immunosuppressive therapy.

3. The lung transplant does not reverse the damage that has been done to the child's other organs, but it does offer a chance of a longer life.

4. The average life span of a patient with CF is mid-30s. The life span has increased over the years with the daily regimens of CPT, exercise, medications and high-calorie, high-protein diets.

TEST-TAKING HINT: Answer 4 can be eliminated because of the word "only." There are very few times in health care when an answer will be "only." Answers 1 and 3 can be eliminated if the test taker has a basic knowledge of the pathophysiology of CF.

6. 1. A barrel-shaped chest is a long-term respiratory problem that occurs as a result of recurrent hyperinflation of alveoli.

2. A chronic productive cough is common as pulmonary damage increases.

3. Bronchiectasis develops in advanced stages of CF.

4. Wheezing respirations and a dry non-productive cough are common early symptoms in CF.

TEST-TAKING HINT: Answer 2 can be eliminated because of the word "chronic." "Chronic" implies that the disease process is advanced rather than in the initial stages. Answers 1 and 3 can be eliminated if the test taker has knowledge of signs and symptoms of advanced lung disease.

7. 1. CF patients who present with constipation usually do not require surgery. They commonly receive a stool softener or an osmotic solution orally to relieve their constipation.

2. IV fluids may be ordered if the patient is NPO for any reason. However, IV fluids do not help relieve the patient's constipation. CF patients with constipation commonly receive a stool softener or an osmotic solution orally to relieve their constipation.

3. CF patients with constipation commonly receive a stool softener or an osmotic solution orally to relieve their constipation.

4. CF patients are not placed on a liquid diet to relieve the constipation. CF patients with constipation commonly receive a stool softener or an osmotic solution orally to relieve their constipation. Once the constipation is relieved, the patient will likely be placed on a low-fat diet and a stool softener.

TEST-TAKING HINT: Answer 1 can be eliminated because surgery is not indicated for constipation.

8. 1. The parents are devastated by the new diagnosis and are likely not ready to hear about the current life expectancy for CF patients. They are in shock and are trying to deal with the new diagnosis, so any additional information will just add to their stress level.

2. The mother had a negative experience with CF in her own family and will likely continue to focus on her past experience with the disease. It may be more effective to give her time to consider her son's diagnosis and present her with information about current treatments and life span in a few days.

3. Listening to the parents is an appropriate intervention. However, having the physician return with additional information will not help these parents at this time. They need time before they are given additional information.

4. The nurse's best intervention is to let the parents express their concerns and fears. The nurse should be available if the parents have any other concerns or questions or if they just need someone with whom to talk.

TEST-TAKING HINT: When parents are given information that their child has a chronic life-threatening disease, they are not capable of processing all the information right away, they need time. The parents are often given more information than they can possibly understand and often just need someone to listen to their concerns and needs.

9. 1. Strict bedrest is not necessary. Children with respiratory illnesses usually self-limit their activity. Parents just need to ensure that their children are getting adequate rest.
   2. It is not necessary to avoid contact with family members. Nasopharyngitis is spread by contact with the secretions, so hand washing is the key to limiting the spread of the virus.
   3. **Infants are nose breathers and often have increased difficulty when they are congested. Nasal saline drops and gentle suctioning with a bulb syringe are often recommended.**
   4. The head of the bed should be elevated in order to help with the drainage of secretions.

TEST-TAKING HINT: The test taker can eliminate answer 4 given a basic understanding of interventions to improve respiratory function.

10. 1. It is common for children to have a decreased appetite when they have a respiratory illness. However, the nurse needs to be sure to instruct the parent that the child take in an adequate amount of fluid in order to stay hydrated.
    2. **It is common for children to have a decreased appetite when they have a respiratory illness. The nurse is appropriately instructing the parent that the child will be fine by taking in an adequate amount of fluid.**
    3. The child may want to eat some favorite foods; however, the child will be fine if an adequate amount of fluid is maintained.
    4. The parent should not force the child to eat; the child's appetite should return in a couple of days.

TEST-TAKING HINT: Answer 4 can be eliminated because one should not force the child to eat. If the word had been "encourage," it would have been a better choice, although still not the best answer. Answer 1 can be eliminated because the nurse did not inform the parent of the importance of maintaining adequate fluid intake.

11. 1. The child may need bedrest. However, the child does need antibiotics to treat the strep infection.
    2. The child does not need the tonsils removed; the child has pharyngitis and strep throat. Surgical removal of the tonsils is done only following recurrent bouts of infection.
    3. **The child will need a 10-day course of penicillin to treat the strep infection. It is essential that the nurse always tell the family that, although the child will feel better in a few days, the entire course of antibiotics must be completed.**
    4. Strep throat can be treated at home with oral penicillin and does not require IV antibiotics and hospitalization.

TEST-TAKING HINT: Answer 2 can be eliminated because it is a treatment for recurrent tonsillitis, not pharyngitis. Answer 1 can be eliminated if the test taker understands that bacterial infections need to be treated with antibiotics.

12. 1. Gargling with warm saline is a recommended treatment to relieve some of the discomfort associated with pharyngitis and is appropriate for a 5-year-old child.
    2. Encouraging ice chips is a recommended treatment to relieve some of the discomfort associated with pharyngitis and is an acceptable choice for a 5-year-old child.
    3. Tylenol is a suggested treatment for relief of discomfort related to pharyngitis for children of all ages.
    4. **Pharyngitis is a self-limiting viral illness that does not require antibiotic therapy. Pharyngitis should be treated with rest and comfort measures, including Tylenol, throat sprays, cold liquids, and popsicles.**

TEST-TAKING HINT: Answers 1, 2, and 3 are comfort measures and are developmentally appropriate for the age of the child. The question requires that the student have knowledge regarding pharyngitis.

13. 1. School systems require that children remain home for 24 hours after having a documented fever. However, in this question the child has been diagnosed with strep throat. Even if the child is fever-free, the child must have completed a 24-hour course of antibiotics before returning to school. Children with strep throat are no longer contagious 24 hours after initiation of antibiotic therapy.

2. **Children with strep throat are no longer contagious 24 hours after initiation of antibiotic therapy.**

3. Children with strep throat are no longer contagious 24 hours after initiation of antibiotic therapy.

4. School systems require that children remain home for 24 hours after having a documented fever. However, in this question the child has been diagnosed with strep throat. Even if the child is fever-free, the child must have completed a 24-hour course of antibiotics before returning to school. Children with strep throat are no longer contagious 24 hours after initiation of antibiotic therapy.

TEST-TAKING HINT: The test taker can eliminate answers 1 and 4 given knowledge of the communicability of strep throat.

14. 1. The patient is complaining of pain so it is not unusual that there is an elevated heart rate and blood pressure. The nurse should address the pain by giving any prn pain medications ordered or calling the physician for an order.

2. Most children will complain after a tonsillectomy. This is expected.

3. Oral intake is usually limited to popsicles, ice chips, and cold liquids following a tonsillectomy. The child is in pain and should not be expected to be eating solid foods 8 hours after surgery.

4. **Excessive swallowing is a sign that the child is swallowing blood. This should be considered a medical emergency, and the physician should be contacted immediately. The child is likely bleeding and will need to return to surgery.**

TEST-TAKING HINT: Answer 1 can be eliminated if the test taker understands the common vital-sign changes that occur when a person is experiencing pain.

15. 1. A child should be restricted to soft foods for the first couple of days postoperatively. Soft foods are recommended because the child will have a sore throat for several days following surgery. Soft foods are also recommended to decrease the risk of bleeding.

2. Most children self-limit their food intake postoperatively. Children can have solids, but soft foods are recommended for the first several postoperative days.

3. Most children prefer to eat cold foods, but they are not restricted to them.

4. **Soft foods are recommended to limit the child's pain and to decrease the risk for bleeding.**

TEST-TAKING HINT: The test taker can eliminate answer 1 by knowing there are usually some dietary restrictions following any surgical procedure.

16. 1. The CBC gives the health-care team information about the child's red and white blood cell count and hemoglobin and hematocrit levels. The CBC indicates if the child has or is developing an infection but nothing about the child's current respiratory status.

2. **The ABG gives the health-care team valuable information about the child's respiratory status: level of oxygenation, carbon dioxide, and blood pH.**

3. The BUN provides information about the patient's kidney function but nothing regarding the patient's respiratory status.

4. The PTT provides information about how long it takes the patient's blood to clot but nothing about the patient's respiratory status.

TEST-TAKING HINT: The test taker can eliminate answers 1, 2, and 4 with a knowledge of common laboratory tests.

17. 1. The nurse needs to know when the child ate last in the event that the child may need to be intubated for severe respiratory distress, but it is not the most vital piece of information in order to best treat the child for the current state of distress.

2. The nurse needs to know if the child was exposed to anything that usually triggers the asthma, but that is not the most important information for treating the child's immediate need.

3. Knowing when the child was admitted last will give the nurse an idea of the severity of the child's asthma, but that is not the most important information for treating the child's immediate need.

4. **The nurse needs to know what medication the child had last and when the child took it in order to know how to begin treatment for the current asthmatic condition.**

TEST-TAKING HINT: Whereas all of the information here is essential, answer 4 gives the most important information. The test taker can eliminate answers 2 and 3 because the responses to these inquiries have no direct impact on the immediate treatment of the child. These two answers give information about the severity of the child's illness but they do not affect the immediate treatment plan. Answer 4 is essential to deciding what medication should be given the child to relieve the current symptoms.

18. 1. It is essential that the child take all of the scheduled asthma medications, but there is no guarantee the child will be fine and be able to play all sports.
    2. **When a child is diagnosed with asthma at an early age, the child is more likely to have significant symptoms on aging.**
    3. Children diagnosed at an early age usually exhibit worse symptoms than those diagnosed later in life.
    4. Children with asthma are encouraged to participate in sports, but they are also instructed to take scheduled bronchodilator medication prior to any sports activity.

TEST-TAKING HINT: The test taker can eliminate answer 4 because not all asthmatics also have exercise-induced asthma necessitating use of a fast-acting bronchodilator before playing.

19. 1. **The parent should always give one puff at a time and should wait 1 minute before administering the second puff.**
    2. A spacer is recommended when administering medications by MDI to children.
    3. The child should be in an upright position when medications are administered by MDI.
    4. The inhaler should always be shaken before administering a dose of the medication.

TEST-TAKING HINT: The test taker evaluates how the parents administer the MDI.

20. 1. Prednisone, a corticosteroid, is often given to children with asthma, but it is not a quick-relief medication. The prednisone will take time to relieve the child's symptoms.
    2. Singulair is an allergy medication that should be taken daily by asthmatics with significant allergies. Allergens are often triggers for asthmatics, so treating the

child for allergies can help avoid an asthma attack. Singulair, however, does not help a child immediately with the symptoms of a particular asthma attack.
    3. **Albuterol is the quick-relief bronchodilator of choice for treating an asthma attack.**
    4. Flovent is a long-term therapy medication for asthmatics and should be used in conjunction with quick-relief medications.

TEST-TAKING HINT: The test taker must know the medications used to treat asthma and which are used in which situations.

21. 1. This child is exhibiting symptoms of mild asthma and should not be seen before the other children.
    2. This child is exhibiting signs of moderate asthma and should be watched but is not the patient of highest priority.
    3. **This child is exhibiting signs of severe asthma. This child should be seen first. The child no longer has wheezes and now has diminished breath signs.**
    4. This child is exhibiting signs of moderate asthma and is not the patient of highest priority.

TEST-TAKING HINT: The test taker can eliminate answers 1, 2, and 4 by knowing that diminished breath sounds are a sign the patient has a worsening condition. The other bit of information that is essential in this problem is the child's age. The younger the child, the faster the respiratory status can diminish.

22. 1. A child of 3 years old is too young to comply with incentive spirometry.
    2. Breathing into a paper bag results in a prolonged inspiratory and expiratory phase.
    3. **Blowing a pinwheel is an excellent means of increasing a child's expiratory phase. Play is an effective means of engaging a child in therapeutic activities. Blowing bubbles is another method to increase the child's expiratory phase.**
    4. Taking deep breaths results in a prolonged inspiratory phase.

TEST-TAKING HINT: The test taker can eliminate answers 1 and 4 by considering the age of the child: 3 years. Play is one of the best ways to engage young children in therapeutic activities.

23. 1. It is better to maintain 30% to 50% humidity in homes of asthmatic children. However, humidifiers are not recommended because they can harbor mold as a result of lack of proper cleaning.
2. Chemical cleaning is not recommended because the chemicals used can be a trigger and actually cause the child to have an asthma attack. The best recommendation is to remove all carpet from the house, if possible.
3. Household pets are not recommended for children with asthma.
4. **Leather furniture is recommended rather than upholstered furniture. Upholstered furniture can harbor large amounts of dust, whereas leather furniture may be wiped off regularly with a damp cloth.**

TEST-TAKING HINT: The test taker can eliminate answer 3 because there is no known way to make a pet allergy-free. Household pets are discouraged for all children with asthma or severe allergies. Answer 2 can be eliminated if the test taker understands that chemical agents are triggers to asthma for many children.

24. 1. A viral illness does not require antibiotics. The patient would need to complete a course of antibiotics for bacterial tonsillitis.
2. Viral tonsillitis is usually a self-limiting disease and does not require a follow-up appointment unless the child's symptoms worsen.
3. **Tylenol is recommended prn for pain relief.**
4. Warm compresses to the neck are not recommended, as they may in fact increase the inflammation. Cold compresses or ice packs are recommended for comfort.

TEST-TAKING HINT: The test taker can eliminate answer 1 by knowing that antibiotics are not given for viral illnesses. Answer 4 can be eliminated by knowing that swelling and inflammation increase with heat. Cold causes vasoconstriction of the vessels, aiding in decreasing the amount of inflammation.

25. 1. Shallow breathing is a late sign of respiratory distress.
2. **Tachypnea is an early sign of distress and is often the first sign of respiratory illness in infants.**
3. Tachycardia is a compensatory response by the body. When a child has respiratory distress and is not oxygenating well, the body increases the heart rate in an attempt to improve oxygenation.
4. Bradycardia is a late sign of respiratory distress.

TEST-TAKING HINT: The test taker must know the signs and symptoms of respiratory distress and be able to recognize those in a patient

26. 1. **Children with mononucleosis are more susceptible to secondary infections. Therefore, they should be limited to visitors within the family, especially during the acute phase of illness.**
2. Children with mononucleosis do not need to be forced to be on bedrest. Children usually self-limit their behavior.
3. Children with mononucleosis do not need a restricted diet. Often they are very tired and are not interested in eating. The nurse and family must ensure that the children are taking in adequate nutrition.
4. Children with mononucleosis usually have decreased appetite, but it is essential that they remain hydrated. There is no reason to restrict fluid.

TEST-TAKING HINT: The test taker can eliminate answers 2 and 3 by understanding mononucleosis. Children with mononucleosis are usually very tired, are not interested in engaging in vigorous activity, and are rarely interested in eating.

27. 1. Children do not need to stay home unless they have a fever. However, the children should be taught to cough or sneeze into their sleeve and to wash their hands after sneezing or coughing.
2. Children should always wash their hands after using the restroom. In order to decrease the spread of influenza, however, it is more important for the children to wash their hands after sneezing or coughing.
3. **It is essential that children wash their hands after any contact with nasopharyngeal secretions.**
4. Children should have a flu shot annually, but that information is best included in an educational session for the parents. There is little that children can do directly to ensure they receive flu shots. Children of this age are often frightened of shots and would not likely pass that information on to their parents.

TEST-TAKING HINT: Answers 1 and 4 can be eliminated because both situations are under parental control.

28. 1. The flu vaccine is recommended for all ages, but the 18-year-old is not the highest priority. A person this age will likely recover without any complications.
2. Children between the ages of 6 and 23 months are at the highest risk for having complications as a result of the flu. Their immune systems are not so developed, so they are at a higher risk for influenza-related hospitalizations.
3. The flu vaccine is recommended for all ages, but the 7-year-old is not the highest priority. A child this age will likely recover without any complications.
4. The flu vaccine should not be given to anyone who is immunocompromised.

TEST-TAKING HINT: The test taker can eliminate answers 1 and 3 by knowing that infants and the elderly are at highest risk for complications related to the flu.

29. **1. Influenza is most contagious 24 hours before and 24 hours after onset of symptoms.**
2. Influenza is most contagious 24 hours before and 24 hours after onset of symptoms.
3. Influenza is most contagious 24 hours before and 24 hours after onset of symptoms.
4. Influenza is most contagious 24 hours before and 24 hours after onset of symptoms.

TEST-TAKING HINT: This is a knowledge-level question and requires the test taker to have knowledge of the communicability of influenza.

30. 1. The child is receiving intravenous fluids, so he is being hydrated. However, this response does not explain to the father why his son cannot eat.
2. Infants are at higher risk of aspiration because their airways are shorter and narrower than those of an adult.
3. Eating burns calories, but if the baby is upset and crying he is also expending energy. Therefore, this is not the best choice of answers.
4. If the child has nasal congestion, that may make it difficult for him to feed. However, the recommendation to parents is to bulb-suction an infant with nasal congestion before feeding.

TEST-TAKING HINT: The test taker can eliminate answer 1 because it does not give the father an explanation of why his son cannot eat.

31. 1. Repeated exposure to smoke damages the cilia in the ear, making the child more prone to ear infections.

2. Children experience fewer ear infections as they age because their immune system is maturing.
3. Removing children's tonsils may not have any effect on their ear infection. Children who have repeated bouts of tonsillitis can have ear infections secondary to the tonsillitis, but there is no indication in this question that the child has a problem with tonsillitis.
4. Children who have repeated ear infections are at a higher risk of having decreased hearing during and between infections. Hearing loss directly affects a child's speech development.

TEST-TAKING HINT: The test taker can eliminate answers 1, 2, and 4 because those options are true.

32. **1. It is essential that parents ensure that their children remain hydrated during a URI. The best way to accomplish this is by giving small amounts of fluid frequently.**
2. Over-the-counter cough and cold medicine is not recommended for any child younger than 6 years.
3. Baby aspirin is never given to children because of the risk of developing Reye syndrome.
4. Over-the-counter cough and cold medicine is not recommended for any child younger than 6 years.

TEST-TAKING HINT: The test taker can eliminate answers 2 and 4 because over-the-counter cold and cough medications are not recommended for infants.

33. 1. The parent should administer all of the medication. Stopping the medication when symptoms subside may not clear up the ear infection and may actually cause more severe symptoms.
2. Antihistamines have not been shown to decrease the number of ear infections a child gets.
3. It is essential that all the medication be given.
4. The child is old enough to participate in the administration of medication but should only do so in the presence of the parents.

TEST-TAKING HINT: Answer 1 can be eliminated because a complete course of antibiotics should always be completed as ordered, no matter what the age of the patient. Answer 4 can be eliminated because children should never be expected

to administer their own medications without supervision by an adult.

34. 1. Singulair is an allergy medication, but it has not been proved to help reduce the number of ear infections a child gets.
2. **Tobacco smoke has been proved to increase the incidence of ear infections. The tobacco smoke damages mucociliary function, prolonging the inflammatory process and impeding drainage through the eustachian tube.**
3. Otitis is not transmitted from one child to another. Otitis is often preceded by a URI, so children who are around other children with URIs may contract one, increasing their chances of developing an ear infection.
4. Wearing a hat outside will have no impact on whether a child contracts an ear infection.

TEST-TAKING HINT: The test taker can eliminate answer 3 by understanding that otitis is not a contagious disease process. Answer 4 can be eliminated if the test taker understands that otitis is not caused by exposing the child to cold air.

35. 1. Surgical intervention is not a first line of treatment. Surgery is usually reserved for children who have suffered from recurrent ear infections.
2. **A 2-year-old who has had multiple ear infections is a perfect candidate for ear tubes. The other issue is that a 2-year-old is at the height of language development, which can be adversely affected by recurrent ear infections.**
3. A 7-year-old who has had two ear infections is not the appropriate candidate. Surgical intervention is usually reserved for children who have suffered from recurrent ear infections.
4. Surgery is not a prophylactic treatment. Just because the sibling has had several ear infections does not suggest that the 3-year-old will also have frequent ear infections. The 3-year-old has not had an ear infection yet.

TEST-TAKING HINT: The test taker must also consider the developmental level of the child in this question. The 2-year-old has had multiple infections and is also at a stage at which language development is essential. If this child is not hearing appropriately, speech will also be delayed. Surgical intervention for otitis is reserved for those who have had recurrent infections.

36. 1. Hearing loss is not an issue that would be discussed following one ear infection. Children with recurrent untreated ear infections are more likely to develop hearing loss.
2. Speech delays are not an issue that would be discussed following one ear infection. Children with recurrent untreated ear infections are more likely to develop some hearing loss, which often results in delayed language development.
3. **When children acquire an ear infection at such a young age, there is an increased risk of recurrent infections.**
4. Surgical intervention is not a first line of treatment. Surgery is usually reserved for children who have suffered from recurrent ear infections.

TEST-TAKING HINT: Answers 1, 2, and 4 can be eliminated if the test taker understands that these are all long-term effects of recurrent ear infections. The question is asking about a single incident of otitis.

37. 1. It is important to educate the family about the signs and symptoms of an ear infection, but that is not the priority at this time. The infant has already been diagnosed with the infection.
2. The parents may need emotional support because they are likely suffering from a lack of sleep because their infant is ill. However, this will not solve their current problems with their infant.
3. **Providing pain relief for the infant is essential. With pain relief, the child will likely stop crying and rest better.**
4. Promoting drainage flow from the ear is important, but providing pain relief is the highest priority.

TEST-TAKING HINT: The test taker needs to consider the needs of the child and the parent at this time. If the pain is controlled, the parents and child will both be in a better state. The other items are all essential in providing care for the child with otitis, but pain relief offers the best opportunity for the child and the parent to return to normal conditions.

38. 1. RSV is not diagnosed by a blood draw.
2. Nasal secretions are tested to determine if a child has RSV.
3. **The child is swabbed for nasal secretions. The secretions are tested to determine if a child has RSV.**
4. Viral cultures are not done very often because it takes several days to receive

results. The culture does not have to be sent to an outside lab for evaluation.

TEST-TAKING HINT: The test taker can eliminate answers 1, 2, and 4 because the child's nasal sections will be swabbed.

39. 1. **Synagis will not help the child who has already contracted the illness. Synagis is an immunization and a method of primary prevention.**
    2. RSV is spread through direct contact with respiratory secretions, so it is a good idea to keep the ill child away from the healthy one.
    3. RSV is spread through direct contact with respiratory secretions, so it is a good idea to have all persons coming in contact with the child wash their hands.
    4. RSV is spread through direct contact with respiratory secretions, so it is a good idea to have ill persons avoid any contact with the children until they are well.

TEST-TAKING HINT: This is a knowledge-level question and requires that the test taker understand how RSV is transmitted and how to prevent the spread of the virus.

40. 1. Most children with RSV can be managed at home. Children 2 years and younger are at highest risk for developing complications related to RSV. Children who were premature, have cardiac conditions, or have chronic lung disease are also at a higher risk for needing hospitalization. The 3-year-old with a congenital heart disease is not the highest risk among this group of patients.
    2. **The younger the child, the greater the risk for developing complications related to RSV. The age and the premature status of this child make the the patient the highest risk.**
    3. Children who were premature, have cardiac conditions, or have chronic lung disease are also at a higher risk for needing hospitalization. This child was a former premature infant but is now 4 years of age.
    4. This child has a tracheostomy, but this is not an indication that the child cannot be managed at home.

TEST-TAKING HINT: The test taker must know who is at greatest risk of complications from RSV. The test taker must also consider that whereas all of these children have some amount of risk for requiring hospitalization, the 2-month-old has two of the noted risk factors. That child is

both a premature baby and a very young infant.

41. 1. Tachypnea, an increase in respiratory rate, should be monitored but is a common symptom of RAD.
    2. Retractions should be monitored, but they are a common symptom of respiratory distress and RAD.
    3. Wheezing should be monitored but is a common symptom of RAD.
    4. **Grunting is a sign of impending respiratory failure and is a very concerning physical finding.**

TEST-TAKING HINT: The test taker can eliminate answers 1, 2, and 3 by knowing the signs and symptoms of respiratory distress. Answers 1, 2, and 3 are normal signs and symptoms of respiratory distress in an infant and can be expected. They warrant frequent respiratory assessment, but they are not the most concerning physical signs.

42. 1. RSV is a viral illness and is not treated with antibiotics.
    2. Steroids are not used to treat RSV.
    3. **Racemic epinephrine promotes mucosal vasoconstriction.**
    4. Tylenol and Motrin can be given to the child for comfort, but they do not improve the child's respiratory status.

TEST-TAKING HINT: This is a knowledge-level question that requires the test taker understand how RSV is treated.

43. 1. **The night air will help decrease sub-glottic edema, easing the child's respiratory effort. The coughing should diminish significantly, and the child should be able to rest comfortably. If the symptoms do not improve after taking the child outside, the parent should have the child seen by a health-care provider.**
    2. There is no immediate need to bring the child to the ER. The child's symptoms will likely improve on the drive to the hospital because of the child's exposure to the night air.
    3. Over-the-counter cough suppressants are not recommended for children because they reduce their ability to clear secretions.
    4. Warm liquids may increase subglottic edema and actually aggravate the child's symptoms. Cool liquids or a popsicle are the best choice.

TEST-TAKING HINT: The test taker must accurately identify that the question is describing a child with croup. The test taker must also have some knowledge of how croup is treated.

44. 1. **This child has signs and symptoms of epiglottitis and should receive immediate emergency medical treatment. The patient has no spontaneous cough and has a frog-like croaking because of a significant airway obstruction.**
    2. This child has signs and symptoms of acute laryngitis and is not in a significant amount of distress.
    3. This child has signs and symptoms of LTB and is not in significant respiratory distress.
    4. This child has signs and symptoms of bacterial tracheitis and should be treated with antibiotics but is not the patient in the most significant amount of distress.

    TEST-TAKING HINT: The test taker must accurately identify that the question is describing a child with epiglottitis. The test taker must also understand that epiglottitis is a pediatric emergency and can cause the child to have complete airway obstruction.

45. 1. Nasopharyngitis is a viral illness and does not require antibiotic therapy.
    2. Children who attend day care are more prone to catching viral illnesses, but it is not the nurse's place to tell the parents not to send their child to day care. Often families do not have a choice about using day care.
    3. **Nursing care for nasopharyngitis is primarily supportive. Keeping the child comfortable during the course of the illness is all the parents can do. Nasal congestion can be relieved using normal saline drops and a bulb suction. Tylenol can also be given for discomfort or a mild fever.**
    4. There is no reason to restrict the child to clear liquids. Many children have a decreased appetite during a respiratory illness, so the most important thing is to keep them hydrated.

    TEST-TAKING HINT: This question requires the test taker to understand how nasopharyngitis is treated.

46. 1. Retractions, low-grade fever, and nasal congestion are common symptoms of a respiratory illness and are not overly concerning.
    2. **When children are sitting in the tripod position, that is an indication they are having difficulty breathing. The child is sitting and leaning forward in order to breathe more easily. Diminished breath sounds indicate that there is fluid in the lungs and are indicative of a worsening condition. A muffled cough indicates that the child has some subglottic edema. This child has several signs and symptoms of a worsening respiratory condition.**
    3. Coarse breath sounds, cough, and fussiness are common signs and symptoms of a respiratory illness.
    4. Restlessness, wheezes, poor feeding, and crying are common signs and symptoms of a respiratory illness.

    TEST-TAKING HINT: The test taker can eliminate answers 1, 3, and 4 if familiar with common signs and symptoms of respiratory illness.

47. 1. A blood test does not indicate a diagnosis of epiglottitis. A CBC may show an increased white blood cell count indicating that the child has some sort of infection.
    2. A throat culture is not done to diagnose epiglottitis. It is contraindicated to insert anything into the mouth or throat of any patient who is suspected of having epiglottitis. Inserting anything into the throat could cause the child to have a complete airway obstruction.
    3. **A lateral neck x-ray is the method used to diagnose epiglottitis definitively. The child is at risk for complete airway obstruction and should always be accompanied by a nurse to the x-ray department.**
    4. Epiglottitis is not diagnosed based on signs and symptoms. A lateral neck film is the definitive diagnosis.

    TEST-TAKING HINT: The test taker can eliminate answers 1, 2, and 4 because epiglottitis is diagnosed by lateral neck films.

48. 1. This child is exhibiting signs and symptoms of epiglottitis and should be kept as comfortable as possible. Agitating the child may cause increased airway swelling and may lead to complete obstruction.
    2. Respiratory treatments often frighten children. This child is exhibiting signs and symptoms of epiglottitis and should be kept as comfortable as possible. Agitating the child may cause increased airway swelling and may lead to complete obstruction.

3. This child is exhibiting signs and symptoms of epiglottitis and should be kept as comfortable as possible. Agitating the child may cause increased airway swelling and may lead to complete obstruction. The child should be allowed to remain on the parent's lap and kept as comfortable as possible until a lateral neck film is obtained.

4. **This child is exhibiting signs and symptoms of epiglottitis and should be kept as comfortable as possible. The child should be allowed to remain in the parent's lap until a lateral neck film is obtained for a definitive diagnosis.**

TEST-TAKING HINT: The test taker must accurately identify that the question is describing a child with epiglottitis. The test taker must understand that agitation in a child with epiglottitis can result in complete airway obstruction.

49. 1. **Epiglottitis is bacterial in nature and requires intravenous antibiotics. A 7- to 10-day course of oral antibiotics is usually ordered following the intravenous course of antibiotics.**
2. Surgery is not the course of treatment for epiglottitis. Epiglottal swelling usually diminishes after 24 hours of intravenous antibiotics.
3. Ribavirin is an antiviral medication that is used to treat RSV.
4. Epiglottitis is bacterial in nature and requires intervention. A course of intravenous antibiotics is indicated for this patient.

TEST-TAKING HINT: Understanding that epiglottitis is bacterial in nature will lead the test taker to choose the correct answer.

50. 1. Epiglottitis is most common in children from 2 to 5 years of age. The onset is very rapid. Telling parents not to blame themselves is not effective. Parents tend to blame themselves for their child's illnesses even though they are not responsible.
2. The nurse should not tell the parent to seek medical attention for any and all signs of illness.
3. Epiglottitis is rapidly progressive and cannot be predicted.
4. **Epiglottitis is rapidly progressive and cannot be predicted.**

TEST-TAKING HINT: When something happens to a child, the parents always blame themselves. Telling them epiglottitis is rapidly progressive may be helpful.

51. 1. All children should be treated as individuals when they are being treated for a particular illness. However, most children exhibit similar symptoms when they have the same diagnosis. Younger children have worse symptoms than older children because their immune systems are less developed.
2. Children have airways that are shorter and narrower than those of an adult. As children age, their airways begin to grow in length and diameter.
3. Children are more prone to ear infections because they have eustachian tubes that are short and wide and lie in a horizontal plane.
4. **Younger children have less developed immune systems and usually exhibit worse symptoms than older children.**

TEST-TAKING HINT: Answer 1 can be eliminated because it does not directly address the mother's question. Answer 2 can be eliminated if the test taker has knowledge of the anatomical structure of a child's airway. Answer 3 can be eliminated because the eustachian tubes have no direct relationship to acquiring croup.

52. 1. The child is exhibiting signs and symptoms of croup and is not in any significant respiratory distress.
2. **The child has stridor, indicating airway edema, which can be relieved by aerosolized racemic epinephrine.**
3. A tracheostomy is not indicated for this child. A tracheostomy would be indicated for a child with a complete airway obstruction.
4. This child is exhibiting signs and symptoms of croup and has no indication of tonsillitis. A tonsillectomy is usually reserved for children who have recurrent tonsillitis.

TEST-TAKING HINT: The test taker must accurately identify that the question is describing a child with croup and know the accepted treatments.

53. 1. Cough suppressants are not recommended for children. Coughing is a protective mechanism, so do not try to stop it.
2. Cough expectorants are not recommended for children younger than 6 years of age. There is no research information that they are effective.
3. Cold and flu medications are not indicated for children younger than 6 years of age as there is no indication they are effective.

4. **Warm fluids, humidifcation, and honey are best treatments for a URI.**

TEST-TAKING HINT: The latest recommendations for treatment of URIs in children are to treat the symptoms because cough medications are not effective.

54. 1. Pneumonia is most frequently caused by viruses but can also be caused by bacteria such as *Streptococcus pneumoniae*.
    2. **Children with bacterial pneumonia are usually sicker than children with viral pneumonia. Children with bacterial pneumonia can be treated effectively, but they require a course of antibiotics.**
    3. Children with viral pneumonia are not usually as ill as those with bacterial pneumonia. Treatment for viral pneumonia includes maintaining adequate oxygenation and comfort measures.
    4. Treatment for viral pneumonia includes maintaining adequate oxygenation and comfort measures.

TEST-TAKING HINT: The test taker must have an understanding of the differences between viral and bacterial infections.

55. 1. These are all common symptoms of pneumonia and should be monitored but do not require hospitalization. Most people with pneumonia are treated at home, with a focus on treating the symptoms and keeping the patient comfortable. Comfort measures include cool mist, CPT, antipyretics, fluid intake, and family support.
    2. **The teen who has been vomiting for several days and is unable to tolerate oral fluids and medication should be admitted for intravenous hydration.**
    3. These are all common symptoms of pneumonia and should be monitored but do not require hospitalization.
    4. These are all common symptoms of pneumonia and should be monitored but do not require hospitalization.

TEST-TAKING HINT: The test taker can eliminate answers 1, 3, and 4 if familiar with the common signs and symptoms of pneumonia.

56. 1. The Trendelenburg position is not effective for improving respiratory difficulty. Patients with pneumonia are usually most comfortable in a semierect position.
    2. **Lying on the left side may provide the patient with the most comfort. Lying on the left splints the chest and reduces the pleural rubbing.**

3. It is most comfortable for the patient to lie on the affected side. Lying on the left splints the chest and reduces the pleural rubbing.
4. Lying in the supine position does not provide comfort for the patient and does not improve the child's respiratory effort.

TEST-TAKING HINT: The test taker can eliminate answers 1 and 4 because neither of them would improve the child's respiratory effort. Both these positions may actually cause the patient increased respiratory distress.

57. 1. The nurse should instruct the parents on signs and symptoms of aspiration pneumonia, but that is not the most beneficial piece of information the nurse can provide. The most valuable information relates to preventing aspiration pneumonia from occurring in the future.
    2. The nurse should instruct the parents on the treatment plan of aspiration pneumonia, but that is not the most beneficial piece of information the nurse can provide. The most valuable information relates to preventing aspiration pneumonia from occurring in the future.
    3. The nurse should instruct the parents on the risks associated with recurrent aspiration pneumonia, but that is not the most beneficial piece of information the nurse can provide. The most valuable information relates to preventing aspiration pneumonia from occurring in the future.
    4. **The most valuable information the nurse can give the parents is how to prevent aspiration pneumonia from occurring in the future.**

TEST-TAKING HINT: The test taker can eliminate answers 1, 2, and 3 because they are all forms of tertiary prevention. Primary prevention is key to maximizing this child's function.

58. 1. A chest x-ray will only show radiopaque items (items that x-rays cannot go through easily), so it is not helpful in determining if the child aspirated a carrot.
    2. **A bronchoscopy will allow the physician to visualize the airway and will help determine if the child aspirated the carrot.**
    3. A blood gas will identify whether the child has suffered any respiratory compromise, but the blood gas cannot definitively determine the cause of the compromise.

4. A sputum culture may be helpful several days later to determine if the child has developed aspiration pneumonia. Aspiration pneumonia may take several days or a week to develop following aspiration.

TEST-TAKING HINT: Answer 1 can be eliminated because items that are not radiopaque (opaque to x-rays) cannot be seen on an x-ray. Answers 3 and 4 can be eliminated because they do not provide confirmation regarding whether the child aspirated.

59. 1. Abdominal thrusts are not recommended for children younger than 1 year.
    2. Inserting a finger in the child's mouth may cause the object to be pushed further down the airway, making it more difficult to remove.
    3. The Heimlich should be performed only on adults.
    4. **The current recommendation for infants younger than 1 year is to administer five back blows followed by five chest thrusts.**

    TEST-TAKING HINT: The test taker can eliminate answers 1, 2, and 3 if familiar with CPR.

60. 1. Teaching the parents signs and symptoms of foreign body aspiration is important, but it is a tertiary means of prevention and will not help the parents prevent the aspiration.
    2. Teaching the parents the therapeutic management of foreign body aspiration is important, but it is a tertiary means of prevention and will not help the parents prevent the aspiration.
    3. **Teaching parents the most common objects aspirated by toddlers will help them the most. Parents can avoid having those items in the household or in locations where toddlers may have access to them.**

4. Teaching the parents the risks associated with foreign body aspiration is important but it is a tertiary means of prevention and will not help the parents prevent the aspiration.

TEST-TAKING HINT: The test taker can eliminate answers 1, 2, and 4 because they are all forms of tertiary prevention. Primary prevention is key to preventing foreign body aspiration.

61. **1, 3, 4, 5.**
    1. **Children with CF have difficulty absorbing nutrients because of the blockage of the pancreatic duct. Pancreatic enzymes cannot reach the duodenum to aid in digestion of food. These children often require up to 150% of the caloric intake of their peers. The nutritional recommendation for CF patients is high-calorie and high-protein.**
    2. A high-fat, high-carbohydrate diet is not recommended for adequate nutrition.
    3. **Exercise is effective in helping CF patients clear secretions.**
    4. **Minimizing pulmonary complications is essential to a better outcome for CF patients. Compliance with CPT, nebulizer treatments, and medications are all components of minimizing pulmonary complications.**
    5. **Medication compliance is a necessary part of maintaining pulmonary and gastrointestinal function.**

    TEST-TAKING HINT: The test taker can eliminate answer 2 because patients are not placed on a high-fat diet.

62. **60 mEq/L.**
    The definitive diagnosis of CF is made when a patient has a sweat chloride test with a chloride level >60 mEq/L. A normal chloride level is <40 mEq/L.

    TEST-TAKING HINT: The test taker must have knowledge of the tests used to identify a diagnosis of CF.

Neurological Disorders

5

KEYWORDS

Absence seizure
Akinetic seizure
Anencephaly
Anterior fontanel
Apgar
Atonic seizure
Brachycephaly
Brudzinski sign
Cerebellum
Coma
Confusion
Consciousness
Craniosynostosis
Cushing triad
Decerebrate posturing
Decorticate posturing
Delirium
Encephalitis
Epidural hematoma
Epilepsy
Hemiplegia
Hydrocephalus

Kernig sign
Ketogenic diet
Leukemia
Malignancy
Meningitis
Meningocele
Myelomeningocele
Neuroblastoma
Neurogenic bladder
Neurogenic shock
Neurological checks
Nuchal rigidity
Obtunded
Pancytopenia
Posturing
Reye syndrome
Seizure
Spina bifida occulta
Subdural hematoma
Ventricle
Ventriculoperitoneal shunt

ABBREVIATIONS

Cerebral palsy (CP)
Cerebrospinal fluid (CSF)
Diabetes insipidus (DI)
Electroencephalogram (EEG)

Intracranial pressure (ICP)
Motor vehicle accident (MVA)
Pediatric intensive care unit (PICU)
Shaken baby syndrome (SBS)

QUESTIONS

1. The nurse is caring for a child who has been in an MVA. The child continues to fall asleep unless her name is called or she is gently shaken. The nurse knows that this state of consciousness is referred to as:
   1. Coma.
   2. Delirium.
   3. Obtunded.
   4. Confusion.

2. The nurse is caring for a 3-year-old female with an altered state of consciousness. The nurse determines that the child is oriented by asking the child to:
   1. Name the president of the United States.
   2. Identify her parents and state her own name.
   3. State her full name and phone number.
   4. Identify the current month but not the date.

3. The nurse is preparing to assess a 6-year-old male with altered consciousness in the PICU. His parents ask if they can stay during his morning assessment. Select the nurse's best response.
   1. "Your child is more likely to answer questions and cooperate with any procedures if you are not present."
   2. "Most children feel more at ease when parents are present, so you are more than welcome to stay at the bedside."
   3. "It is our policy to ask parents to leave during the first assessment of the shift."
   4. "Many children fear that their parents will be disappointed if they do not do well with procedures, so we recommend that no parents be present at this time."

4. The nurse is caring for a 9-year-old female who is unconscious in the PICU. The child's mother has been calling her name repeatedly and gently shaking her shoulders in an attempt to wake her up. The nurse notes that the child is flexing her arms and wrists while bringing her arms closer to the midline of her body. The child's mother asks, "What is going on?" Select the nurse's best response.
   1. "I think your daughter hears you, and she is attempting to reach out to you."
   2. "Your child is responding to you; please continue trying to stimulate her."
   3. "It appears that your child is having a seizure."
   4. "Your child is demonstrating a reflex that indicates she is overwhelmed with the stimulation she is receiving."

5. The nurse is caring for a 6-month-old infant with a diagnosis of hydrocephalus. Which of the following signs best indicates increased ICP in this child?
   1. Sunken anterior fontanel.
   2. Complaints of blurred vision.
   3. High-pitched cry.
   4. Increased appetite.

6. The nurse is preparing to give preoperative teaching to the parents of an infant with hydrocephalus. The nurse knows that the most common treatment for hydrocephalus includes the surgical placement of a shunt connecting which of the following?
   1. The ventricle of the brain to the peritoneum.
   2. The ventricle of the brain to the right atrium of the heart.
   3. The ventricle of the brain to the lower esophagus.
   4. The ventricle of the brain to the small intestine.

7. The nurse receives a phone call from the parents of a 9-year-old female who is complaining of a headache and blurry vision. The child has been healthy but has a history of hydrocephalus and received a ventriculoperitoneal shunt at the age of 1 month. The parents also state that she is not acting like herself, is irritable, and sleeps more than she used to. They ask the nurse what they should do. Select the nurse's best response.
   1. "Give her some acetaminophen, and see if her symptoms improve. If they do not improve, bring her to the pediatrician's office."
   2. "It is common for girls to have these symptoms, especially prior to beginning their menstrual cycle. Give her a few days, and see if she improves."
   3. "You are probably worried that she is having a problem with her shunt. This is very unlikely as it has been working well for 9 years."
   4. "You should immediately bring her to the emergency room as these may be symptoms of a shunt malfunction."

8. The nurse is working in the PICU caring for an infant who has just returned from having a ventriculoperitoneal shunt placed. Which position initially will be most beneficial for this child?
   1. Semi-Fowler in an infant seat.
   2. Flat in the crib.
   3. Trendelenburg.
   4. In the crib with the head elevated to 90 degrees.

9. A child is being evaluated in the emergency room for a possible diagnosis of meningitis. The nurse is assisting with the lumbar puncture and notes that the CSF is cloudy. The nurse is aware that cloudy CSF most likely means:
   1. Viral meningitis.
   2. Bacterial meningitis.
   3. No infection, as CSF is usually cloudy.
   4. Sepsis.

10. The nurse is caring for a child who is being admitted with a diagnosis of meningitis. The child's plan of care includes the following: administration of intravenous antibiotics, administration of maintenance intravenous fluids, placement of a Foley catheter, and obtaining cultures of spinal fluid and blood. Select the procedure the nurse should do first.
    1. Administration of intravenous antibiotics.
    2. Administration of maintenance intravenous fluids.
    3. Placement of a Foley catheter.
    4. Send the spinal fluid and blood cultures to the laboratory.

11. The nurse is caring for a 6-month-old infant diagnosed with meningitis. When she places the infant in the supine position and flexes his neck, she notes that the infant flexes his knees and hips. The nurse knows that this is referred to as:
    1. Brudzinski sign.
    2. Cushing triad.
    3. Kernig sign.
    4. Nuchal rigidity.

12. A toddler is being admitted to the hospital with a diagnosis of bacterial meningitis. Select the best room assignment for the patient.
    1. A semiprivate room with a roommate who also has bacterial meningitis.
    2. A semiprivate room with a roommate who has bacterial meningitis but has received intravenous antibiotics for more than 24 hours.
    3. A private room that is dark and quiet with minimal stimulation.
    4. A private room that is bright and colorful and has developmentally appropriate activities available.

13. The nurse is caring for a child who has just been admitted to the pediatric floor with a diagnosis of bacterial meningitis. When reviewing the child's plan of care, which of the following orders would the nurse question?
   1. Maintain isolation precautions until 24 hours after receiving intravenous antibiotics.
   2. Intravenous fluids at 1½ times regular maintenance.
   3. Neurological checks every 4 hours.
   4. Administer acetaminophen for temperatures higher than 38°C (100.4°F).

14. The nurse is caring for a 1-year-old female who has just been diagnosed with viral encephalitis. The parents ask if their child will be admitted. Select the nurse's best response.
   1. "Your child will likely be sent home because encephalitis is usually caused by a virus and not bacteria."
   2. "Your child will likely be admitted to the pediatric floor for intravenous antibiotics and observation."
   3. "Your child will likely be admitted to the PICU for close monitoring and observation."
   4. "Your child will likely be sent home because she is only 1 year old. We tend to see fewer complications and a shorter disease process in the younger child."

15. The nurse is providing education concerning Reye syndrome to a mothers' group. She knows that further education is needed when a mother states:
   1. "I will have my children immunized against varicella and influenza."
   2. "I will make sure not to give my child any products containing aspirin when my child is ill."
   3. "Because I do not give my child aspirin, my child will probably never get Reye syndrome, but if that happens, it will be a very mild case."
   4. "Children with Reye syndrome are admitted to the hospital."

16. The nurse is caring for a child with Reye syndrome in the PICU. At noon, the nurse notes that the child is comatose with sluggish pupils. When stimulated, the child demonstrates decerebrate posturing. At 2 p.m., the nurse notes that the child remains unchanged except that the child now demonstrates decorticate posturing when stimulated. The nurse concludes that:
   1. The child's condition is worsening and progressing to a more advanced stage of Reye syndrome.
   2. The child's condition is worsening, and the child may likely experience cardiac and respiratory failure.
   3. The child's condition is improving and progressing to a less advanced stage of Reye syndrome.
   4. The child's condition remains unchanged as posturing reflexes are similar.

17. The nurse is caring for a child with Reye syndrome stage III. The child is comatose with sluggish pupils. The child is currently maintaining his own respirations, and all vital signs are within normal range. In order to treat a common manifestation, what medication would the nurse expect to have readily available?
   1. Lasix.
   2. Insulin.
   3. Glucose.
   4. Morphine.

18. The nurse is caring for a child with meningitis. The parents call for the nurse as "something is wrong." When the nurse arrives, she notes that the child is having a generalized tonic-clonic seizure. Which of the following should the nurse do first?
   1. Administer blow-by oxygen and call for additional help.
   2. Reassure the parents that seizures are common in children with meningitis.
   3. Call a code and ask the parents to leave the room.
   4. Assess the child's temperature and blood pressure.

19. A 5-year-old female has been diagnosed with a seizure disorder. Her teacher noticed that she has been having episodes where she drops her pencil and simply appears to be daydreaming. This is most likely called:
   1. An absence seizure.
   2. An akinetic seizure.
   3. A non-epileptic seizure.
   4. A simple spasm seizure.

20. The school nurse is called to the preschool classroom to evaluate a child. He has been noted to have periods where he suddenly falls and appears to be weak for a short time after the event. The preschool teacher asks what she should do. Select the nurse's best response.
   1. "Have the parents follow up with his pediatrician as this is likely an atonic seizure."
   2. "Find out if there have been any new stressors in his life, as it could be attention-seeking behavior."
   3. "Have the parents follow up with his pediatrician as this is likely an absence seizure."
   4. "The preschool years are a time of rapid growth, and many children appear clumsy. It would be best to watch him, and see if it continues."

21. The nurse is discussing a ketogenic diet with a family. The nurse knows that this diet is sometimes used with children who have had little success with anticonvulsant medication. The diet that produces anticonvulsant effects from ketosis consists of:
   1. High fat and low carbohydrates.
   2. High fat and high carbohydrates.
   3. Low fat and low carbohydrates.
   4. Low fat and high carbohydrates.

22. The nurse is working in the emergency room when an ambulance arrives with a 9-year-old male who has been having a generalized seizure for 35 minutes. The paramedics have provided blow-by oxygen and monitored vital signs. The patient does not have intravenous access yet. Which of the following medications should the nurse anticipate administering first?
   1. Establish an intravenous line, and administer intravenous lorazepam.
   2. Administer rectal diazepam.
   3. Administer an oral glucose gel to the side of the child's mouth.
   4. Place a nasogastric tube, and administer oral diazepam.

23. The nurse is providing discharge teaching to the parents of a toddler who has experienced a febrile seizure. The nurse knows that clarification is needed when the mother says:
   1. "My child will likely have another seizure."
   2. "My child's 7-year-old brother is also at high risk for a febrile seizure."
   3. "I'll give my child acetaminophen when ill to prevent the fever from rising too high too rapidly."
   4. "Most children with febrile seizures do not require seizure medicine."

24. The nurse is caring for a 5-year-old female recently diagnosed with epilepsy. She is being evaluated for anticonvulsant medication therapy. The nurse knows that the child will likely be placed on which kind of regimen?
   1. Two to three oral anticonvulsant medications so that dosing can be low and side effects minimized.
   2. One oral anticonvulsant medication to observe effectiveness and minimize side effects.
   3. One rectal gel to be administered in the event of a seizure.
   4. A combination of oral and intravenous anticonvulsant medications to ensure compliance.

25. The nurse is providing discharge instructions to the parents of a 13-year-old girl who has been diagnosed with epilepsy. Her parents ask if there are any activities that she should avoid. Select the nurse's best response.
    1. "She should avoid swimming, even with a friend."
    2. "She should avoid being in a car at night."
    3. "She should avoid any strenuous activities."
    4. "She should not return to school right away as her peers will likely cause her to feel inadequate."

26. An 8-year-old child is attending a Cub Scout camp picnic. He has a history of epilepsy and has had generalized seizures since the age of 3. The child falls to the ground and has a generalized seizure. Which of the following is the best action for the nurse to take during the child's seizure?
    1. Administer the child's rescue dose of oral valium.
    2. Loosen the child's clothing, and call for help.
    3. Place an oral tongue blade in the child's mouth to prevent aspiration.
    4. Carry the child to the infirmary to call 911 and start an intravenous line.

27. The nurse is caring for a child who has sustained a closed-head injury. The nurse knows that brain damage can be caused by which of the following factors?
    1. Increased perfusion to the brain and increased metabolic needs of the brain.
    2. Decreased perfusion to the brain and decreased metabolic needs of the brain.
    3. Increased perfusion to the brain and decreased metabolic needs of the brain.
    4. Decreased perfusion of the brain and increased metabolic needs of the brain.

28. The emergency room nurse is caring for a 5-year-old child who fell off his bike and sustained a closed-head injury. The child is currently awake and alert, but his mother states that he "passed out" for approximately 2 minutes. The mother appears highly anxious and is very tearful. The child was not wearing a helmet. Which of the following statements is a priority for the nurse at this time?
    1. "Was anyone else injured in the accident?"
    2. "Tell me more about the accident."
    3. "Did he vomit, have a seizure, or display any other behavior that was unusual when he woke up?"
    4. "Why was he not wearing a helmet?"

29. The emergency room nurse is caring for an unconscious 6-year-old girl who has had a severe closed-head injury and notes the following changes in her vital signs. Her heart rate has dropped from 120 to 55, her blood pressure has increased from 110/44 to 195/62, and her respirations are becoming more irregular. After calling the physician, which of the following should the nurse expect to do?
    1. Call for additional help, and prepare to administer mannitol.
    2. Continue to monitor the patient's vital signs, and prepare to administer a bolus of isotonic fluids.
    3. Call for additional help, and prepare to administer an antihypertensive.
    4. Continue to monitor the patient, and administer supplemental oxygen.

30. The nurse is caring for a 2-year-old male in the PICU with a head injury. The child is comatose and unresponsive at this time. The parents ask if he needs pain medication. Select the nurse's best response.
    1. "Pain medication is not necessary as he is unresponsive and cannot feel pain."
    2. "Pain medication may interfere with his ability to respond and may mask any signs of improvement."
    3. "Pain medication is necessary to promote comfort."
    4. "Although pain medication is necessary for comfort, we use it cautiously as it increases the demand for oxygen."

31. The nurse is caring for a 6-year-old female with a skull fracture who is unconscious and has severely increased ICP. The nurse notes the child's temperature to be 104°F (40°C). Which of the following should the nurse do first?
    1. Place a cooling blanket on the child.
    2. Administer Tylenol via nasogastric tube.
    3. Administer Tylenol rectally.
    4. Place ice packs in the child's axillary areas.

32. The nurse is caring for a 16-year-old female who remains unconscious 24 hours after sustaining a closed-head injury in an MVA. She responds to deep painful stimulation with decorticate posturing. The child has an intracranial monitor that shows periodic increased ICP. All other vital signs remain stable. Select the most appropriate nursing action.
    1. Encourage the child's peers to visit and talk to the child about school and other pertinent events.
    2. Encourage the child's parents to hold her hand and speak loudly to her in an attempt to help her regain consciousness.
    3. Attempt to keep a normal day/night pattern by keeping the child in a bright lively environment during the day and dark quiet environment at night.
    4. Attempt to keep the environment dark and quiet, and encourage minimal stimulation.

33. A 2-month-old infant is brought to the emergency room after experiencing a seizure. The nurse notes that the infant appears lethargic with very irregular respirations and periods of apnea. The parents report that the child is no longer interested in feeding and that, prior to the seizure, the infant rolled off the couch. What additional testing should the nurse immediately prepare for?
    1. Computed tomography scan of the head and dilation of the eyes.
    2. Computed tomography scan of the head and EEG.
    3. Close monitoring of vital signs.
    4. X-rays of all long bones.

34. The nurse knows that young infants are at risk for injury from SBS because:
    1. Anterior fontanel is open.
    2. Insufficient musculoskeletal support and a disproportionate head-to-body ratio.
    3. Immature vascular system with veins and arteries that are more superficial.
    4. Immature myelination of the nervous system.

35. An infant is born with a sac protruding through the spine. The sac contains CSF, a portion of the meninges, and nerve roots. The nurse knows that this is referred to as:
    1. Meningocele.
    2. Myelomeningocele.
    3. Spina bifida occulta.
    4. Anencephaly.

36. The nurse is caring for a neonate who has just been diagnosed with a meningocele. The parents ask what to expect. Which of the following is the nurse's best response?
    1. "After initial surgery to close the defect, most children experience no neurological dysfunction."
    2. "Surgery to close the sac will be postponed until the infant has grown and has enough skin to form a graft."
    3. "After the initial surgery to close the defect, the child will likely have motor and sensory deficits."
    4. "After the initial surgery to close the defect, the child will likely have future problems with urinary and bowel continence."

37. The nurse is caring for an infant with a myelomeningocele. The parents ask the nurse why the nurse keeps measuring the baby's head circumference. Select the nurse's best response:
    1. "We measure all babies' heads to ensure that their growth is on track."
    2. "Babies with myelomeningocele are at risk for hydrocephalus, which can show up with an increase in head circumference."
    3. "Because your baby has an opening on the spinal cord, your infant is at risk for meningitis, which can show up with an increase in head circumference."
    4. "Many infants with myelomeningocele have microcephaly, which can show up with a decrease in head circumference."

38. The most common complication associated with myelomeningocele is:
    1. Learning disability.
    2. Urinary tract infection.
    3. Hydrocephalus.
    4. Decubitus ulcers and skin breakdown.

39. The nurse is caring for a newborn infant who has just been diagnosed with a myelomeningocele. Which of the following is included in the child's plan of care?
    1. Place the child in the prone position with a sterile dry dressing over the defect. Slowly begin oral gastric feeds to prevent the development of necrotizing enterocolitis.
    2. Place the child in the prone position with a sterile dry dressing over the defect. Begin intravenous fluids to prevent dehydration.
    3. Place the child in the prone position with a sterile moist dressing over the defect. Slowly begin oral gastric feeds to prevent the development of necrotizing enterocolitis.
    4. Place the child in the prone position with a sterile moist dressing over the defect. Begin intravenous fluids to prevent dehydration.

40. The parents of a 12-month-old female with a neurogenic bladder ask the nurse if their child will always have to be catheterized. Select the nurse's best response.
    1. "Your child will never feel when her bladder is full, so she will always have to be catheterized. Because she is female, she will always need assistance."
    2. "As your child ages, she will likely be able to sense when her bladder is full and will be able to empty it on her own."
    3. "Although your child will not be able to feel when her bladder is full, she can learn to urinate every 4 to 6 hours and therefore not require catheterizations."
    4. "Your child will never be able to completely empty her bladder spontaneously, but there are other options to traditional catheterization. An opening can be made surgically through the abdomen, thus allowing the parents and child to be able to place a catheter into the opening."

41. The nurse is caring for a 9-year-old with myelomeningocele who has just had surgery to release a tight ligament to the lower extremity. Which of the following does the nurse include in the child's postoperative plan of care?
    1. Encourage the child to resume a regular diet, beginning slowly with bland foods that are easily digested, such as bananas.
    2. Encourage the child to blow balloons to increase deep breathing and avoid postoperative pneumonia.
    3. Assist the child to change positions to avoid skin breakdown.
    4. Provide education on dietary requirements to prevent obesity and skin breakdown.

42. A 6-month-old infant male has just been diagnosed with craniosynostosis. He is being evaluated for reconstructive surgery. The infant's father asks the nurse for more information about the surgery. Select the nurse's best response.
    1. "The surgery is done for cosmetic reasons and is without many complications."
    2. "The surgery is important to allow the brain to grow properly. Although most children do well, serious complications can occur, so your child will be closely observed in the intensive care unit."
    3. "The surgery is important to allow the brain to grow properly. Most surgeons wait until the child is 3 years old to minimize potential complications."
    4. "The surgery is mainly done for cosmetic reasons, and most surgeons wait until the child is 3 years old as the head has finished growing at that time."

43. A 6-month-old male has been diagnosed with positional brachycephaly. The nurse is providing teaching about the use of a helmet for his therapy. Which of the following statements indicate that his parents understand the education?
    1. "We will keep the helmet on him when he is awake and remove it only for bathing and sleeping."
    2. "He will start wearing the helmet when he is closer to 12 months, as he will be more upright and mobile."
    3. "He will wear the helmet 23 hours every day."
    4. "Most children need to wear the helmet for 6 to 12 months."

44. The nurse is caring for a child with CP. The nurse knows that since the 1960s the incidence of CP has:
    1. Increased.
    2. Decreased.
    3. Remained the same.
    4. Has decreased due to early misdiagnosis.

45. The nurse is caring for several children. She knows that which of the following children is at increased risk for CP?
    1. An infant born at 34 weeks with an Apgar score of 6 at 5 minutes.
    2. A 17-day-old infant with sepsis.
    3. A 24-month-old child who has experienced a febrile seizure.
    4. A 5-year-old with a closed-head injury after falling off a bike.

46. The nurse is working in the pediatric developmental clinic. Which of the children requires continued follow-up because of behaviors suspicious of CP?
    1. A 1-month-old who demonstrates the startle reflex when a loud noise is heard.
    2. A 6-month-old who always reaches for toys with the right hand.
    3. A 14-month-old who has not begun to walk.
    4. A 2-year-old who has not yet achieved bladder control during waking hours.

47. The nurse is caring for a 13-month-old with meningitis. The child has experienced increased ICP and multiple seizures. The child's parents ask if the child is likely to develop CP. Select the nurse's best response.
    1. "When your daughter is stable, she'll undergo computed tomography and magnetic resolution imaging. The physicians will be able to let you know if she has CP."
    2. "Most children do not develop CP at this late age."
    3. "Your child will be closely monitored after discharge, and a developmental specialist will be able to make the diagnosis."
    4. "Most children who have had complications of meningitis develop some amount of CP."

48. The nurse is caring for a 2-month-old male infant who is at risk for CP due to extreme low birth weight and prematurity. There is a multidisciplinary team caring for him. His parents ask why there is a speech therapist involved in his care. Select the nurse's best response.
    1. "Your child is likely to have speech problems because of his early birth. Involving the speech therapist at this point will ensure vocalization at a developmentally appropriate age."
    2. "The speech therapist will help with tongue and jaw movements to assist with babbling."
    3. "The speech therapist will help with tongue and jaw movements to assist with feeding."
    4. "It is the hospital routine to involve as many members of the health-care team in your child's care so that we will know if he has any unmet needs."

49. The nurse is giving morning medications to a 4-year-old female who has just had a surgical procedure to release her hamstrings. The child has a history of CP. When the nurse prepares to administer baclofen, the child's parents ask what the medication is for. Select the nurse's best response.
    1. "It is a medication that will help decrease the pain from her surgery."
    2. "It is a medication that will prevent her from having seizures."
    3. "It is a medication that will help control her spasms."
    4. "It is a medication that will help with bladder control."

50. A 3-year-old male with CP has just been fitted for braces and is beginning physical therapy to assist with ambulation. His parents ask why he needs the braces when he was crawling without any assistive devices. Select the nurse's best response:
    1. "The CP has progressed, and he now needs more assistance to ambulate."
    2. "As your child ages and grows, the CP can manifest in different ways, and different muscle groups can need more assistance."
    3. "Most children with CP need braces to help with ambulation."
    4. "We have found that when children with CP use braces, they are less likely to fall."

51. The parents of a 12-month-old with CP ask the nurse if they should teach their child sign language because he has not begun any vocalization yet. The nurse bases her response on which of the following?
    1. Sign language may be a very beneficial way to help children with CP communicate.
    2. Sign language may cause confusion and further delay verbalization.
    3. Most children with CP will have great difficulty learning sign language.
    4. Sign language may be beneficial, but it would be best to wait until the child is closer to the preschool age.

52. The parents of a 2-year-old with CP are learning how to feed their child and avoid aspiration. When reviewing the teaching plan, the nurse should question which of the following?
    1. Place the food on the tip of the tongue, as the child will be less likely to choke.
    2. Place the child in an upright position during feedings.
    3. Feed the child soft and blended foods.
    4. Feed the child slowly.

53. The nurse is caring for a 5-year-old male with CP. His weight is in the fifth percentile, and he has been hospitalized for aspiration pneumonia. His parents are anxious and state that they do not want a G-tube put in. Which of the following would be the nurse's best response?
    1. "A G-tube will help your son gain weight and reduce his risk for future hospitalizations due to pneumonia."
    2. "G-tubes are very easy to care for and will make feeding time easier for your family."
    3. "Are you concerned that you will not be able to care for his G-tube?"
    4. "Tell me your thoughts about G-tubes."

54. The nurse is caring for a 4-month-old infant who was diagnosed with a neuroblastoma. The nurse knows that this particular child's prognosis is:
1. Excellent, as a neuroblastoma is always cured.
2. Excellent, as infants with a neuroblastoma have the best prognosis.
3. Poor, as infants with a neuroblastoma rarely survive.
4. Variable, depending on where the site of origin is.

55. The nurse is caring for a 6-year-old female with a neuroblastoma. The girl has metastasis to the bone marrow and has been diagnosed with pancytopenia. Which of the following should be included in her care?
1. Administration of red blood cells.
2. Limit school attendance to less than 4 hours daily.
3. Administration of Coumadin.
4. Encourage a diet high in fresh fruits and vegetables.

56. The nurse is caring for a 3-year-old with neuroblastoma. The child's parents ask the nurse what the typical signs and symptoms are at first. Select the nurse's best answer.
1. "Most children complain of abdominal fullness and difficulty urinating."
2. "Many children in the early stages of a neuroblastoma have joint pain and walk with a limp."
3. "The signs and symptoms vary depending on where the tumor is located, but typical symptoms include weight loss, abdominal distention, and fatigue."
4. "The signs and symptoms are fairly consistent regardless of the location of the tumor. They include fatigue, hunger, weight gain, and abdominal fullness."

57. The nurse is working in the pediatric cancer center caring for a group of children with brain tumors. Which of the following children would have likely experienced a delay in diagnosis?
1. A 3-month-old, as signs and symptoms would not have been readily apparent.
2. A 5-month-old, as signs and symptoms would not have been readily suspected.
3. A school-age child, as signs and symptoms could have been misinterpreted.
4. An adolescent, as signs and symptoms could have been ignored and denied.

58. A 5-year-old female has been diagnosed with a midline brain tumor. In addition to showing signs of increased ICP, she has been voiding large amounts of very dilute urine. Which of the following medications does the nurse expect to administer?
1. Mannitol.
2. Vasopressin.
3. Lasix.
4. Dopamine.

59. The nurse is caring for a 30-month-old female receiving radiation therapy for a brain tumor. The parents ask if their child will likely have any learning disabilities in the future. Select the nurse's best answer.
1. "All children who receive radiation have some amount of learning disability. As long as they receive extra tutoring, they usually do well in school."
2. "Because your daughter is so young, she will likely do well and have no problems in the future."
3. "Response varies with each child, but younger children who receive radiation tend to have some amount of learning disability later in life."
4. "Response varies with each child, but younger children who receive radiation tend to have fewer problems later in life than older children."

60. The nurse is working in the emergency room caring for a 10-year-old who was in an MVA. The child is currently on a backboard with a cervical collar in place. The child is diagnosed with a cervical fracture. Which of the following would the nurse expect to find in the child's plan of care?
    1. Remove the cervical collar, keep the backboard in place, and administer high-dose methlyprednisolone.
    2. Continue with all forms of spinal stabilization, and administer high-dose methylprednisolone and ranitidine.
    3. Remove the backboard and cervical collar, and prepare for halo traction placement.
    4. Remove the cervical collar and backboard, place the child on spinal precautions, and administer high-dose methylprednisolone and ranitidine.

61. Which of the following has the potential to alter a child's level of consciousness? Select all that apply.
    1. Metabolic disorders.
    2. Trauma.
    3. Hypoxic episode.
    4. Dehydration.
    5. Endocrine disorders.

1. 1. Coma describes a state of consciousness in which the child is not responsive to any stimulation, including painful stimulation.
   2. Delirium describes a state of consciousness in which the child is extremely confused and anxious.
   3. **Obtunded describes a state of consciousness in which the child has a limited response to the environment and can be aroused by verbal or tactile stimulation.**
   4. Confusion describes a state of consciousness in which the child is not oriented to person, place, and time.

   TEST-TAKING HINT: The test taker needs to be familiar with terms describing states of consciousness.

2. 1. Most 3-year-olds are not capable of naming the president.
   2. **Asking the 3-year-old to identify her parents and state her name is a developmentally appropriate way to assess orientation.**
   3. Many 3-year-olds are not familiar with their phone numbers or may not be able to share this information during a stressful time, such as hospitalization.
   4. Many 3-year-olds do not know the current month.

   TEST-TAKING HINT: The test taker needs to be familiar with the concept of consciousness and applying developmental theories to specific age groups.

3. 1. School-age children feel more comfortable when parents are present and are therefore more likely to cooperate with a neurological assessment.
   2. **Parents should be encouraged to remain with their child for mutual comfort.**
   3. Describing a policy is not sufficient and does not give the parents enough information.
   4. School-age children feel more comfortable when parents are present and are therefore more likely to cooperate with a neurological assessment.

   TEST-TAKING HINT: The test taker needs to be familiar with growth and development of children and applying theories to specific clinical situations.

4. 1. The child is demonstrating a reflex called posturing. The parent should not be given any false hope that the child is responding at a higher level than is truly occurring.
   2. The posturing reflex often indicates irritability, and the child should not continue to receive stimulation.
   3. Posturing is a reflex, not a seizure.
   4. **Posturing is a reflex that often indicates that the child is receiving too much stimulation.**

   TEST-TAKING HINT: The test taker needs to be familiar with caring for the comatose child and what causes posturing.

5. 1. The anterior fontanel is usually raised and bulging in infants with increased ICP.
   2. The infant is not able to comprehend blurred vision or make any statements.
   3. **A high-pitched cry is often indicative of increased ICP in infants.**
   4. The infant with increased ICP usually has a poor appetite and does not feed well.

   TEST-TAKING HINT: The test taker needs to be familiar with hydrocephalus and how increased ICP is manifested in infants. Answer 2 can be eliminated because an infant cannot specifically verbalize.

6. 1. **The ventriculoperitoneal is the most common shunt used to treat hydrocephalus.**
   2. Although ventriculoatrial shunts can be used, they are not used nearly as often as ventriculoperitoneal shunts.
   3. The ventricle of the brain is not shunted to the lower esophagus.
   4. The ventricle of the brain is not shunted to the small intestine.

   TEST-TAKING HINT: The test taker needs to be familiar with treatments for hydrocephalus.

7. 1. These are symptoms of a shunt malfunction and should be evaluated immediately.
   2. Although these symptoms may be associated with the start of a girl's menstrual cycle, they are symptoms of a shunt malfunction and require immediate evaluation.
   3. A shunt can malfunction at any point and should be evaluated when signs of increased ICP become evident.
   4. **These are symptoms of a shunt malfunction and should be evaluated immediately.**

   TEST-TAKING HINT: The test taker should recognize these symptoms as signs of a shunt malfunction and can eliminate answers 1, 2, and 3 because they do not address the situation as an emergency.

8. 1. A semi-Fowler position in an infant seat may allow the ventricles to drain too rapidly in the immediate postoperative period.
   2. **Flat in the crib is the position usually used initially, with the angle gradually increasing as the child tolerates.**
   3. The Trendelenburg position is not used immediately after ventriculoperitoneal shunt placement.
   4. The head elevated to 90 degrees will allow the ventricle of the brain to drain too quickly.

   TEST-TAKING HINT: The test taker should note the word "initially" and consider why the position would be immediately beneficial. Answer 3 can be eliminated because that particular position could increase ICP.

9. 1. The CSF in viral meningitis is usually clear.
   2. **The CSF in bacterial meningitis is usually cloudy.**
   3. The CSF in healthy children is usually clear.
   4. Sepsis is an infection of the bloodstream.

   TEST-TAKING HINT: The test taker can eliminate answer 4 because an infection of the bloodstream would not be detected in the CSF.

10. 1. Administration of intravenous antibiotics should not be started until after all cultures have been obtained.
    2. Administration of maintenance IV fluids can wait until after the cultures have been obtained.
    3. Placement of a Foley catheter is not a priority procedure.
    4. **Cultures of spinal fluid and blood should be obtained, followed by administration of intravenous antibiotics.**

    TEST-TAKING HINT: The test taker needs to think about priority of care. Answer 3 can be immediately eliminated, as it is not a priority. Answer 4 should be considered a priority, as antibiotics should not be started before the cultures have been sent.

11. 1. **Brudzinski sign occurs when the child responds to a flexed neck with an involuntary flexion of the hips and/or knees.**
    2. Cushing triad is a sign of increased ICP and is manifested with an increase in systolic blood pressure, decreased heart rate, and irregular respirations or apnea.
    3. Kernig sign occurs when there is resistance or pain in response to raising the child's flexed leg.

    4. Nuchal rigidity occurs when there is a resistance to neck flexion.

    TEST-TAKING HINT: The test taker should be familiar with terms used to describe meningeal irritation.

12. 1. The child with bacterial meningitis should be placed in a private room isolated from all other patients. Bacterial meningitis is caused by many pathogens, and patients should be isolated from each other.
    2. The child with bacterial meningitis should be placed in a private room isolated from all other patients. Bacterial meningitis is caused by many pathogens, and patients should be isolated from each other.
    3. **A quiet private room with minimal stimulation is ideal as the child with meningitis should be in a quiet environment to avoid cerebral irritation.**
    4. A bright room with developmental activities may cause irritation and increase ICP.

    TEST-TAKING HINT: The test taker should consider what contributes to cerebral irritation and should not be influenced by the developmental requirements of a healthy toddler.

13. 1. Isolation precautions must be maintained for at least the first 24 hours of intravenous antibiotic therapy.
    2. **Intravenous fluids at 1½ times regular maintenance could cause fluid overload and lead to increased ICP.**
    3. Neurological checks are usually made at least every 4 hours.
    4. Acetaminophen is usually administered when the child has a fever, as increased temperature can lead to increased ICP.

    TEST-TAKING HINT: The test taker should consider the answers and eliminate those that may increase ICP. Intravenous fluids are often given at less than maintenance unless the child is hemodynamically unstable.

14. 1. Although encephalitis is usually seen after viral infection, the child is usually admitted for close observation.
    2. Intravenous antibiotics are not given to the child with viral encephalitis.
    3. **The young child with encephalitis should be admitted to a PICU where close observation and monitoring are available. The child should be observed for signs of increased ICP and for cardiac and respiratory compromise.**

4. The child should not be discharged as she needs to be observed for complications. As a general rule, younger children tend to have more complications and require a PICU admission.

TEST-TAKING HINT: The test taker should be familiar with the diagnosis and treatment of encephalitis. The test taker should not be influenced by the word "viral" but should realize that the sequelae of encephalitis require close monitoring in an ICU environment.

15. 1. Having a child immunized helps prevent the viral illnesses from occurring, thereby decreasing the likelihood of Reye syndrome.
    2. **The administration of aspirin or products containing aspirin have been associated with the development of Reye syndrome.**
    3. Although Reye syndrome is rare, it continues to be a serious illness with the potential for rapid deterioration of the patient.
    4. Children with Reye syndrome are always admitted to the hospital as there is a strong possibility for complications and rapid deterioration.

TEST-TAKING HINT: The test taker should be aware that aspirin administration in children with viruses has been linked to Reye syndrome.

16. 1. Decorticate posturing is seen with a less advanced stage of Reye syndrome and likely indicates that the child's condition is improving.
    2. The child's condition is improving; therefore, cardiac and respiratory failure are less likely.
    3. **Progressing from decerebrate to decorticate posturing usually indicates an improvement in the child's condition.**
    4. Decorticate posturing is associated with inflammation above the brainstem, whereas decerebrate posturing is associated with inflammation in the brainstem.

TEST-TAKING HINT: The test taker needs to be familiar with posturing reflexes and their significance.

17. 1. A common manifestation is increased ICP, which is treated with an osmotic diuretic. Lasix is a loop diuretic.
    2. A common manifestation is hypoglycemia. Insulin does not treat hypoglycemia, but decreases the blood sugar instead.

3. **A common manifestation is hypoglycemia, which is treated with the administration of intravenous glucose.**
4. Morphine is a narcotic used for pain relief. It should be used with caution as it can lead to respiratory depression.

TEST-TAKING HINT: The test taker needs to be aware that increased ICP is a very common manifestation of Reye syndrome and can therefore eliminate any answers that do not treat increased ICP. The test taker can also eliminate answers 2 and 4 because they do not treat hypoglycemia, which is another common manifestation of Reye syndrome.

18. 1. **The child experiencing a seizure usually requires more oxygen as the seizure increases the body's metabolic rate and demand for oxygen. The seizure may also affect the child's airway, causing the child to be hypoxic. It is always appropriate to give the child blow-by oxygen immediately. The nurse should remain with the child and call for additional help.**
    2. It is important to reassure the parents, but giving the child oxygen and calling for additional support is the priority of care.
    3. It is not necessary to call a code unless the child experiences a cardiac or respiratory arrest. Research indicates that encouraging parents to remain with the child in emergency situations benefits both the child and family.
    4. It is important to monitor and observe the child during a seizure, but it is very difficult to obtain a blood pressure from a seizing child. The priority of care involves administering oxygen and calling for additional help.

TEST-TAKING HINT: The test taker needs to prioritize care and choose answer 1 because it will help maintain the airway. Answer 3 could immediately be eliminated because the child is having a seizure, not a cardiac arrest.

19. 1. **Absence seizures occur frequently and last less than 30 seconds. The child experiences a brief loss of consciousness where she may have a change in activity. These children rarely fall, but they may drop an object. The condition is often confused with daydreaming.**
    2. Akinetic seizures occur when the young child experiences a brief loss of consciousness and postural tone and falls to the

ground. The child quickly regains consciousness.

3. A non-epileptic seizure is a seizure that occurs secondary to another disorder, such as a fever or increased ICP.

4. A simple spasm seizure is not a diagnosis.

TEST-TAKING HINT: "Daydreaming" is the classic description of an absence seizure.

20. 1. **An atonic seizure is characterized by a loss of muscular tone, whereby the child may fall to the ground.**

2. It is important to evaluate the child for life stressors, but suspected seizure activity needs immediate evaluation.

3. An absence seizure is characterized by a change in activity whereby the child appears to be daydreaming or staring straight ahead. The child usually continues basic simple movements but loses an awareness of surroundings.

4. The preschool years are a not a time of rapid growth. Many children in this age group appear clumsy, but suspected seizure activity needs immediate evaluation.

TEST-TAKING HINT: The test taker should recognize the description as seizure activity and, therefore, could immediately eliminate answers 3 and 4.

21. 1. **High fat and low carbohydrates are the components of the ketogenic diet.**

2. High fat and high carbohydrates are the components of the ketogenic diet.

3. Low fat and low carbohydrates are the components of the ketogenic diet.

4. Low fat and high carbohydrates are the components of the ketogenic diet.

TEST-TAKING HINT: The test taker needs to be familiar with the components of a ketogenic diet.

22. 1. It is very difficult and time-consuming to establish an intravenous line on a child who is experiencing a generalized seizure. Rectal diazepam is first administered in an attempt to stop the seizure long enough to establish a line, and then medication is administered intravenously.

2. **Rectal diazepam is first administered in an attempt to stop the seizure long enough to establish an IV, and then IV medication is administered.**

3. Although the child may become hypoglycemic due to increased metabolic demands, stopping the seizure with rectal diazepam is the first priority. Medication is not placed in the mouth of a child

experiencing a generalized seizure as it increases the risk of injury and aspiration.

4. Stopping the seizure with rectal diazepam takes priority over placing a nasogastric tube.

TEST-TAKING HINT: The test taker needs to consider the current situation and the level of difficulty establishing intravenous access in a child experiencing a generalized seizure.

23. 1. Children who experience a febrile seizure are likely to experience another febrile seizure.

2. **Most children over the age of 5 years do not have febrile seizures.**

3. Antipyretics are administered to prevent the child's temperature from rising too rapidly.

4. Most children are not prescribed anticonvulsant medication after experiencing a febrile seizure.

TEST-TAKING HINT: There is an increased risk in siblings, but the 7-year-old child is above the usual age of febrile seizures.

24. 1. Although many children with epilepsy require more than one medication to achieve seizure control, it is recommended that only one medication be begun at a time so that the child's reaction to the specific medication can be observed.

2. **One medication is the preferred way to achieve seizure control. The child is monitored for side effects and drug levels.**

3. Rectal gels are used to stop a seizure once it has begun; they are not used to prevent seizures.

4. The route of choice for the prevention of seizures is oral. There is no reason to assume that compliance will be an issue prior to beginning anticonvulsant therapy.

TEST-TAKING HINT: The test taker should eliminate answer 4 because IV medications are not included in the initial home medication regimen.

25. 1. Swimming does not need to be avoided as long as there is someone else with her to call for help in the event of an emergency.

2. **The rhythmic reflection of other car lights can trigger a seizure in some children.**

3. There is no reason to avoid strenuous activity.

4. It is important for adolescents to be with their peers in order to reach developmental milestones.

TEST-TAKING HINT: The test taker should consider the answers that can lead to a seizure. Answer 2 is the only answer that includes a common trigger.

26. 1. Nothing should be placed in the child's mouth as he is at risk for aspiration. Rescue valium is usually administered rectally.
    2. **The nurse should remain with the child and observe the seizure. The child should be protected from his environment, and clothing should be loosened.**
    3. A tongue blade should never be placed in the child's mouth, as it can cause injury or increase the risk of aspiration.
    4. The nurse should remain with the child and call for help. An 8-year-old child can be injured if carried during a seizure.

TEST-TAKING HINT: The test taker should eliminate answers 1 and 3 because nothing should ever be placed in the mouth of a child having a seizure.

27. 1. The child who has a closed-head injury has decreased perfusion to the brain and increased metabolic needs that lead to ischemia and brain damage.
    2. The child who has a closed-head injury has decreased perfusion to the brain and increased metabolic needs that lead to ischemia and brain damage.
    3. The child who has a closed-head injury has decreased perfusion to the brain and increased metabolic needs that lead to ischemia and brain damage.
    4. **Decreased perfusion of the brain and increased metabolic needs of the brain.**

TEST-TAKING HINT: The test taker needs to be familiar with the mechanics of a head injury.

28. 1. It is not a priority of care to find out if anyone else was injured.
    2. Although open-ended questions are important, the nurse needs specific information, and the anxious parent may need to be guided during triage assessment.
    3. **Asking specific questions will give the nurse the information needed to determine the level of care for the child.**
    4. Although it is important to provide safety education, this information should be given in a nonjudgmental manner at a point when the parents and child are less stressed.

TEST-TAKING HINT: The test taker needs to consider the role of a triage nurse. Specific information needs to be obtained

quickly. Answer 4 can be eliminated because it implies judgment and does not help the current situation.

29. 1. **Cushing triad is characterized by a decrease in heart rate, an increase in blood pressure, and changes in respirations. The triad is associated with severely increased ICP. Mannitol is an osmotic diuretic that helps decrease the increased ICP.**
    2. The child's vital signs need to be monitored, but a fluid bolus will increase the circulating volume and lead to an increase in the child's ICP. Fluid boluses are necessary in cases of shock but must be administered carefully and the child closely observed.
    3. An antihypertensive will not help decrease the ICP.
    4. The child will benefit from supplemental oxygen, but it will not help decrease the ICP.

TEST-TAKING HINT: The test taker should recognize the signs of Cushing triad. If not recognized, the child's condition should be seen as deteriorating and emergent. Answer 2 and 4 can be eliminated because they are only partially correct.

30. 1. Even if the child is unresponsive, the child can still feel pain.
    2. If pain medication is administered cautiously, the child can still be monitored, and signs of improvement will be evident.
    3. **Pain medication promotes comfort and ultimately decreases ICP.**
    4. Pain medication decreases the demand for oxygen.

TEST-TAKING HINT: The test taker needs to consider the presence and significance of pain in the unresponsive child. Answer 1 can be immediately eliminated because the unresponsive child does feel pain.

31. 1. **A cooling blanket will help cool the child quickly and at a controlled temperature.**
    2. Tylenol should be administered after the cooling blanket has been applied. Tylenol is an effective medication, but a cooling blanket will begin to be effective before the medication is absorbed.
    3. Tylenol should be administered after the cooling blanket has been applied. Tylenol is an effective medication, but a cooling blanket will begin to be effective before the medication is absorbed.

4. Ice packs will cause the child to shiver, which will increase oxygen consumption and possibly increase ICP. Shivering can also cause the child to experience a rebound increase in temperature.

TEST-TAKING HINT: The test taker should consider the cause of the increased temperature and how to cool the child quickly. Answer 4 should be eliminated because ice packs are no longer recommended to treat increased temperatures.

32. 1. Although peers play an important role in the adolescent's development, this particular patient is at risk for increased ICP and should have decreased stimulation.
   2. Loud speaking may cause the child's ICP to increase.
   3. A bright, lively environment may lead to increased ICP.
   4. **A dark, quiet environment and minimal stimulation will decrease oxygen consumption and ICP.**

TEST-TAKING HINT: The test taker should consider the causes of ICP and select answers that will not increase ICP. Answers 1, 2, and 3 cause an increase in ICP and should be eliminated.

33. 1. **A computed tomography scan of the head will reveal trauma. Dilating the eyes is performed to check for retinal hemorrhages that are seen in an infant who has experienced SBS.**
   2. An EEG is not usually done as a priority test in an infant displaying symptoms of SBS.
   3. Although close monitoring of vital signs are important, further testing is required.
   4. X-rays of all long bones may be performed to rule out any old or new fractures, but CT and pupil examinations are the priority for this patient.

TEST-TAKING HINT: The test taker should consider child abuse (SBS) as the story does not match the injury. The pupils are always dilated to rule out SBS.

34. 1. An open anterior fontanel allows for swelling, therefore decreasing the risk of injury.
   2. **Insufficient musculoskeletal support and a disproportionate head places the infant at risk because the head cannot be supported during a shaking episode.**
   3. Superficial veins and arteries do not place the infant at a higher risk for injury.

4. Although the myelination is immature, the immature musculoskeletal support places the infant at risk.

TEST-TAKING HINT: Answer 4 should be eliminated because superficial vessels do not lead to SBS.

35. 1. A meningocele is a sac that contains a portion of the meninges and the CSF.
   2. **A myelomeningocele is a sac that contains a portion of the meninges, the CSF, and the nerve roots.**
   3. Spinal bifida occulta is a failure of the vertebral arches to fuse. There is no sac, and no defect is visible.
   4. Anencephaly occurs when the brain does not develop above the brainstem.

TEST-TAKING HINT: The test taker could eliminate answer 4 because anencephaly is a brainstem abnormality and does not involve the spine.

36. 1. **Because a meningocele does not contain any nerve endings, most children experience no neurological problems after surgical correction.**
   2. Corrective surgery is done as soon as possible to minimize the risk of infection.
   3. Because a meningocele does not contain any nerve endings, most children experience no neurological problems after surgical correction.
   4. Because a meningocele does not contain any nerve endings, most children experience no neurological problems after surgical correction.

TEST-TAKING HINT: The test taker should consider the risks of infection and immediately eliminate answer 2 because the surgery is not postponed but performed as soon as possible.

37. 1. Although it is important to measure the head circumference of all babies, children with myelomeningocele are at increased risk for hydrocephalus, which can be manifested with an increase in head circumference.
   2. **Children with myelomeningocele are at increased risk for hydrocephalus, which can be manifested with an increase in head circumference.**
   3. Although a defect in the spine can be a portal of entry for infection, children with myelomeningocele often have hydrocephalus as well.
   4. Children with myelomeningocele are not at risk for microcephaly.

TEST-TAKING HINT: The test taker should consider the diagnosis and choose a response that best fits the current diagnosis.

38. 1. Some children with myelomeningocele experience learning disabilities, but it is not the most common complication.
    2. **Urinary tract infections are the most common complication of myelomeningocele. Nearly all children with myelomeningocele have a neurogenic bladder that leads to incomplete emptying of the bladder and subsequent urinary tract infections. Frequent catheterization also increases the risk of urinary tract infection.**
    3. Many children with myelomeningocele experience hydrocephalus, but it is not the most common complication.
    4. Children with myelomeningocele are at risk for skin breakdown and decubitus ulcers, but they are not the most common complications.

    TEST-TAKING HINT: The test taker needs to be familiar with the complications of myelomeningocele. Neurogenic bladder is the most common complication, so the test taker should be led to select answer 2.

39. 1. Placing the child in the prone position is correct. A dry dressing may adhere to the defect, causing irritation.
    2. A dry dressing may adhere to the defect, causing irritation.
    3. Oral gastric feedings are not usually started unless there is going to be a delay in surgery. The defect is usually corrected immediately to avoid infection.
    4. **The child is placed in the prone position to avoid any pressure on the defect. A sterile moist dressing is placed over the defect to keep it as clean as possible. Intravenous fluids are begun after the surgery.**

    TEST-TAKING HINT: The test taker should consider the location of the defect and eliminate answer 1. Answer 2 should be eliminated as a dry dressing could cause irritation.

40. 1. The child with a neurogenic bladder will never be able to spontaneously empty it completely. Most girls learn to self-catheterize at a young age.
    2. The child with a neurogenic bladder will never be able to spontaneously empty it completely.

3. Placing the child with a neurogenic bladder on a bladder training program is not helpful, as the child with a neurogenic bladder will never be able to spontaneously empty it completely.
4. **A vesicostomy is an example of an option for children with myelomeningoceles where alternatives to traditional catheterizations are created.**

TEST-TAKING HINT: The test taker should recognize that the neurogenic bladder in a child with myelomeningocele is irreversible, and answers 2 and 3 should be eliminated.

41. 1. Children with myelomeningocele are prone to latex allergies and therefore should not eat bananas.
    2. Children with myelomeningocele are prone to latex allergies and therefore should not be exposed to balloons.
    3. **Preventing skin breakdown is important in the child with myelomeningocele, as pressure points are not felt easily.**
    4. It is always important to provide education on dietary needs, but it is not the priority in the immediate postoperative period.

    TEST-TAKING HINT: The test taker should consider that children with myelomeningocele are prone to latex allergies and therefore should eliminate answers 1 and 2.

42. 1. Although there is a cosmetic benefit, the surgery is done to reconstruct the skull to allow the brain to grow properly. There are potential complications associated with this surgery, such as increased ICP.
    2. **The surgery is done to reconstruct the skull to allow the brain to grow properly. Because there are potential complications associated with this surgery, such as increased ICP, the child is usually closely observed in the PICU.**
    3. The surgery is not usually postponed as it will allow for brain growth.
    4. The surgery is not usually postponed as it will allow for brain growth.

    TEST-TAKING HINT: The test taker should consider the importance of allowing room for brain growth. Answers 3 and 4 can be eliminated because the surgery is performed sooner than later.

43. 1. The infant needs to wear the helmet 23 hours daily. It is removed for bathing, but not sleeping.
    2. The helmet is most effective when the child is younger, as the bones in the skull

are more malleable. The child is less likely to need the helmet when upright and mobile as there is less pressure in one area.

  3. **The helmet is worn 23 hours every day and removed only for bathing.**
  4. Most children wear the helmet for 3 months.

TEST-TAKING HINT: The test taker should recognize that the helmet is worn 23 hours daily and can eliminate answers 1, 2, and 4.

44. 1. **The incidence of CP has increased partly due to the increased survival of extreme low-birth-weight and premature infants.**
  2. The incidence of CP has increased since the 1960s.
  3. The incidence of CP has increased since the 1960s.
  4. There is no evidence to suggest that CP has been diagnosed erroneously.

TEST-TAKING HINT: The test taker should consider the causes of CP and be led to answer 1 because technology has increased the survival rate of low-birth-weight and premature infants. The test taker should resist the temptation to select answer 2 because it has not decreased like many disorders.

45. 1. There is an increased incidence of CP when the infant has an Apgar score of 3 or less at 5 minutes.
  2. **Any infection of the central nervous system increases the infant's risk of CP.**
  3. A febrile seizure does not increase the risk of CP.
  4. Although head trauma can increase the risk of CP, the school-age child is not likely to develop CP from falling off a bike.

TEST-TAKING HINT: The test taker should consider the risks for CP. Answers 3 and 4 should be eliminated because these symptoms are least likely to lead to CP.

46. 1. The startle reflex is expected in an infant 1 month old.
  2. **The clinical characteristic of hemiplegia can be manifested by the early preference of one hand. This may be an early sign of CP.**
  3. Although many children walk before the age of 14 months, it is not considered a motor delay to not have achieved this milestone at this point.
  4. Many 2-year-olds have not achieved bladder control.

TEST-TAKING HINT: The test taker should be familiar with normal developmental milestones and eliminate answers 1, 3, and 4 because they are all developmentally appropriate.

47. 1. CP is diagnosed based on clinical characteristics and developmental findings. It is not diagnosed with any type of radiological examination.
  2. Although most cases of CP are developed during the neonatal period, some children can develop CP at a later age.
  3. **The child will be given a chance to recover and will be monitored closely before a diagnosis is made.**
  4. Although many children develop CP after having complications of meningitis, many do not. Although the parents should not be given false hope, they should not be led to lose hope for a complete recovery.

TEST-TAKING HINT: The test taker should be led to answer 3 because it explains the process and does not state that the child definitely will or will not develop CP.

48. 1. The nurse cannot assume that the child will have speech difficulties. Speech therapy does not guarantee vocalization at a developmentally appropriate age.
  2. Although speech therapy will assist with babbling at a later age, its primary purpose is to assist with feeding.
  3. **It is important to involve speech therapy to strengthen tongue and jaw movements to assist with feeding. The infant who is at risk for CP may have weakened and uncoordinated tongue and jaw movements.**
  4. Members of a multidisciplinary team become involved in a child's care based on specific needs, not hospital routine.

TEST-TAKING HINT: The test taker should immediately eliminate answer 4 because it does not consider the child's individual needs.

49. 1. Baclofen is not given for postoperative pain control.
  2. Baclofen is not given for seizures.
  3. **Baclofen is given to help control the spasms associated with CP.**
  4. Baclofen is not given for bladder control.

TEST-TAKING HINT: The test taker needs to be familiar with the medication baclofen.

50. 1. CP is a nonprogressive disorder.
  2. **CP can be manifested in different ways as the child grows. It does not progress,**

but its clinical manifestations may change.

3. Children with CP have different abilities and needs. CP can result in mild to severe motor deficits; therefore, one treatment regimen cannot be used or recommended for all children.

4. Although braces may assist some children with ambulation, they will not be useful in all cases.

TEST-TAKING HINT: The test taker can eliminate answers 3 and 4 because generalizations cannot be made regarding CP. Each child has different abilities and disabilities.

51. 1. **Sign language may help the child with CP communicate and ultimately decrease frustration. Children with CP may have difficulty verbalizing because of weak tongue and jaw muscles. They may be able to have sufficient motor skills to communicate with their hands.**

2. Sign language does not cause confusion and may help reinforce vocabulary and vocalization.

3. CP is manifested differently in all children; therefore, generalizations cannot be made.

4. The earlier sign language is taught, the more it will be beneficial.

TEST-TAKING HINT: The test taker can immediately eliminate answer 3 because it makes a generalization. All forms of language are beneficial and well tolerated by the children, especially young children.

52. 1. **The food should be placed far back in the mouth to avoid tongue thrust.**

2. The child should be placed in an upright position.

3. Soft and blended foods minimize the risk of aspiration.

4. Allowing the child time to feed minimizes the risk of aspiration.

TEST-TAKING HINT: The test taker should consider which methods will decrease the risk of aspiration. Answers 2, 3, and 4 all decrease the risk of choking and should be eliminated because the question asks, "Which shows that more education is needed?"

53. 1. Sharing information may not be helpful if the family is not ready to listen.

2. Sharing information may not be helpful if the family is not ready to listen.

3. The family may have other concerns that would be communicated through an open-ended question.

4. **An open-ended question will encourage family members to share what they know and potentially clear any misconceptions.**

TEST-TAKING HINT: The test taker should consider the principles of therapeutic communication. Answer 4 is an open-ended question that will not be perceived as judgmental and should elicit the most information.

54. 1. Neuroblastoma is not always cured and can be fatal depending on the stage at diagnosis, site of origin, and the age of the child.

2. **Infants younger than 1 year have the best prognosis.**

3. Infants younger than 1 year have the best prognosis.

4. Although the prognosis varies with the site of origin, infants have the most favorable outcome.

TEST-TAKING HINT: The question requires the test taker to be familiar with the prognosis of neuroblastoma.

55. 1. **Red blood cells will be needed to increase the red blood cell count.**

2. The child should not be around groups of people due to the potential of exposure to infection.

3. Blood thinners are not given to the child with a decreased platelet count.

4. Fresh fruits and vegetables should be avoided as they may contain microorganisms that can lead to infection in the child with a low white blood cell count.

TEST-TAKING HINT: The test taker should consider all components of pancytopenia and select the answer that will not harm the child. Answers 3 and 4 should be immediately eliminated because they both increase infection.

56. 1. Although abdominal fullness is often seen, difficulty urinating is not a common symptom.

2. Bone manifestations are a sign of bone metastasis, which is not seen in the early stages of neuroblastoma.

3. **The signs and symptoms vary depending on where the tumor is located, but typical symptoms include weight loss, abdominal distention, and fatigue.**

4. The signs and symptoms vary according to the location of the tumor. Generally, hunger and weight gain are not seen.

TEST-TAKING HINT: The test taker should eliminate answer 2 because bone metastases are a late sign, and the test taker is looking for initial signs.

57. 1. **In infants, signs and symptoms may not be readily apparent as the open fontanel allows for expansion.**
    2. Although brain tumors are not suspected in infants, a delay in diagnosis is most likely due to the open fontanel, allowing some expansion to go unnoticed.
    3. Signs and symptoms may be misinterpreted, but increased ICP will become apparent.
    4. Signs and symptoms may be denied, but increased ICP will become apparent.

TEST-TAKING HINT: The test taker should consider growth and development in answering this question. The anterior fontanel allows for brain expansion, therefore delaying the discovery of signs and symptoms of a brain tumor.

58. 1. The child is experiencing diabetes insipidus, a common occurrence in children with midline brain tumors. Mannitol is an osmotic diuretic that will not treat diabetes insipidus.
    2. **The child is experiencing diabetes insipidus, a common occurrence in children with midline brain tumors. Vasopressin is a hormone that is used to help the body retain water.**
    3. The child is experiencing diabetes insipidus, a common occurrence in children with midline brain tumors. Lasix is a diuretic that will not treat diabetes insipidus.
    4. The child is experiencing diabetes insipidus, a common occurrence in children with midline brain tumors. Dopamine is a beta-adrenergic agonist that is not used to treat diabetes insipidus.

TEST-TAKING HINT: The test taker should be familiar with diabetes insipidus. The question describes its symptoms. Diabetes insipidus commonly occurs in children with midline brain tumors. The test taker can eliminate answers 1 and 3 because they increase dieresis, which needs to be avoided.

59. 1. Not all children who receive radiation experience learning disabilities.
    2. Younger children tend to experience more learning difficulties than older children.

3. **Although variable, younger children tend to experience more learning difficulties than older children.**
4. Although variable, younger children tend to experience more learning difficulties than older children.

TEST-TAKING HINT: The test taker should be familiar with radiation therapy. The test taker should be led to answers 3 and 4 because they both state that difficulties are variable.

60. 1. The cervical collar should not be removed. In addition to the methylprednisolone, ranitidine should be administered to prevent gastric ulcer formation.
    2. **All forms of spinal stabilization should be continued while methylprednisolone and Zantac are administered.**
    3. The backboard and cervical collar should not be removed until after the halo traction has been applied.
    4. The cervical collar should not be removed.

TEST-TAKING HINT: The test taker should be familiar with spinal cord injuries. The test taker should eliminate any answer stating the cervical collar be removed, such as 1, 3, and 4.

61. 1, 2, 3, 4, 5.
    1. **Many metabolic disorders are associated with hypoglycemia. The hypoglycemic child experiences a decreased level of consciousness as the brain does not have stores of glucose.**
    2. **Trauma can lead to generalized brain swelling with resultant increased ICP.**
    3. **Hypoxemia leads to a decreased level of consciousness as the brain is intolerant to the lack of oxygen.**
    4. **Dehydration can lead to inadequate perfusion to the brain, which can result in a decreased level of consciousness.**
    5. **Endocrine disorders often result in a decreased level of consciousness as they can lead to hypoglycemia, which is poorly tolerated by the brain.**

TEST-TAKING HINT: Metabolic disorders, trauma, hypoxic episodes, dehydration, and endocrine disorders are examples of disorders that can alter a child's level of consciousness by either increasing ICP or decreasing the perfusion of blood to the brain.

Cardiovascular Disorders

6

KEYWORDS

Bacterial endocarditis
Cardiac demand
Defects with decreased pulmonary flow

Defects with increased pulmonary flow
Obstructive defects

ABBREVIATIONS

Angiotensin receptor blockers (ARB)
Aortic stenosis (AS)
Atrial septal defect (ASD)
Atrioventricular canal (AVC)
Bacterial endocarditis (BE)
Blood pressure (BP)
Cardiac output (CO)
Cardiovascular accident (CVA)
Coarctation of the aorta (COA)
Congenital heart defect (CHD)
Congestive heart failure (CHF)

Heart rate (HR)
Kawasaki disease (KD)
Left sternal border (LSB)
Patent ductus arteriosus (PDA)
Pulmonic stenosis (PS)
Rheumatic fever (RF)
Supraventricular tachycardia (SVT)
Systemic vascular resistance (SVR)
Tetralogy of Fallot (TOF)
Ventricular septal defect (VBD)

QUESTIONS

1. A child with a history of cardiac surgery requires an annual electrocardiogram. What can the electrocardiogram detect? Select all that apply.
   1. Ischemia.
   2. Injury.
   3. CO.
   4. Dysrhythmias.
   5. SVR.
   6. Occlusion pressure.
   7. Conduction delay.

2. A newborn is diagnosed with a CHD. The test results reveal that the lumen of the duct between the aorta and pulmonary artery remains open. This defect is known as

   _____ .

3. The parent of an infant newly diagnosed with TOF is asking the nurse which defects are involved. Select all that apply.
   1. VSD.
   2. Right ventricular hypertrophy.
   3. Left ventricular hypertrophy.
   4. PS.
   5. Pulmonic atresia.
   6. Overriding aorta.
   7. PDA.

4. A 10-year-old child is recovering from a severe sore throat. The caregiver now states that the child complains of chest pain. The nurse observes that the child has swollen joints, nodules on the fingers, and a rash on the chest. The likely cause of this syndrome is _____.

5. An infant with CHF is receiving digoxin to enhance myocardial function. What should the nurse assess prior to administering the medication?
   1. Yellow sclera.
   2. Apical pulse rate.
   3. Cough.
   4. Liver function test.

6. Which statement by the mother of an infant boy with CHF who is being sent home on digoxin indicates she needs further education on the care of her child?
   1. "I will give him the medication at regular 12-hour intervals."
   2. "If he vomits, I will not give him a make-up dose."
   3. "If I miss a dose, I will not give an extra dose, but keep him on his same schedule."
   4. "I will mix the digoxin in some of his formula to make it taste better for him."

7. A 1-year-old child is being prepared for a cardiac catheterization procedure. Which of the following findings about the child might delay the procedure?
   1. 30th percentile for weight.
   2. Severe diaper rash.
   3. Allergy to soy.
   4. Oxygen saturation of 91% on room air.

8. The nurse is caring for a child who has undergone cardiac catheterization. During the recovery phase, the nurse notices the dressing is saturated with bright red blood and a 6-inch circle of blood on the crib sheet. The nurse's first action is to:
   1. Call the interventional cardiologist.
   2. Notify the cardiac catheterization laboratory that the child will be returning.
   3. Apply a bulky pressure dressing over the present dressing.
   4. Apply direct pressure 1 inch above the puncture site.

9. The nurse is caring for an infant with CHF. The following are interventions to decrease cardiac demands on the infant. Select all that apply.
   1. Allow parents to hold and rock their child.
   2. Feed only when the infant is crying.
   3. Keep the child uncovered to promote low body temperature.
   4. Make frequent position changes.
   5. Feed the child when sucking the fists.
   6. Change bed linens only when necessary.
   7. Organize nursing activities.

10. Indomethacin may be given to close what CHD in newborns? _____

11. For the child with hypoplastic left heart syndrome, what drug may be given to allow the PDA to remain open until surgery? _____

12. The nurse is examining a 5-year-old boy who has diarrhea and fever. The caregiver states that the boy is normally active and healthy. On examination, the nurse hears a murmur at the LSB. The caregiver asks why the pediatrician has never said anything about it. The nurse explains:
    1. "The pediatrician is not a cardiologist."
    2. "Murmurs are difficult to detect, especially in children."
    3. "The fever increased the intensity of the murmur."
    4. "We need to refer the child to an interventional cardiologist."

13. While assessing a newborn with respiratory distress, the nurse auscultates a machine-like heart murmur. Other findings are a wide pulse pressure, periods of apnea, increased $PaCO_2$, and decreased PO_2. The nurse suspects that the newborn has:
    1. Pulmonary hypertension.
    2. A PDA.
    3. A VSD.
    4. Bronchopulmonary dysplasia.

14. A child has been diagnosed with KD. The parents are asking questions about the child's outcome. The nurse explains the most serious complications. Select all that apply.
    1. Coronary thrombosis.
    2. Coronary stenosis.
    3. Coronary artery aneurysm.
    4. Hypocoagulability.
    5. Decreased sedimentation rate.
    6. Hypoplastic left heart syndrome.

15. The nurse is caring for a 3-year-old boy whose caregiver noticed that his eyes are reddened with no discharge, and his palms and soles of the feet are red, swollen, and peeling. Upon examination, the nurse's assessment includes dry, cracked lips and a "strawberry tongue." The nurse most likely suspects _____.

16. The nurse is caring for a school-aged boy with KD. A student nurse who is on the unit asks if there are medications to treat this disease. The nurse's response to the student nurse is:
    1. Immunoglobulin G and aspirin.
    2. Immunoglobulin G and ACE inhibitors.
    3. Immunoglobulin E and heparin.
    4. Immunoglobulin E and ibuprofen.

17. CHDs are classified by which of the following? Select all that apply.
    1. Cyanotic defect.
    2. Acyanotic defect.
    3. Defects with increased pulmonary blood flow.
    4. Defects with decreased pulmonary blood flow.
    5. Mixed defects.
    6. Obstructive defects.
    7. Pansystolic murmurs.

18. A 2-month-old with TOF is seen in your clinic for a check-up. During the examination, the child develops severe respiratory distress and becomes cyanotic. The nurse's first action should be to:
    1. Lay the child flat to promote hemostasis.
    2. Lay the child flat with legs elevated to increase blood flow to the heart.
    3. Sit the child on the parent's lap, with legs dangling, to promote venous pooling.
    4. Hold the child in knee-chest position to decrease venous blood return.

19. Hypoxic spells in the infant with CHD can cause which of the following? Select all that apply.
    1. Polycythemia.
    2. Blood clots.
    3. CVA.
    4. Developmental delays.
    5. Viral pericarditis.
    6. Brain damage.
    7. Alkalosis.

20. The 6-month-old who has a "tet spell" could have the CHD defect of decreased pulmonary blood flow called _____.

21. The nurse is caring for a toddler who has been hospitalized for 2 days with vomiting due to gastroenteritis. During morning assessment, she is sleeping and difficult to wake up. Assessment reveals vital signs of a regular HR of 220 beats per minute, respiratory rate of 30 per minute, BP of 84/52, and capillary refill of 3 seconds. Which dysrhythmia does the nurse suspect in this child?
    1. Rapid pulmonary flutter.
    2. Sinus bradycardia.
    3. Rapid atrial fibrillation.
    4. Supraventricular tachycardia.

22. BP screenings to detect end-organ damage should be done routinely beginning at what age?
    1. Birth.
    2. 3 years.
    3. 8 years.
    4. 13 years.

23. A 4-year-old is diagnosed with Wilm tumor. What associated manifestation does the nurse expect?
    1. Atrial fibrillation.
    2. Hypertension.
    3. Endocarditis.
    4. Hyperlipidemia.

24. A 15-year-old female who is sexually active is diagnosed with secondary hypertension. She admits to intermittent use of birth control. Which of the following drugs should not be used to control her BP?
    1. Beta blockers.
    2. Calcium channel blockers.
    3. ACE inhibitors.
    4. Diuretics.

25. A 16-year-old male is diagnosed with hypertension. His laboratory values are hemoglobin B 16 g/dL, hematocrit level 43%, sodium 139 mEq/L, potassium 4.4 mEq/L, and total cholesterol of 220 mg/dL. Which of the following drugs would increase his total cholesterol?
    1. Beta blockers.
    2. Calcium channel blockers.
    3. ACE inhibitors.
    4. Diuretics.

26. The _____ serves as the septal opening between the atria of the fetal heart.

27. While looking through the chart of an infant with a CHD of decreased pulmonary blood flow, the nurse would expect what laboratory finding?
    1. Decreased platelet count.
    2. Polycythemia.
    3. Decreased ferritin level.
    4. Shift to the left.

28. The nurse is caring for a 9-month-old who was born with a CHD. Assessment reveals an HR of 160, capillary refill of 4 seconds, bilateral crackles, and sweat on the scalp. These are signs of _____.

29. The following are examples of acquired heart disease. Select all that apply.
    1. Infective endocarditis
    2. Hypoplastic left heart syndrome.
    3. RF.
    4. Cardiomyopathy.
    5. KD.
    6. Transposition of the great vessels.

30. The nurse is caring for a preschool female diagnosed with CHF. She is receiving maintenance doses of digoxin and furosemide. She is rubbing her eyes when she is looking at the lights in the room, and her HR is 70 beats per minute. The nurse suspects which laboratory finding?
    1. Hypokalemia.
    2. Hypomagnesemia.
    3. Hypocalcemia.
    4. Hypophosphatemia.

31. A 2-month-old is being treated with furosemide for CHF. Which of the following plans would also be appropriate in helping to control the CHF?
    1. Promoting fluid restriction.
    2. Feeding a low-salt formula.
    3. Feeding in semi-Fowler position.
    4. Encouraging breast milk.

32. In which of the following CHDs would the nurse need to take upper and lower extremity BPs?
    1. Transposition of the great vessels.
    2. AS.
    3. COA.
    4. TOF.

33. A 10-year-old has undergone a cardiac catheterization. At the end of the procedure, the nurse should first assess:
    1. Pain.
    2. Pulses.
    3. Hemoglobin and hematocrit levels.
    4. Catheterization report.

34. Which statement by the mother of a male toddler with RF shows she has good understanding of the care of her child?
    1. "I will apply heat to his swollen joints to promote circulation."
    2. "I will have him do gentle stretching exercises to prevent contractures."
    3. "I will give him the aspirin that is ordered for pain and inflammation."
    4. "I will apply cold packs to his swollen joints to reduce pain."

35. The school-aged female for whom you are caring has been diagnosed with valvular disease following RF. During patient teaching, you discuss the child's long-term prophylactic therapy with antibiotics for dental procedures, surgery, and childbirth. The parents indicate they understand when they say:
    1. "She will need to take the antibiotics until she is 18 years old."
    2. "She will need to take the antibiotics for 5 years after the last attack."
    3. "She will need to take the antibiotics for 10 years after the last attack."
    4. "She will need to take the antibiotics for the rest of her life."

36. A child born with Down syndrome should be evaluated for what associated cardiac manifestation?
    1. CHD.
    2. Systemic hypertension.
    3. Hyperlipidemia.
    4. Cardiomyopathy.

37. A child with a CHD undergoes the Norwood procedure. This procedure is used to correct:
    1. Transposition of the great vessels.
    2. Hypoplastic left heart syndrome.
    3. TOF.
    4. PDA.

38. The nurse is caring for a 4-year-old female with a Glasgow Coma Scale of 3, HR of 88 beats per minute and regular, respiratory rate of 22, BP of 78/52, and blood sugar of 35 mg/dL. The nurse asks the caregiver about accidental ingestion of what drug?
    1. Calcium channel blocker.
    2. Beta blocker.
    3. ACE inhibiter.
    4. ARB.

39. A 6-year-old is receiving aspirin therapy for KD. Exposure to what illnesses should be a cause to discontinue therapy and substitute dipyridamole (Persantine)?
    1. Chickenpox or flu.
    2. *E. coli* or staphylococcus.
    3. Mumps or streptococcus A.
    4. Streptococcus A or staphylococcus.

40. The nurse is caring for an 8-year-old girl whose parents indicate she has developed spastic movements of her extremities and trunk, facial grimace, and speech disturbances. They state it seems worse when she is anxious and does not occur when she is sleeping. The nurse questions the parents about what recent illness?
    1. KD.
    2. RF.
    3. Malignant hypertension.
    4. Atrial fibrillation.

41. The nurse in the pediatric telemetry unit has been reviewing heart rhythms in children. The most common dysrhythmia in pediatrics is:
    1. Ventricular tachycardia.
    2. Sinus bradycardia.
    3. Supraventricular tachycardia.
    4. First-degree heart block.

42. A nursing action that promotes ideal nutrition in an infant with CHF is:
    1. Feeding formula that is supplemented with additional calories.
    2. Allowing the infant to nurse at each breast for 20 minutes.
    3. Providing large feedings every 5 hours.
    4. Using firm nipples with small openings to slow feedings.

43. An 18-month-old with a myelomeningocele is going to undergo a cardiac catheterization. The mother expresses concern about the use of dye in the procedure. The child does not have any allergies listed on the medical record. In addition to the concern for an iodine allergy, what other allergy should the nurse bring to the attention of the catheterization staff?
    1. Soy.
    2. Latex.
    3. Penicillin.
    4. Dairy.

44. The nurse is caring for a 1-year-old who has been diagnosed with CHF. Treatment began 3 days ago and has included digoxin and furosemide. The child no longer has retractions, lungs are clear and equal bilaterally, and HR is 96 beats per minute while the child sleeps. The nurse is confident that the child has diuresed successfully and has good renal perfusion when the nurse notes the child's urine output is:
    1. 0.5 cc/kg/hr
    2. 1 cc/kg/hr
    3. 30 cc/hr
    4. 1 oz/hr

45. A 3-month-old has been diagnosed with a VSD. The flow of blood through the heart with this type of defect is:
    1. Right to left.
    2. Equal between the two chambers.
    3. Left to right.
    4. Bypassing the defect.

46. The nurse is caring for a 3-month-old with a VSD. The physicians have decided not to repair it surgically. The parents express concern that this is not best for their child and ask why their daughter will not have an operation. The nurse's best response to the parents is:
    1. "It is always helpful to get a second opinion about any serious condition like this."
    2. "Your daughter's defect is small and will likely close on its own by the time she is 2 years old."
    3. "It is common for the physicians to wait until an infant develops respiratory distress before they do the surgery because of the danger."
    4. "With a small defect like this, we will wait until the child is 10 years old to do the surgery."

47. A 5-month-old has been diagnosed with an ASD. The flow of blood through the heart with this type of defect is:
    1. Right to left.
    2. Equal between the two chambers.
    3. Left to right.
    4. Bypassing the defect.

48. An infant has been diagnosed with an ASD, or AVC defect. The flow of blood through the heart with this type of defect is:
    1. Right to left.
    2. Equal between the two chambers.
    3. Bypassing the defect.
    4. In either direction.

49. Parents report that their 6-year-old has been seen by the school nurse for dizziness that occurred when standing in line for recess and homeroom since the start of the school term. The child now reports that she would rather sit and watch her friends play hopscotch because she cannot count out loud and jump at the same time. When the nurse asks the child if her chest ever hurts, she says yes. Based on this history, the nurse suspects that she has:
    1. VSD.
    2. AS.
    3. Mitral valve prolapse.
    4. Tricuspid atresia.

50. The school nurse has been following an 8-year-old female who comes to the office frequently. She has come mainly for vague complaints of dizziness and headache. Today, she is brought after fainting in the cafeteria following a nosebleed. Her BP is 122/85, and her radial pulses are bounding. Calling for the ambulance, the nurse suspect she has:
    1. Transposition of the great vessels.
    2. COA.
    3. AS.
    4. PS.

51. Which medication should the nurse give to a patient who is diagnosed with transposition of the great vessels?
    1. Ibuprofen.
    2. Betamethasone.
    3. Prostaglandin E.
    4. Indocin.

52. Which statement by the mother of a patient with RF shows she has an understanding of prevention in her other children?
    1. "Whenever one of them gets a sore throat, I will give that child an antibiotic."
    2. "There is no treatment. It must run its course."
    3. "If their culture is positive for group A streptococcus, I will give them their antibiotic."
    4. "If their culture is positive for staphylococcus A, I will give them their antibiotic."

53. Which patient could require feeding by gavage?
    1. A patient with KD in the acute phase.
    2. A toddler with repair of transposition of the great vessels.
    3. An infant with CHF.
    4. A school-ager with RF and chorea.

54. What two physiological changes occur as a result of hypoxemia in CHF?
    1. Polycythemia and clubbing.
    2. Anemia and barrel chest.
    3. Increased white blood cells and low platelets.
    4. Elevated erythrocyte sedimentation rate and peripheral edema.

55. Aspirin has been ordered for the child with RF in order to:
    1. Keep the PDA open.
    2. Reduce joint inflammation.
    3. Decrease swelling of strawberry tongue.
    4. Treat ventricular hypertrophy of endocarditis.

56. Gamma globulin is being given to a 1-year-old being treated for KD. Which of the following vaccines must be delayed for 11 months after the administration of gamma globulin?
    1. Diphtheria, tetanus, and pertussis.
    2. Hepatitis B.
    3. Inactivated polio virus.
    4. Measles, mumps, and rubella.

57. The mother of a toddler reports that the baby's father has just had a myocardial infarction. Because of this information, the nurse recommends the child have a(n):
    1. Electrocardiogram.
    2. Lipid profile.
    3. Echocardiogram.
    4. Cardiac catheterization.

58. During play, a toddler with a history of TOF might assume which of the following positions?
   1. Sitting.
   2. Supine.
   3. Squatting.
   4. Left lateral recumbent.

59. Heart transplant may be indicated for a child with which of the following symptoms?
   1. Severe heart failure and PDA.
   2. Severe heart failure and VSD.
   3. Severe heart failure and hypoplastic left heart syndrome.
   4. Severe heart failure and PS.

60. Family discharge teaching has been effective when the parents of a female toddler diagnosed with KD states:
   1. "The arthritis in her knees is permanent. She will need knee replacements."
   2. "I will give her a pain reliever for her peeling palms and soles of her feet."
   3. "I know she will be irritable for 2 months after her symptoms started."
   4. "I will continue with high doses of Tylenol for her inflammation."

61. Which of the following assessments indicate that the parents of a 7-year-old are following the prescribed treatment for CHF?
   1. HR of 56 beats per minute.
   2. Elevated red blood cell count.
   3. 50th percentile height and weight for age.
   4. Urine output of 0.5 cc/kg/hr.

1. 1, 2, 4, 7.
   1. An electrocardiogram can indicate ischemia of the heart muscle.
   2. An electrocardiogram can indicate injury to the heart muscle.
   3. An electrocardiogram does not indicate CO.
   4. An electrocardiogram can show dysrhythmias.
   5. An electrocardiogram does not show SVR.
   6. An electrocardiogram does not show occlusion pressures.
   7. An electrocardiogram does show conduction delays.

   TEST-TAKING HINT: The electrocardiogram checks the electrical system of the heart, not the mechanical system. CO is mechanical; occlusion pressure does not have to do with the electrocardiogram; and SVR measures pressures in the peripheral system.

2. PDA.

   TEST-TAKING HINT: This is a defect with increased pulmonary flow. It should close in the first few weeks of life.

3. 1, 2, 4, 6.
   1. TOF is a congenital defect with ventricular septal defect, right ventricular hypertrophy, pulmonary valve stenosis, and overriding aorta.
   2. TOF is a congenital defect with ventricular septal defect, right ventricular hypertrophy, pulmonary valve stenosis, and overriding aorta.
   3. TOF is a congenital defect with ventricular septal defect, right ventricular hypertrophy, pulmonary valve stenosis, and overriding aorta.
   4. TOF is a congenital defect with ventricular septal defect, right ventricular hypertrophy, pulmonary valve stenosis, and overriding aorta.
   5. TOF is a congenital defect with ventricular septal defect, right ventricular hypertrophy, pulmonary valve stenosis, and overriding aorta.
   6. TOF is a congenital defect with ventricular septal defect, right ventricular hypertrophy, pulmonary valve stenosis, and overriding aorta.
   7. PDA is not one of the defects in tetralogy of Fallot.

   TEST-TAKING HINT: Tetralogy of Fallot has four defects. Pulmonary stenosis causes decreased pulmonary flow.

4. To make the diagnosis of RF, major and minor criteria are used. Major criteria include carditis, subcutaneous nodules, erythema marginatum, chorea, and arthritis. Minor criteria include fever and previous history of RF.

   TEST-TAKING HINT: It is an inflammatory disease caused by group A beta-hemolytic streptococcus.

5. 1. Yellow sclera has nothing to do with CHF. It is seen in patients with liver disease.
   2. The apical pulse rate is ordered because digoxin decreases the HR, and if the HR is <60 digoxin should not be administered.
   3. Cough would not be assessed before administration. It is more commonly seen in patients who have been prescribed ACE inhibitors.
   4. Liver function tests are not assessed before digoxin is administered. Digoxin can lower HR and cause dysrhythmias.

   TEST-TAKING HINT: The test taker should know that yellow sclera and liver function tests have nothing to do with digoxin. Cough could be associated with ACE inhibitors.

6. 1. This is appropriate for digoxin administration.
   2. This is appropriate for digoxin administration.
   3. This is appropriate for digoxin administration.
   4. If the medication is mixed in his formula, and he refuses to drink the entire amount, the digoxin dose will be inadequate.

   TEST-TAKING HINT: What if the child does not drink all the formula?

7. 1. This may be a reason the child needs the catheterization.
   2. A child with severe diaper rash has potential for infection if the interventionist makes the standard groin approach.
   3. Shellfish, not soy, is an allergy concern.
   4. This may be a reason the child needs the catheterization.

   TEST-TAKING HINT: Consider the risk for infection as a delaying factor.

8. 1. This is not an appropriate action.
   2. This is not an appropriate action.

3. This can be done after number 4.
4. **Applying direct pressure 1 inch above the puncture site will localize pressure over the vessel site.**

TEST-TAKING HINT: Consider the risk for volume depletion.

9. **1, 4, 5, 6, 7.**
   1. **Rocking by the parents will comfort the infant and decrease demands.**
   2. The infant would not be fed when crying because crying increases cardiac demands. The infant might choke if the nipple is placed in the mouth and the child inhales when trying to swallow.
   3. Keep the child normothermic to reduce metabolic demands.
   4. **Frequent position changes will decrease the risk for infection by avoiding immobility with its potential for skin breakdown.**
   5. **An infant sucking the fists could indicate hunger.**
   6. **Change bed linens only when necessary to avoid disturbing the child.**
   7. **Organize nursing activities to avoid disturbing the child.**

TEST-TAKING HINT: Do all that can be done to decrease demands on the child.

10. **PDA.**

TEST-TAKING HINT: Prostaglandins allow the duct to remain open; thus, a prostaglandin inhibitor, such as Indocin or ibuprofen, can help close the duct. Consider the defect with increased pulmonary blood flow.

11. **Prostaglandin E.**

TEST-TAKING HINT: Prostaglandin E maintains ductal patency to promote blood flow until the Norwood procedure is begun. Consider the opposite of wanting to close the PDA.

12. 1. This is not a collegial response.
   2. The increased CO of the fever increases the intensity of the murmur, making it easier to hear.
   3. **The increased CO of the fever increases the intensity of the murmur, making it easier to hear.**
   4. This child does not need to see an interventionist cardiologist. The murmur needs to be diagnosed first, and then a treatment plan would be developed.

TEST-TAKING HINT: Consider the pathophysiology of fever.

13. 1. Pulmonary hypertension is a pulmonary condition, which does not create a heart murmur.
   2. **The main identifier in the stem is the machine-like murmur, which is the hallmark of a PDA.**
   3. A VSD does not produce a machine-like murmur.
   4. Bronchopulmonary dysplasia is a pulmonary condition, which does not create a heart murmur.

TEST-TAKING HINT: Know murmur sounds.

14. **1, 2, 3.**
   1. **Thrombosis, stenosis, and aneurysm affect blood vessels. The child with KD has hypercoagulability and an increased sedimentation rate due to inflammation.**
   2. **Thrombosis, stenosis, and aneurysm affect blood vessels. The child with KD has hypercoagulability and an increased sedimentation rate due to inflammation.**
   3. **Thrombosis, stenosis, and aneurysm affect blood vessels. The child with KD has hypercoagulability and an increased sedimentation rate due to inflammation.**
   4. The child with KD has hypercoagulability and an increased sedimentation rate due to inflammation.
   5. The child with KD has hypercoagulability and an increased sedimentation rate due to inflammation.
   6. Hypoplastic left heart syndrome is a CHD and has no relation to KD.

TEST-TAKING HINT: KD is an inflammation of small- and medium-sized blood vessels.

15. **KD.**

TEST-TAKING HINT: Classic signs of KD include red eyes with no discharge; dry, cracked lips; strawberry tongue; and red, swollen and peeling palms and soles of the feet. Incidence of KD is higher in males than females. The strongest indicator for this disease is the hallmark strawberry tongue.

16. 1. **High-dose immunoglobulin G and salicylate therapy for inflammation are the current treatment for KD.**
   2. Immunoglobulin G is correct, but ACE inhibitors are incorrect for treatment.
   3. Heparin may be used for the child with an aneurysm, but not immunoglobulin E.

4. Immunoglobulin E and ibuprofen are not correct.

TEST-TAKING HINT: Consider anti-inflammatory medications for treatment.

17. 3, 4, 5, 6.
    1. Heart defects are no longer classified as cyanotic or acyanotic.
    2. Heart defects are no longer classified as cyanotic or acyanotic.
    3. **Heart defects are now classified as defects with increased or decreased pulmonary blood flow.**
    4. **Heart defects are now classified as defects with increased or decreased pulmonary blood flow.**
    5. **Heart defects are now classified as defects with increased or decreased pulmonary blood flow.**
    6. **Heart defects are now classified as defects with increased or decreased pulmonary blood flow.**
    7. A murmur may be heard with a CHD, but a murmur does not classify the defect.

TEST-TAKING HINT: Know the new classifications, not the older ones.

18. 1. Laying the child flat would increase preload, increasing blood to the heart, therefore making respiratory distress worse.
    2. Laying the child flat with legs elevated would increase preload, increasing blood to heart, therefore making respiratory distress worse.
    3. Sitting the child on the parent's lap with legs dangling might possibly help, but it would not be as effective as the knee-chest position in occluding the venous return.
    4. **The increase in the SVR would increase afterload and increase blood return to the pulmonary artery.**

TEST-TAKING HINT: The test taker should choose the response that decreases the preload in this patient.

19. 1, 2, 3, 4, 6.
    1. Hypoxia causes polycythemia, which can lead to increased blood viscosity, which can lead to blood clots and a stroke.
    2. Hypoxia causes polycythemia, which can lead to increased blood viscosity, which can lead to blood clots and a stroke.
    3. Hypoxia causes polycythemia, which can lead to increased blood viscosity, which can lead to blood clots and a stroke.
    4. **Developmental delays can be caused by multiple hospitalizations and surgeries.**

The child usually catches up to the appropriate level.
   5. Hypoxia can increase the risk for bacterial endocarditis, not viral pericarditis.
   6. **Brain damage can be caused by hypoxia, blood clots, and stroke.**
   7. Hypoxic episodes cause acidosis, not alkalosis.

TEST-TAKING HINT: Consider hypoxia and hemoglobin B and hematocrit level.

20. TOF.
    The nickname is in the stem.

TEST-TAKING HINT: Know the defect classifications.

21. 1. This is not a real dysrhythmia.
    2. Sinus bradycardia is a slow rate for the child's age.
    3. Rapid atrial fibrillation is an irregular rhythm.
    4. **SVT is often above 200 and a result of dehydration, which a vomiting child could have. The rapid rate causes a low CO, resulting in the low BP and prolonged capillary refill.**

TEST-TAKING HINT: The HR is regular and very rapid for a child of any age. The child has been vomiting, which can result in dehydration.

22. 1. Birth is too early and often not reliable due to patient movement.
    2. **Age 3 years is the recommended age to establish a baseline BP in a normal healthy child.**
    3. Age 8 years is too late to detect early damage.
    4. Age 13 years is too late to detect early damage.

TEST-TAKING HINT: What age group would catch systemic hypertension early before end-organ damage could begin?

23. 1. Wilm tumor does not affect or cause this condition.
    2. **Because Wilm tumor sits on the kidney, it can be associated with secondary hypertension. It does not affect or cause the other conditions.**
    3. Wilm tumor does not affect or cause this condition.
    4. Wilm tumor does not affect or cause this condition.

TEST-TAKING HINT: Where is the Wilm tumor located?

24. 1. ACE inhibitors and angiotensin II receptor blockers can cause birth defects. The others are not teratogenic.
2. ACE inhibitors and angiotensin II receptor blockers can cause birth defects. The others are not teratogenic.
3. **ACE inhibitors and angiotensin II receptor blockers can cause birth defects. The others are not teratogenic.**
4. ACE inhibitors and angiotensin II receptors can cause birth defects. The others are not teratogenic.

TEST-TAKING HINT: The test taker needs to know which of these drugs are teratogenic.

25. 1. **Beta blockers are used with caution in patients with hyperlipidemia, hyperglycemia and impotence.**
2. Calcium channel blockers do not affect these blood levels.
3. ACE inhibitors do not affect these blood levels.
4. Diuretics do not affect these blood levels.

TEST-TAKING HINT: The test taker needs to know side effects of drugs.

26. **Foramen ovale.**

TEST-TAKING HINT: The foramen ovale is the septal opening between the atria of the fetal heart. The test taker needs to know basic fetal circulation.

27. 1. The nurse should expect a decreased platelet count in an infant with a CHD of decreased pulmonary blood flow.
2. **Polycythemia is the result of the body attempting to increase the oxygen supply in the presence of hypoxia by increasing the total number of red blood cells to carry the oxygen.**
3. Ferritin measures the amount of iron stored in the body and not affected by decreased pulmonary blood flow.
4. "Shift to the left" refers to an increase in the number of immature white blood cells.

TEST-TAKING HINT: The test taker needs to know what laboratory values hypoxia can affect.

28. **CHF.**

TEST-TAKING HINT: All of these are signs of pump failure. The infant is likely to have diaphoresis only on the scalp. The signs are not unlike those of an adult with this condition.

29. **1, 3, 4, 5.**
1. **Infective endocarditis is an example of an acquired heart problem.**
2. Hypoplastic left heart syndrome is a CHD.
3. **RF is an acquired heart problem.**
4. **Cardiomyopathy is an acquired heart problem.**
5. **KD is an acquired heart problem.**
6. Transposition of the great vessels is a CHD.

TEST-TAKING HINT: "Acquired" means occurring after birth and seen in an otherwise normal and healthy heart.

30. 1. **The rubbing of the child's eyes may mean that she is seeing halos around the lights, indicating digoxin toxicity. The HR, slow for her age, also indicates digoxin toxicity. A decrease in serum potassium because of the furosemide can increase the risk for digoxin toxicity.**
2. Hypomagnesemia does not affect digoxin and is not related to the child rubbing her eyes.
3. Hypocalcemia does not affect digoxin and is not related to the child rubbing her eyes.
4. Hypophosphatemia does not affect digoxin and is not related to the child rubbing her eyes.

TEST-TAKING HINT: The test taker needs to know that furosemide causes the loss of potassium and can cause digoxin toxicity.

31. 1. The nurse would not need to restrict fluids, as the child likely would not be getting overloaded with oral fluids.
2. The infant likely will have sodium depletion because of the chronic diuretic use; the infant needs a normal source of sodium, so low-sodium formula would not be used.
3. **The infant has a great deal of difficulty feeding with CHF, so even getting the maintenance fluids is a challenge. The infant is fed in the more upright position so fluid in the lungs can go to the base of the lungs, allowing better expansion.**
4. Breast milk has slightly less sodium than formula, and the child needs a normal source of sodium because of the diuretic.

TEST-TAKING HINT: Infants are not able to concentrate urine well and may have sodium depletion, so they need a normal source of sodium.

32. 1. BPs would not need to be taken in both the upper and lower extremities in transposition of the great vessels. The aorta and pulmonary arteries are in opposite positions, which does not change the BP readings.
2. AS is a narrowing of the aortic valve, which does not affect the BP in the extremities.
3. **With COA there is narrowing of the aorta, which increases pressure proximal to the defect (upper extremities) and decreases pressure distal to the defect (lower extremities). There will be high BP and strong pulses in the upper extremities and lower-than-expected BP and weak pulses in the lower extremities.**
4. TOF is a congenital cardiac problem with four defects that do not affect the BP in the extremities.

TEST-TAKING HINT: **The test taker must know the anatomy of the defects and what assessments are to be made in each one.**

33. 1. Pain needs to be assessed post procedure but is not the priority.
2. **Checking for pulses, especially in the canulated extremity, would assure perfusion to that extremity and is the priority post procedure.**
3. Hemoglobin and hematocrit levels would be checked post procedure if the child had bled very much during or after the procedure.
4. The catheterization report would be of interest to know what was determined from the procedure. This would also be good to check on the patient post procedure.

TEST-TAKING HINT: **The test taker would know that the priority is assessing the cannulated extremity checking for adequate perfusion.**

34. 1. During the acute phase, limit any manipulation of the joint, and avoid heat or cold.
2. During the acute phase, limit any manipulation of the joint, and avoid heat or cold.
3. **Aspirin is the drug of choice for treatment of RF.**
4. During the acute phase, limit any manipulation of the joint, and avoid heat or cold.

TEST-TAKING HINT: **The test taker should know that aspirin is the drug of choice and that manipulation of the joint should be limited during the acute phase.**

35. 1. This could be true for a patient with a less severe form of RF.
2. This could be true for a patient with a less severe form of RF.
3. This could be true for a patient with a less severe form of RF.
4. **Valvular involvement indicates significant damage, so antibiotics would be taken for the rest of her life.**

TEST-TAKING HINT: **The test taker would know that the severity of the damage to the heart valves determines how long prophylaxic antibiotics will be administered.**

36. 1. **CHD is found often in children with Down syndrome.**
2. This is not associated with Down syndrome.
3. This is not associated with Down syndrome.
4. This is not associated with Down syndrome.

TEST-TAKING HINT: **A child with a syndrome, such as Down, is likely to have other abnormalities.**

37. 1. Transposition of the great vessels requires different surgical procedures.
2. **The Norwood procedure is specific to hypoplastic left heart syndrome.**
3. TOF requires different surgical procedures.
4. PDA requires different surgical procedures.

TEST-TAKING HINT: **Review surgical treatment of CHD.**

38. 1. Calcium channel blockers decrease the force of cardiac contraction and slow the electrical conduction of the heart, resulting in slowing of the HR. The HR is normal in this child.
2. **The beta blocker not only affects the heart and lungs but also blocks the beta sites in the liver, reducing the amount of glycogen available for use, causing hypoglycemia. The lower HR and BP also suggest ingestion of a cardiac medication.**
3. ACE inhibiters block the conversion of a protein from its inactive to its active form. The protein causes constriction of small blood vessels, which raises BP. By blocking this protein, BP is lowered.
4. Angiotensin receptor blockers relax blood vessels, which lowers BP and makes it easier for the heart to pump blood.

TEST-TAKING HINT: Know the drug's side effects. In this case, the glucose is blocked.

39. 1. **Both chickenpox and influenza are viral in nature, so consider stopping the aspirin because of the danger of Reye syndrome.**
    2. *E. coli* and staphylococcus are not viral, so Reye syndrome is not a factor.
    3. Mumps and streptococcus A mumps are caused by a virus; because streptococcus A is a bacterium, Reye syndrome is not a factor.
    4. Streptococcus A and staphylococcus are not viral, so Reye syndrome is not a factor.

TEST-TAKING HINT: Consider Reye syndrome when the patient is taking aspirin and has a viral infection.

40. 1. KD does not result in this condition, called chorea or St. Vitus dance.
    2. **Chorea is often a manifestation of RF, especially in children, with a higher incidence in females.**
    3. Malignant hypertension does not result in this condition, called chorea or St. Vitus dance.
    4. Atrial fibrillation is not an illness.

TEST-TAKING HINT: The test taker can eliminate answer 1 because KD can cause damage to coronary arteries.

41. 1. Ventricular tachycardia is uncommon in children.
    2. Sinus bradycardia is uncommon in children.
    3. **Supraventricular tachycardia is most common in children.**
    4. First-degree heart block is uncommon in children.

TEST-TAKING HINT: Consider a tachycardiac rhythm.

42. 1. **Formula can be supplemented with extra calories, either from a commercial supplement, such as Polycose, or from corn syrup. Calories in formula would increase from 20 kcal/oz to 30 kcal/oz or more.**
    2. The infant would get too tired while feeding, while increasing cardiac demand. Limit feeding to a half hour.
    3. Smaller feedings more often, such as every 2 to 3 hours, would decrease cardiac demand.
    4. Soft nipples that are easy for the infant to suck would make for less work getting nutrition.

TEST-TAKING HINT: Allow the child to get the most nutrition most effectively.

43. 1. Children with spina bifida (myelomeningocele) often have a latex allergy. It is best assumed that they do, unless proved otherwise. The catheter balloon is often made of latex, and all personnel caring for the patient should be made aware of the allergy.
    2. **Children with spina bifida (myelomeningocele) often have a latex allergy. It is best assumed that they do, unless proved otherwise. The catheter balloon is often made of latex, and all personnel caring for the patient should be made aware of the allergy.**
    3. Children with spina bifida (myelomeningocele) often have a latex allergy. It is best assumed that they do, unless proved otherwise. The catheter balloon is often made of latex, and all personnel caring for the patient should be made aware of the allergy.
    4. Children with spina bifida (myelomeningocele) often have a latex allergy. It is best assumed that they do, unless proved otherwise. The catheter balloon is often made of latex, and all personnel caring for the patient should be made aware of the allergy.

TEST-TAKING HINT: Material that composes the balloon catheter is made of latex, which is a common allergy in a child with a myelomeningocele.

44. 1. This is incorrect because 0.5 cc/kg/hr is below the normal pediatric output.
    2. **Normal pediatric urine output is 1 cc/kg/hr.**
    3. This is incorrect because 30 cc/hr is above the normal pediatric output.
    4. This is incorrect because 1 oz/hr is above the normal pediatric output.

TEST-TAKING HINT: The test taker needs to know that normal urine output for a child is 1 cc/kg/hr.

45. 1. **The pressures in the left side of the heart are greater, causing the flow of blood to be from an area of higher pressure to lower pressure, or left to right, increasing the pulmonary blood flow with the extra blood.**
    2. The pressures in the left side of the heart are greater, causing the flow of blood to be from an area of higher pressure to lower pressure, or left to right, increasing the pulmonary blood flow with the extra blood.

3. The pressures in the left side of the heart are greater, causing the flow of blood to be from an area of higher pressure to lower pressure, or left to right, increasing the pulmonary blood flow with the extra blood.

4. The pressures in the left side of the heart are greater, causing the flow of blood to be from an area of higher pressure to lower pressure, or left to right, increasing the pulmonary blood flow with the extra blood.

TEST-TAKING HINT: The test taker should know that the classification for this defect is left to right.

46. 1. This is not a collegial response, and the nurse should explain to the parents why an operation is not necessary now.
2. **Usually a VSD will close on its own within the first year of life.**
3. It is not common for physicians to wait until respiratory distress develops because that puts the infant at greater risk for complications. The defect is small and will likely close on its own.
4. Small defects usually close on their own within the first year.

TEST-TAKING HINT: Know the various treatments depending on size of the defect. VSD is the most common CHD.

47. 1. The pressures in the left side of the heart are greater, causing the flow of blood to be from an area of higher pressure to lower pressure, or left to right, increasing the pulmonary blood flow with the extra blood.
2. The pressures in the left side of the heart are greater, causing the flow of blood to be from an area of higher pressure to lower pressure, or left to right, increasing the pulmonary blood flow with the extra blood.
3. **The pressures in the left side of the heart are greater, causing the flow of blood to be from an area of higher pressure to lower pressure, or left to right, increasing the pulmonary blood flow with the extra blood.**
4. The pressures in the left side of the heart are greater, causing the flow of blood to be from an area of higher pressure to lower pressure, or left to right, increasing the pulmonary blood flow with the extra blood.

TEST-TAKING HINT: What is the CHD classification of ASD?

48. 1. The blood flow generally is left to right.
2. There is blood flow between all the chambers.
3. The blood flow is dependent on the pulmonary and systemic circulations.
4. **The blood flow can be in any direction but generally is left to right.**

TEST-TAKING HINT: What is the CHD classification of AVC?

49. 1. Murmur and CHF are often found in infancy.
2. **AS can progress, and the child can develop exercise intolerance that can be better when resting.**
3. Mitral valve prolapse causes a murmur and palpitations, often in adulthood.
4. Tricuspid atresia causes hypoxemia in infancy.

TEST-TAKING HINT: What does each of the last words of the defects mean, and what do those cause?

50. 1. Transposition of the great vessels does not cause these symptoms.
2. **In the older child, COA causes dizziness, headache, fainting, elevated blood pressure, and bounding radial pulses.**
3. AS does not cause these symptoms.
4. PS does not cause these symptoms.

TEST-TAKING HINT: The test taker should recognize that the child's BP is elevated and her pulses are bounding, which are symptoms of COA.

51. 1. Ibuprofen blocks prostaglandins, which would speed up the closing of the PDA.
2. Betamethasone blocks prostaglandins, which would speed up the closing of the PDA.
3. **Prostaglandin E inhibits closing of the PDA, which connects the aorta and pulmonary artery.**
4. Indocin is used to treat osteoarthritis and gout.

TEST-TAKING HINT: The test taker would know that children who have transposition of the great vessels also have another cardiac defect, and the common one is PDA.

52. 1. **Do not use an antibiotic if the disease is not bacterial in origin. Some sore throats are viral.**
2. RF is caused by group A beta-hemolytic streptococcus, and the drug of choice is penicillin. RF is a bacterial infection and is treated by antibiotic.

3. **RF is caused by a streptococcus infection, not by staphylococcus.**
4. RF is cause by a streptococcus infection, not by staphylococcus.

TEST-TAKING HINT: The test taker needs to know the cause of RF and how it is treated.

53. 1. A patient with KD in the acute phase does not need to be gavage-fed.
    2. Transposition of the great vessels should be repaired before the toddler years, so that child would not need to be gavage-fed.
    3. **The child may experience increased cardiac demand while feeding. Feedings by gavage eliminate that work and still provide high-calorie intake for growth.**
    4. An RF patient with St. Vitus dance (chorea) does not need to be gavage-fed. Most of these children do not have CHF.

TEST-TAKING HINT: The test taker should consider how gavage feedings would affect the work of the heart. Hypoxemia stimulates erythropoietin, which causes the polycythemia. This is an attempt to increase oxygen by having more red blood cells to carry the oxygen. The clubbing of the fingers is a result of the polycythemia and hypoxemia.

54. 1. **The hypoxemia stimulates erythropoiesis, which causes polycythemia, in an attempt to increase oxygen by having more red blood cells carry oxygen. Clubbing of the fingers is a result of the polycythemia and hypoxemia.**
    2. Anemia and barrel chest do not occur as a result of hypoxemia. Hypoxemia stimulates the production of erythropoietin to increase the number of red blood cells to carry more oxygen. The barrel chest is the result of air trapping.
    3. Increased white blood cells occur as the result of an infection, not hypoxemia. Hypoxemia does not cause a decreased number of platelets.
    4. An elevated erythrocyte sedimentation rate is the result of inflammation in the body. Peripheral edema can be caused by CHF.

TEST-TAKING HINT: The test taker could eliminate answers 2, 3, and 4 by knowing that they do not cause hypoxemia in CHF.

55. 1. Aspirin is not used to treat this condition. A PDA does not occur with RF.

2. **Joint inflammation is experienced in RF; aspirin therapy helps with inflammation and pain.**
3. Strawberry tongue is manifested in KD; aspirin is not used to treat this disease.
4. Aspirin is not used to treat this condition.

TEST-TAKING HINT: Know the manifestations of RF.

56. 1. Diphtheria, tetanus, and pertussis can be given following administration of gamma globulin. These are killed vaccines, and the only vaccines not administered would be live vaccines such as measles, mumps, rubella.
    2. Hepatitis B can be administered following gamma globulin. Live vaccines are held for at least 11 months.
    3. Inactivated polio virus can be given following gamma globulin administration. Live vaccines are held for 11 months.
    4. **The body might not produce the appropriate number of antibodies following gamma globulin infusion. Also, delay the varicella vaccine for 11 months.**

TEST-TAKING HINT: The test taker needs to know which vaccines are killed and which are live.

57. 1. Current recommendations are for a lipid profile in children over 2 years with a first- or second-degree relative with stroke, myocardial infarction, angina, or sudden cardiac death. Also screen if parent, sibling, or grandparent has cholesterol of 240 mg/dL or greater.
    2. **Current recommendations are for a lipid profile in children over 2 years with a first- or second-degree relative with stroke, myocardial infarction, angina, or sudden cardiac death. Also screen if parent, sibling, or grandparent has cholesterol of 240 mg/dL or greater.**
    3. Current recommendations are for a lipid profile in children over 2 years with a first- or second-degree relative with stroke, myocardial infarction, angina, or sudden cardiac death. Also screen if parent, sibling, or grandparent has cholesterol of 240 mg/dL or greater.
    4. Current recommendations are for a lipid profile in children over 2 years with a first- or second-degree relative with stroke, myocardial infarction, angina, or sudden cardiac death. Also screen if parent, sibling, or grandparent has cholesterol of 240 mg/dL or greater.

TEST-TAKING HINT: Think about the cause of the father's MI.

58. 1. The toddler will naturally assume this position to decrease preload by occluding venous flow from the lower extremities and increasing afterload. Increasing SVR in this position increases pulmonary blood flow. This occurs with squatting.
2. The toddler will naturally assume this position to decrease preload by occluding venous flow from the lower extremities and increasing afterload. Increasing SVR in this position increases pulmonary blood flow. This occurs with squatting.
3. The toddler will naturally assume this position to decrease preload by occluding venous flow from the lower extremities and increasing afterload. Increasing SVR in this position increases pulmonary blood flow.
4. The toddler will naturally assume this position to decrease preload by occluding venous flow from the lower extremities and increasing afterload. Increasing SVR in this position increases pulmonary blood flow.

TEST-TAKING HINT: The child self-assumes this position during the spell.

59. 1. Severe heart failure can be an indication if quality of life is decreased.
2. Severe heart failure can be an indication if quality of life is decreased.
3. Hypoplastic left heart syndrome is treated by allowing the child to die, which is controversial, the Norwood procedure, or heart transplant.
4. Severe heart failure can be an indication if quality of life is decreased.

TEST-TAKING HINT: Consider severe heart failure and which complex of CHD.

60. 1. Arthritis in KD is always temporary.
2. Peeling palms and feet are painless.
3. Children can be irritable for 2 months after the symptoms of the disease start.
4. Tylenol is never given in high doses due to liver failure, and it is not an anti-inflammatory. Aspirin is given in high doses for KD.

TEST-TAKING HINT: Look for specifics in the stem.

61. 1. HR of 56 beats per minute is likely due to digoxin toxicity.
2. Elevated count of red blood cells indicate polycythemia secondary to hypoxemia.
3. The 50th percentile height and weight for age shows good growth and development, indicating good nutrition and perfusion.
4. Urine output of 0.5 cc/kg/hr indicate that furosemide is not being given as ordered; the output is too low.

TEST-TAKING HINT: The test taker should know the expected responses of medications used to treat CHF.

Hematological or Immunological Disorders

7

KEYWORDS

Aplastic anemia
Beta-thalassemia (Cooley anemia or thalassemia major)
Central nervous system prophylaxis
Chelation therapy
Factor VIII deficiency
Hemarthrosis
Hemophilia A
Hodgkin disease
Immunosuppressive
Intrathecal chemotherapy
Leukemia
Mucositis
Neuroblastoma
Neutropenia

Non-Hodgkin lymphoma
Osteosarcoma
Pancytopenia
Polycythemia
Polycythemia vera
Purpura
Reed-Sternberg cells
Sickle cell disease (sickle cell anemia)
Splenic sequestration
Thrombocytopenia
Vaso-occlusive crises
Von Willebrand disease
Wilms tumor

ABBREVIATIONS

Acute lymphoblastic leukemia (ALL)
Cytomegalovirus (CMV)
Idiopathic thrombocytopenic purpura (ITP)
Pneumocystis carinii pneumonia or Pneumocystic pneumonia (PCP)

Severe combined immunodeficiency disease (SCID)
Vanillylmandelic acid (VMA)

QUESTIONS

1. The nurse is taking care of a child with sickle cell disease. The nurse is aware that which of the following problems is (are) associated with sickle cell disease? Select all that apply.
   1. Polycythemia.
   2. Hemarthrosis.
   3. Aplastic crisis.
   4. Thrombocytopenia.
   5. Splenic sequestration.
   6. Vaso-occlusive crisis.

2. An 18-month-old male is brought to the clinic by his mother. His height is in the 50th percentile, and weight is in the 80th percentile. The child is pale. The physical examination is normal, but his hematocrit level is 20%. Which of the following questions should assist the nurse in making a diagnosis? Select all that apply.
   1. "How many bowel movements a day does your child have?"
   2. "How much did your baby weigh at birth?"
   3. "What does your child eat every day?"
   4. "Has the child been given any new medications?"
   5. "How much milk does your child drink per day?"

3. Which of the following factors need(s) to be included in a teaching plan for a child with sickle cell anemia? Select all that apply.
   1. The child needs to be taken to a physician when sick.
   2. The parent should make sure the child sleeps in an air-conditioned room.
   3. Emotional stress should be avoided.
   4. It is important to keep the child well hydrated.
   5. It is important to make sure the child gets adequate nutrition.

4. A nurse is caring for a 5-year-old with sickle cell vaso-occlusive crisis. Which of the following orders should the nurse question? Select all that apply.
   1. Position the child for comfort.
   2. Apply hot packs to painful areas.
   3. Give Demerol 25 mg intravenously every 4 hours as needed for pain.
   4. Restrict oral fluids.
   5. Apply oxygen per nasal cannula to keep oxygen saturations above 94%.

5. A nurse is caring for a child with von Willebrand disease. The nurse is aware that which of the following is a (are) clinical manifestation(s) of von Willebrand disease? Select all that apply.
   1. Bleeding of the mucous membranes.
   2. The child bruises easily.
   3. Excessive menstruation.
   4. The child has frequent nosebleeds.
   5. Elevated creatinine levels.
   6. The child has a factor IX deficiency.

6. A child with hemophilia A fell and injured a knee while playing outside. The knee is swollen and painful. Which of the following measures should be taken to stop the bleeding? Select all that apply.
   1. The extremity should be immobilized.
   2. The extremity should be elevated.
   3. Warm moist compresses should be applied to decrease pain.
   4. Passive range-of-motion exercises should be administered to the extremity.
   5. Factor VIII should be administered.

7. Which of the following activities should a nurse suggest for a client diagnosed with hemophilia? Select all that apply.
   1. Swimming.
   2. Golf.
   3. Hiking.
   4. Fishing.
   5. Soccer.

8. Which of the following describe(s) ITP? Select all that apply.
   1. ITP is a congenital hematological disorder.
   2. ITP causes excessive destruction of platelets.
   3. Children with ITP have normal bone marrow.
   4. Platelets are small in ITP.
   5. Purpura is observed in ITP.

9. The nurse is caring for a child who is receiving a transfusion of packed red blood cells. The nurse is aware that if the child had a hemolytic reaction to the blood, the signs and symptoms would include which of the following? Select all that apply.
   1. Fever.
   2. Rash.
   3. Oliguria.
   4. Hypotension.
   5. Chills.

10. The nurse is caring for a child with leukemia. The nurse should be aware that children being treated for leukemia may experience which of the following complications? Select all that apply.
    1. Anemia.
    2. Infection.
    3. Bleeding tendencies.
    4. Bone deformities.
    5. Polycythemia.

11. Which of the following is a (are) reason(s) to do a spinal tap on a child with a diagnosis of leukemia? Select all that apply.
    1. Rule out meningitis.
    2. Assess the central nervous system for infiltration.
    3. Give intrathecal chemotherapy.
    4. Determine increased intracranial pressure.
    5. Stage the leukemia.

12. Nausea and vomiting are common adverse effects of radiation and chemotherapy. Which of the following measures should the nurse implement to help with the nausea and vomiting? Select all that apply.
    1. Give an antiemetic 30 minutes prior to the start of therapy.
    2. Continue the antiemetic as ordered until 24 hours after the chemotherapy is complete.
    3. Remove food that has a lot of odor.
    4. Keep the child on a nothing-by-mouth status.
    5. Wait until the nausea begins to start the antiemetic.

13. Which of the following can be manifestations of leukemia in a child? Select all that apply.
    1. Leg pain.
    2. Fever.
    3. Excessive weight gain.
    4. Bruising.
    5. Enlarged lymph nodes.

14. Which of the following can lead to a possible diagnosis of human immunodeficiency virus in a child? Select all that apply.
    1. Repeated respiratory infections.
    2. Intermittent diarrhea.
    3. Excessive weight gain.
    4. Irregular heartbeat.
    5. Poor weight gain.

15. A nurse is caring for a 15-year-old who has just been diagnosed with non-Hodgkin lymphoma. Which of the following should the nurse include in teaching the parents about this lymphoma? Select all that apply.
    1. The malignancy originates in the lymphoid system.
    2. The presence of Reed-Sternberg cells in the biopsy is considered diagnostic.
    3. Mediastinal involvement is typical.
    4. The disease is diffuse rather than nodular.
    5. Treatment includes chemotherapy and radiation.

16. The nurse is caring for a child with sickle cell anemia who has a vaso-occlusive crisis. Which of the following interventions should improve tissue perfusion?
    1. Limiting oral fluids.
    2. Administering oxygen.
    3. Administering antibiotics.
    4. Administrating analgesics.

17. The nurse is caring for a child with sickle cell disease who is scheduled to have a splenectomy. What information should the nurse explain to the parents regarding the reason for a splenectomy?
    1. To decrease potential for infection.
    2. To prevent splenic sequestration.
    3. To prevent sickling of red blood cells.
    4. To prevent sickle cell crisis.

18. Which of the following analgesics is most effective for a child with sickle cell pain crisis?
    1. Demerol.
    2. Aspirin.
    3. Morphine.
    4. Excedrin.

19. The nurse is caring for a child with sickle cell anemia who is scheduled to have an exchange transfusion. What information should the nurse teach the family?
    1. The procedure is done to prevent further sickling during a vaso-occlusive crisis.
    2. The procedure reduces side effects from blood transfusions.
    3. The procedure is a routine treatment for sickle cell crisis.
    4. Once the child's spleen is removed, it is necessary to do exchange transfusions.

20. A nurse instructs the parent of a child with sickle cell anemia about factors that might precipitate a pain crisis in the child. Which of the following factors identified by the parent as being able to cause a pain crisis indicates a need for further instruction?
    1. Infection.
    2. Overhydration.
    3. Stress at school.
    4. Cold environment.

21. A 10-year-old with severe factor VIII deficiency falls, injures an elbow, and is brought to the ER. The nurse should prepare which of the following?
    1. An injection of factor VIII.
    2. An intravenous infusion of factor VIII.
    3. An injection of desmopressin.
    4. An intravenous infusion of platelets.

22. Which of the following will be abnormal in a child with the diagnosis of hemophilia?
    1. The platelet count.
    2. The hemoglobin level.
    3. The white blood cell count.
    4. The partial thromboplastin time.

23. A nurse is reviewing home care instruction with the parent of a child diagnosed with hemophilia. Which of the following activities should the nurse suggest to the parent as a safe activity for the child?
    1. Baseball.
    2. Swimming.
    3. Soccer.
    4. Football.

24. Which of the following measures should the nurse teach the parent of a child with hemophilia to do first if the child sustains an injury to a joint causing bleeding?
    1. Give the child a dose of Tylenol.
    2. Immobilize the joint, and elevate the extremity.
    3. Apply heat to the area.
    4. Administer factor per the home care protocol.

25. Which of the following measures should be implemented for a child with von Willebrand disease who has a nosebleed?
    1. Apply pressure to the nose for at least 10 minutes.
    2. Have the child lie supine and quiet.
    3. Avoid packing of the nostrils.
    4. Encourage the child to swallow frequently.

26. A nurse educator is providing a teaching session for the nursing staff. Which of the following individuals is at greatest risk for developing beta-thalassemia (Cooley anemia)?
    1. A child of Mediterranean descent.
    2. A child of Mexican descent.
    3. A child whose mother has chronic anemia.
    4. A child of American descent who has a low intake of iron.

27. A nurse is doing discharge education with a parent who has a child with beta-thalassemia (Cooley anemia). The nurse informs the parent that the child is at risk for which of the following conditions?
    1. Hypertrophy of the thyroid.
    2. Polycythemia vera.
    3. Thrombocytopenia.
    4. Chronic hypoxia and iron overload.

28. The nurse is caring for a child diagnosed with thalassemia major who is receiving the first chelation therapy. What information should the nurse teach the parent regarding the therapy?
    1. Decreases the risk of bleeding.
    2. Eliminates excess iron.
    3. Prevents further sickling of the red blood cells.
    4. Provides an iron supplement.

29. The nurse is caring for a child with ITP with a platelet count of 5000/mm^3. Which of the following should the nurse administer?
    1. Platelets.
    2. Intravenous immunoglobulin.
    3. Packed red blood cells.
    4. White blood cells.

30. Which test provides a definitive diagnosis of aplastic anemia?
    1. Complete blood count with differential.
    2. Bone marrow aspiration.
    3. Serum IgG levels.
    4. Basic metabolic panel.

31. The nurse is caring for a child with a diagnosis of ALL who is receiving chemotherapy. The nurse notes that the child's platelet count is 20,000/mcL. Based on this laboratory finding, what information should the nurse provide to the child and parents?
    1. A soft toothbrush should be used for mouth care.
    2. Isolation precautions should be started immediately.
    3. The child's vital signs, including blood pressure, should be monitored every 4 hours.
    4. All visitors should be discouraged from coming to see the family.

32. A 5-year-old is admitted to the hospital with complaints of leg pain and fever. On physical examination, the child is pale and has bruising over varies area of the body. The physician suspects that the child has ALL. The nurse informs the parent that the diagnosis will be confirmed by which of the following?
    1. Lumbar puncture.
    2. White blood cell count.
    3. Bone marrow aspirate.
    4. Bone scan.

33. The nurse is caring for a 10-year-old with leukemia who is receiving chemotherapy. The child is on neutropenic precautions. Friends of the child come to the desk and ask for a vase for flowers they have picked from their garden. Which of the following is the best response?
    1. "I will get you a special vase that we use on this unit."
    2. "The flowers from your garden are beautiful but should not be placed in the room at this time."
    3. "As soon as I can wash a vase, I will put the flowers in it and bring it to the room."
    4. "Get rid of the flowers immediately. You could harm the child."

34. The nurse is discharging a child who has just received chemotherapy for neuroblastoma. Which of the following statements made by the child's parent indicates a need for additional teaching?
    1. "I will inspect the skin often for any lesions."
    2. "I will do mouth care daily and monitor for any mouth sores."
    3. "I will wash my hands prior to caring for my child."
    4. "I will take a rectal temperature daily and report a temperature greater than 101°F (38.3°C) immediately to the physician."

35. The child for whom you are caring is to have a bone marrow aspiration. Which intervention should the nurse implement after the procedure?
    1. Ask the child to remain in a supine position.
    2. Place the child in an upright position for 4 hours.
    3. Keep the child nothing by mouth for 6 hours.
    4. Administer analgesics as needed for pain.

36. The nurse is caring for a child who is newly diagnosed with leukemia. When discussing the medical treatment plan for this child with the parents, the nurse informs them that the central nervous system needs to be protected from the invasion of malignant cells. Which of the following should be done to protect the central nervous system?
    1. Cranial and spinal radiation.
    2. Intravenous steroid therapy.
    3. Intrathecal chemotherapy.
    4. High-dose intravenous chemotherapy.

37. A child with leukemia is receiving chemotherapy and is complaining of nausea. The nurse has been giving the scheduled antiemetic. Which of the following should the nurse do when the child is nauseated?
    1. Encourage low-protein foods.
    2. Encourage low-caloric foods.
    3. Offer the child's favorite foods.
    4. Offer cool, clear liquids.

38. Children with cancer often have a body image disturbance related to hair loss, moon face, or debilitation. Which of the following interventions is most appropriate?
    1. Encourage them to wear a wig similar to their own hairstyle.
    2. Emphasize the benefits of the therapy they are receiving.
    3. Have them play only with other children with cancer.
    4. Use diversional techniques to avoid discussing changes in the body because of the chemotherapy.

39. The nurse receives a call from a parent of a child with leukemia in remission. The parent says the child has been exposed to chickenpox. The child has never had chickenpox. Which of the following responses is most appropriate for the nurse?
    1. "You need to monitor the child's temperature frequently and call back if the temperature is greater than 101°F (38.3°C)."
    2. "At this time there is no need to be concerned."
    3. "You need to bring the child to the clinic for a chickenpox immunoglobulin vaccine."
    4. "Your child will need to be isolated for the next 2 weeks."

40. The nurse is caring for a child being treated for ALL. Laboratory results indicate that the child has a white blood cell count of 5000, with 5% polys and 3% bands. Which of the following responses is most appropriate?
    1. The absolute neutrophil count is 400/mm³, and the child is neutropenic.
    2. The absolute neutrophil count is 5800/ mm³, and the child is not neutropenic.
    3. The absolute neutrophil count is 4000/ mm³, and the child is not neutropenic.
    4. The absolute neutrophil count is 800/ mm³, and the child is neutropenic.

41. Children who become immunosuppressed from chemotherapy need to be protected from infection. Which of the following is the best method to prevent the spread of infection?
    1. Administer antibiotics prophylactically to the children.
    2. Have people wash their hands prior to contact with the children.
    3. Assign the same nurses to care for the children each day.
    4. Limit visitors to family members only.

42. The mother of a child who is newly diagnosed with ALL asks the nurse "What is the prognosis?" Which of the following is correct regarding prognostic factors for determining survival for such a child?
    1. The initial white blood cell count on diagnosis.
    2. The race of the child.
    3. The amount of time needed to initiate treatment.
    4. The allergy history of the child.

43. A child diagnosed with leukemia is receiving allopurinol as part of the treatment plan. The parents asks why their child is receiving this medication. What information about the medication should the nurse provide?
    1. Helps reduce the uric acid level caused by cell destruction.
    2. Used to make the chemotherapy work better.
    3. Given to reduce the nausea and vomiting associated with chemotherapy.
    4. Helps decrease pain in the bone marrow.

44. Prednisone is given to children who are being treated for leukemia. Why is this medication given as part of the treatment plan?
    1. Enhances protein metabolism.
    2. Enhances sodium excretion.
    3. Increases absorption of the chemotherapy.
    4. Destroys abnormal lymphocytes.

45. Which of the following best describes the action of chemotherapeutic agents used in the treatment of cancer in children?
    1. Suppress the function of normal lymphocytes in the immune system.
    2. Are alkylating agents and are cell-specific.
    3. Cause a replication of DNA and are cell-specific.
    4. Interrupt cell cycle, thereby causing cell death.

46. A child has completed treatment for leukemia and comes to the clinic with the parents for a checkup. The parents express to the nurse that they are glad their child has been cured of cancer and is safe from getting cancer later in life. Which of the following should the nurse consider in responding?
    1. Childhood cancer usually instills immunity to all other cancers.
    2. Children surviving one cancer are at higher risk for a second cancer.
    3. The child may have a remission of the leukemia but is immune to all other cancers.
    4. As long as the child continues to take steroids, there will be no other cancers.

47. A teen is seen in clinic for a possible diagnosis of Hodgkin disease. The nurse is aware that which of the following symptoms should make the physicians suspect Hodgkin disease?
    1. Fever, fatigue, and pain in the joints.
    2. Anorexia with weight loss.
    3. Enlarged, painless, and movable lymph nodes in the cervical area.
    4. Enlarged liver with jaundice.

48. Which of the following confirms a diagnosis of Hodgkin disease in a 15-year-old?
    1. Reed-Sternberg cells in the lymph nodes.
    2. Blast cells in the blood.
    3. Lymphocytes in the bone marrow.
    4. VMA in the urine.

49. The parent of a teen with a diagnosis of Hodgkin disease asks what the child's prognosis will be with treatment. What information should the nurse give to the parent and child?
    1. Clinical staging of Hodgkin disease will determine the treatment; long-term survival for all stages of Hodgkin disease is excellent.
    2. There is a considerably better prognosis if the client is diagnosed early and is between the ages of 5 and 11 years.
    3. The prognosis for Hodgkin disease depends on the type of chemotherapy.
    4. The only way to obtain a good prognosis is by chemotherapy and bone marrow transplant.

50. The nurse is caring for a child who is receiving extensive radiation as part of the treatment for Hodgkin disease. What intervention should be implemented?
    1. Administer pain medication prior to the child's going to radiation therapy.
    2. Assess the child for neuropathy since this is a common side effect.
    3. Provide adequate rest, as the child may experience excessive malaise and lack of energy.
    4. Encourage the child to eat a low-protein diet while on radiation therapy.

51. The parent of a 4-year-old brings the child to the clinic and tells the nurse the child's abdomen is distended. After a complete examination, a diagnosis of Wilms tumor is suspected. Which of the following is most important when doing a physical examination on this child?
    1. Avoid palpation of the abdomen.
    2. Assess the urine for the presence of blood.
    3. Monitor vital signs, especially the blood pressure.
    4. Obtain an accurate height and weight.

52. The parent of a child diagnosed with Wilms tumor asks the nurse what the treatment plan will be. The nurse explains the usual protocol for this condition. Which information should the nurse give to the parent?
    1. The child will have chemotherapy and, after that has been completed, radiation.
    2. The child will need to have surgery to remove the tumor.
    3. The child will go to surgery for removal of the tumor and the kidney and will then start chemotherapy.
    4. The child will need radiation and later surgery to remove the tumor.

53. The nurse expects which of the following clinical manifestations in a child diagnosed with SCID?
    1. Prolonged bleeding.
    2. Failure to thrive.
    3. Fatigue and malaise.
    4. Susceptibility to infection.

54. What are the clinical manifestations of non-Hodgkin lymphoma?
    1. Basically the same as those in Hodgkin disease.
    2. Depends on the anatomic site and extent of involvement.
    3. Those that affect the abdomen, as non-Hodgkin lymphoma is a fast-growing cancer in very young children.
    4. Changes that occur in the lower extremities.

55. When caring for a child with lymphoma, the nurse needs to be aware of which of the following?
    1. The same staging system is used for lymphoma and Hodgkin disease.
    2. The aggressive chemotherapy with central nervous system prophylaxis will give the child a good prognosis.
    3. All children with lymphoma need a bone marrow transplant for a good prognosis.
    4. Despite high-dose chemotherapy, the prognosis is very poor for most children with a diagnosis of lymphoma.

56. Where is the primary site of origin of the tumor in children who have neuroblastoma?
    1. Bone.
    2. Kidneys.
    3. Abdomen.
    4. Liver.

57. Which of the following is the most common opportunistic infection in children infected with human immunodeficiency virus?
    1. CMV.
    2. Encephalitis.
    3. Meningitis.
    4. Pneumocystic pneumonia.

58. Which of the following laboratory tests will be ordered for an infant whose parent is human immunodeficiency virus–positive in order to determine the presence of the human immunodeficiency virus antigen?
    1. CD4 cell count.
    2. Western blot.
    3. IgG levels.
    4. p24 antigen assay.

59. The nurse is instructing the parent of a child with human immunodeficiency virus infection about immunizations. Which of the following should the nurse tell the parent?
    1. Hepatitis B vaccine will not be given to this child.
    2. Members of the family should be cautioned not to receive the varicella vaccine.
    3. The child will need to have a Western blot test done prior to all immunizations.
    4. Pneumococcal and influenza vaccines are recommended.

60. The parent of a 2-year-old who is human immunodeficiency virus–infected questions the nurse about placing the child in day care. Which of the following is the best response?
    1. The child should not go to day care until older, because there is a high risk for transmission of the disease.
    2. The child can be admitted to day care without restrictions and should be allowed to participate in all activities.
    3. The child can go to day care but should avoid physical activity.
    4. The child may go to day care, but the parent must inform all the parents at the day care that the child is human immunodeficiency virus–infected.

ANSWERS AND RATIONALES

1. 3, 5, 6.
  1. Polycythemia is seen in children with chronic hypoxia, such as cyanotic heart disease.
  2. Hemarthrosis is commonly seen in children with hemophilia.
  3. Aplastic crisis is associated with sickle cell anemia.
  4. Thrombocytopenia is associated with idiopathic thrombocytopenia purpura.
  5. Splenic sequestration is associated with sickle cell anemia.
  6. Vaso-occlusive crisis is the most common problem in children with sickle cell disease.

TEST-TAKING HINT: Review the definition of terms. That will eliminate the other choices.

2. 3, 5.
  1. Because the child has a low hematocrit level, the child most likely has anemia. Anemia in a child is usually of nutritional origin. Iron-deficiency anemia is the most common nutritional anemia. This is important information but not necessary to make the diagnosis of iron-deficiency anemia.
  2. Knowing birth weight can help determine if the child is following his or her own curve on the growth chart.
  3. A diet history is necessary to determine the nutritional status of the child and if the child is getting sufficient sources of iron.
  4. Knowing if the child is taking any new medication is good but is not necessary to make the diagnosis of iron-deficiency anemia.
  5. By asking how much milk the child consumes, the nurse can determine if the child is filling up on milk and then not wanting to take food.

TEST-TAKING HINT: The most common anemia in children and in toddlers is iron-deficiency anemia, frequently due to drinking too much milk and not eating enough iron-rich foods

3. 1, 3, 4, 5.
  1. The goal of therapy with children is to prevent the sickling process.
  2. A cold environment causes vasoconstriction, which needs to be prevented to get good tissue perfusion.
  3. Seek medical attention for illness to prevent the child from going into a crisis.
  4. The child needs good hydration and nutrition to maintain good health.
  5. The child needs good hydration and nutrition to maintain good health.

TEST-TAKING HINT: Focus on how to prevent a sickle cell crisis.

4. 3, 4.
  1. Medical treatment of sickle cell crises is directed toward preventing hypoxia. Tissue hypoxia is very painful, so placing the child in a position of comfort is important.
  2. Hot packs help relieve pain because they cause vasodilatation, which allows increased blood flow and decreased hypoxia.
  3. Tissue hypoxia is very painful. Narcotics such as morphine are usually given for pain when the child is in a crisis. Demerol should be avoided because of the risk for demerol-induced seizures.
  4. The child should receive hydration because when the child is in crisis, the abnormal S-shaped red blood cells clump, causing tissue hypoxia and pain.
  5. Providing oxygen when the oxygen saturation decreases helps treat the hypoxia.

TEST-TAKING HINT: Focus on the pathophysiology of a vaso-occlusive crisis. Keep in mind measures that decrease tissue hypoxia.

5. 1, 2, 3, 4.
  1. Von Willebrand disease is a hereditary bleeding disorder characterized by deficiency of or defect in a protein. The disorder causes adherence of platelets to damaged endothelium and a mild deficiency of factor VIII. One of the manifestations of this disease is bleeding of the mucous membranes.
  2. Bruising is a common manifestation of this disease.
  3. Excessive menstruation may be a manifestation of this disease.
  4. Frequent nosebleeds is a common manifestation of this disease.
  5. There is no increase in creatinine in this disease.
  6. Von Willebrand disease is a mild factor VIII deficiency, not a factor IX deficiency.

TEST-TAKING HINT: Focus on the diagnosis. Von Willebrand disease is a minor deficiency of factor VIII, so the clinical manifestations will be less severe.

6. 1, 2, 5.
    1. Measures are needed to induce vasocon-striction and stop the bleeding, including immobilization of the extremity.
    2. Measures are needed to induce vaso-constriction and stop the bleeding. Treatment should include elevating the extremity.
    3. Measures are needed to induce vasocon-striction and stop the bleeding. Treatment should include an application of cold compression.
    4. Measures are needed to induce vasocon-striction and stop the bleeding. Treatment should include factor replacement.
    5. Hemophilia A is a deficiency in factor VIII, which causes delay in clotting when there is a bleed.

    TEST-TAKING HINT: Focus on the disease process and measures to stop bleeding.

7. 1, 2, 3, 4.
    1. Children with hemophilia should be encouraged to take part in noncontact activities that allow for social, psycho-logical, and physical growth, such as swimming.
    2. Children with hemophilia should be encouraged to take part in noncontact activities that allow for social, psycho-logical, and physical growth, such as golf
    3. Children with hemophilia should be encouraged to take part in noncontact activities that allow for social, psycho-logical, and physical growth, such as hiking.
    4. Children with hemophilia should be encouraged to take part in noncontact activities that allow for social, psycho-logical, and physical growth, such as fishing.
    5. Contact sports like soccer should be discouraged.

    TEST-TAKING HINT: Soccer is the only contact sport listed, so the other answers can be selected.

8. 2, 3, 5.
    1. ITP is an acquired hematological condition that is characterized by excessive destruc-tion of platelets, purpura, and normal bone marrow along with increase in large, yellow platelets.
    2. ITP is characterized by excessive destruction of platelets.
    3. The bone marrow is normal in children with ITP.
    4. Platelets are large, not small.

5. ITP is characterized by purpuras, which are areas of hemorrhage under the skin.

TEST-TAKING HINT: Review the pathophysiology of ITP to determine the manifestations of the disease.

9. 1, 3, 4.
    1. Hemolytic reactions include fever, pain at insertion site, hypotension, renal failure, tachycardia, oliguria, and shock.
    2. Febrile reactions are fever and chills. Allergic reactions include hives, itching and respiratory distress.
    3. Hemolytic reactions include fever, pain at insertion site, hypotension, renal failure, tachycardia, oliguria, and shock.
    4. Hemolytic reactions include fever, pain at insertion site, hypotension, renal failure, tachycardia, oliguria, and shock.
    5. Febrile reactions are fever and rash. Allergic reactions include rash, hives, and respiratory distress.

    TEST-TAKING HINT: Review the signs and symptoms of hemolytic reaction, febrile reaction, and allergic reaction. Under-standing the causes of the reactions will help identify the symptoms.

10. 1, 2.
    1. Anemia is caused by decreased production of red blood cells.
    2. Infection risk in leukemia is secondary to the neutropenia.
    3. Bleeding tendencies are from decreased platelet production.
    4. There are no bone deformities with leukemia, but there is bone pain from the proliferation of cells in the bone marrow.
    5. Polycythemia is an increase in red blood cells.

    TEST-TAKING HINT: Review the pathophysiology of leukemia to determine the clinical problems.

11. 2, 3.
    1. There is no need to do it to rule out meningitis unless the patient has symptoms of meningitis.
    2. A spinal tap is done to assess the central nervous system by obtaining a specimen that can determine presence of leukemic cells.
    3. Chemotherapy can also be given with a spinal tap.

4. Leukemia is not staged, and there should not be an indication to determine increased intracranial pressure.

5. Leukemia is not staged. A spinal tap would be done to determine if leukemic cells are present in the central nervous system.

TEST-TAKING HINT: Review the central nervous system involvement with leukemia.

12. **1, 2, 3.**
   1. **The first dose should be given 30 minutes prior to the start of the therapy.**
   2. **Antiemetic should be administered around the clock until 24 hours after the chemotherapy is completed.**
   3. **It is also helpful to remove foods with odor so the smell of the food does not make the child nauseous.**
   4. The child should be allowed to take food and fluids as tolerated.
   5. Antiemetics are most beneficial if given before the onset of nausea and vomiting.

TEST-TAKING HINT: Review measures to prevent nausea and vomiting.

13. **1, 2, 4, 5.**
   1. **The proliferation of cells in the bone marrow can cause leg pain.**
   2. **Fever is a result of the neutropenia.**
   3. There is usually a decrease in weight, because the child will feel sick and not as hungry.
   4. **A decrease in platelets causes the bruising.**
   5. **The lymph nodes are enlarged from the infiltration of leukemic cells**

TEST-TAKING HINT: Review the consequences of depressed bone marrow, and relate them to the clinical manifestations.

14. **1, 2, 5.**
   1. **Symptoms of human immunodeficiency virus include poor weight gain, intermittent diarrhea, frequent respiratory infections, and inability to tolerate feedings. The symptoms present based on the underlying cellular immunodeficiency-related disease.**
   2. **Symptoms of human immunodeficiency virus include poor weight gain, intermittent diarrhea, frequent respiratory infections, and inability to tolerate feedings. The symptoms present based on the underlying cellular immunodeficiency-related disease.**
   3. Symptoms of human immunodeficiency virus include poor weight gain, intermittent

diarrhea, frequent respiratory infections, and inability to tolerate feedings. The symptoms present based on the underlying cellular immunodeficiency-related disease.

4. Irregular heart rate is not associated with human immunodeficiency virus.

5. **Symptoms of human immunodeficiency virus include poor weight gain, intermittent diarrhea, frequent respiratory infections, and inability to tolerate feedings.**

TEST-TAKING HINT: Review symptoms of HIV that should lead to a differential diagnosis.

15. **1, 3, 4, 5.**
   1. **Non-Hodgkin disease originates in the lymphoid system.**
   2. Reed-Sternberg cells are diagnostic for Hodgkin disease.
   3. **Mediastinal involvement is typical.**
   4. **The disease is diffuse rather than nodular.**
   5. **Treatment includes chemotherapy and radiation.**

TEST-TAKING HINT: Identify the differences between lymphoma and Hodgkin disease.

16. 1. Children with sickle cell anemia need to be well hydrated to promote hemodilution.
   2. **Oxygen prevents hypoxia, helping to prevent acidosis that could lead to increased sickling.**
   3. The child may need antibiotics for infection, not for the sickle cell anemia.
   4. Analgesics are used for pain control.

TEST-TAKING HINT: In sickle cell anemia, the tissues need to be well oxygenated, and measures need to be taken to decrease sickling and increase tissue perfusion.

17. 1. The cells involved with sickle cell anemia are red blood cells, so a decrease in infection would not be correct.
   2. **Splenic sequestration is a life-threatening situation in children with sickle cell anemia. Once a child is considered to be at high risk of splenic sequestration or has had this in the past, the spleen will be removed.**
   3. Removal of the spleen will not prevent sickling, as it will not change the disease condition.
   4. The child will still have sickle cell disease and can still have sickle cell crises.

TEST-TAKING HINT: Review splenic sequestration and when a child can go into sickle cell crisis.

18. 1. Demerol should not be used as it may potentiate seizures.
    2. Aspirin should not be used in children with a viral infection because of the risk for Reye syndrome.
    3. **Morphine is the drug of choice for a child with sickle cell crises. Usually the child is started on oral doses of Tylenol with codeine. When that does not decrease pain, stronger narcotics are prescribed.**
    4. Excedrin contains aspirin.

    TEST-TAKING HINT: One needs to consider using narcotics when a child has sickle cell crises, as tissue hypoxia can cause severe pain.

19. 1. **Exchange transfusion reduces the number of circulating sickle cells and slows down the cycle of hypoxia, thrombosis, and tissue ischemia.**
    2. Exchange transfusion does not decrease risk of a transfusion reaction. Every time a transfusion is done, the child continues to be at risk for a reaction.
    3. This is not a routine procedure performed when the number of sickle cells is elevated and the child is at high risk for thrombosis.
    4. After a splenectomy, transfusions still need to be done depending on the client's hemoglobin level.

    TEST-TAKING HINT: Consider the reasons transfusions are given with sickle cell clients.

20. 1. An infection can cause a child to go into crisis.
    2. **Overhydration does not cause a crisis.**
    3. Emotional stress can cause a child to go into crisis.
    4. A cold environment causes vasoconstriction, which could lead to crisis.

    TEST-TAKING HINT: Because sickle cell anemia may be precipitated by infection, dehydration, trauma, hypoxia or stress, use the process of elimination to determine the need for further instruction.

21. 1. Factor VIII is not given intramuscularly.
    2. **The child is treated with intravenous factor VIII to replace the missing factor and help stop the bleeding.**
    3. Desmopressin is given to stimulate factor VIII production, and it is given intravenously.
    4. Platelets are not affected in hemophilia.

    TEST-TAKING HINT: Focus on the diagnosis of hemophilia: a deficiency in factor VIII causes continued bleeding with an injury.

22. 1. Platelet function is normal in hemophilia.
    2. There is no change in hemoglobin with a diagnosis of hemophilia. The hemoglobin will drop with bleeding.
    3. The white blood cell count does not change with hemophilia.
    4. **The abnormal laboratory results in hemophilia are related to decreased clotting function. Partial thromboplastin time is prolonged.**

    TEST-TAKING HINT: Use the process of elimination to determine the test that indicates a decrease in clotting.

23. 1. Baseball is an activity that may produce joint injury that can cause bleeding.
    2. **Swimming provides good exercise and is least likely to cause any injury.**
    3. Soccer is an activity that may cause injury resulting in bleeding.
    4. Football is a contact sport that can cause injury and bleeding.

    TEST-TAKING HINT: Children with hemophilia need to avoid contact sports or activities that can cause injury resulting in bleeding.

24. 1. Tylenol helps with the pain but does not stop the bleeding.
    2. Elevating and immobilizing the extremity are good interventions as they decrease blood flow. Factor should be administered first, however.
    3. Cold, not heat, should be applied to promote vasoconstriction.
    4. **Administration of factor should be the first intervention if home-care transfusions have been initiated.**

    TEST-TAKING HINT: Treatment of hemophilia is to provide factor replacement as soon as possible after a bleed has started. Application of cold, elevation of extremities, and application of pressure for 10 to 15 minutes are all good interventions after the factor is given.

25. 1. **Applying pressure to the nose may stop the bleeding. In von Willebrand disease, there is an increased tendency to bleed from mucous membranes, leading to nosebleeds commonly from the anterior part of the nasal septum.**
    2. The child should sit up and lean forward to avoid aspiration of blood.
    3. Packing the nose with cotton may be used to stop bleeding, but be careful when the cotton is removed as it may dislodge the clot.

4. Swallowing will cause the child to swallow the blood, which then can cause vomiting.

TEST-TAKING HINT: Focus on the most common areas of bleeding in von Willebrand disease and on how to treat the bleeding.

26. 1. **Beta-thalassemia is an inherited recessive disorder that is found primarily in individuals of Mediterranean descent. The disease has also been reported in Asian and African populations.**
    2. It is not found often in the Mexican population.
    3. This is a hereditary disease that causes chronic anemia. The mother should have had thalassemia for this answer to be correct.
    4. This disorder has nothing to due with iron deficiency.

TEST-TAKING HINT: Use the process of elimination, knowing that the disorder is a hereditary disorder of Mediterranean descent.

27. 1. The thyroid is not involved in beta-thalassemia.
    2. Polycythemia vera refers to excessive red blood cell production, which can result in thrombosis.
    3. There is no increase in platelets in beta-thalassemia.
    4. **In beta-thalassemia there is increased destruction of red blood cells, causing anemia. This results in chronic anemia and hypoxia. The children are treated with multiple blood transfusions, which can cause iron overload and damage to major organs.**

TEST-TAKING HINT: Focus on the pathophysiology of the disease. Then, by process of elimination, the effect of the disease on the body can be identified.

28. 1. There are no bleeding tendencies in thalassemia major (beta-thalassemia or Cooley anemia), and chelation does not affect clotting.
    2. **Chelation therapy is used to rid the body of excess iron stores that result from frequent blood transfusions.**
    3. There is no sickling of red blood cells in thalassemia, and chelation therapy has no direct effect on red blood cells.
    4. Chelation does not provide an iron supplement.

TEST-TAKING HINT: Focus on the treatment of beta-thalassemia and how chelation therapy works.

29. 1. In ITP, destruction of platelets is caused from what is believed to be an immune response, so giving additional platelets would only result in new platelets being destroyed.
    2. **Intravenous immunoglobulin is given because the cause of platelet destruction is believed to be an autoimmune response to disease-related antigens. Treatment is usually supportive. Activity is restricted at the onset because of the low platelet count and risk for injury that could cause bleeding.**
    3. Red blood cells are not an effective treatment for ITP.
    4. White blood cells are not an effective treatment for ITP. White blood cell infusion is rarely done with any disease process.

TEST-TAKING HINT: Focus on the cause of ITP and which cells are affected.

30. 1. A complete blood count with differential indicates pancytopenia but does not reveal what is occurring in the bone marrow.
    2. **Definitive diagnosis is determined from bone marrow aspiration, which demonstrates the conversion of red bone marrow to yellow, fatty marrow.**
    3. Serum IgG levels do not diagnose aplastic anemia, which does not seem to have an immune cause.
    4. A basic metabolic panel tests for metabolic disorders.

TEST-TAKING HINT: Focus on the fact that aplastic anemia is a failure in the bone marrow that causes pancytopenia, so analysis of the bone marrow would confirm the diagnosis.

31. 1. **Because the platelet count is decreased, there is a significant risk of bleeding, especially in soft tissue. The use of the soft toothbrush should help prevent bleeding of the gums.**
    2. A low platelet count does not indicate a need to start isolation.
    3. There is always a need to monitor the child frequently, but the low platelet count puts the child at risk for bleeding.
    4. In caring for children, always screen visitors, but there is no need to restrict visitation unless something is found on the screening.

TEST-TAKING HINT: Identify that the platelet count is low and can cause bleeding. The plan of care should include measures to protect the child from bleeding.

32. 1. A lumbar puncture is done to look for blast cells in the spinal fluid, which indicate central nervous system disease. It is also done to administer intrathecal chemotherapy, as the chemotherapy that will be given does not pass through the blood brain barrier.
2. An altered white blood cell count occurs as a result of the disease, but it does not make the diagnosis, as many diseases can alter the white blood cell count.
3. **The diagnostic test that confirms the diagnosis of leukemia is microscopic examination of the bone marrow aspirate.**
4. Bone scans do not confirm the diagnosis of a disease that occurs in the bone marrow.

TEST-TAKING HINT: The key to answering this question is the phrase "confirming the diagnosis."

33. 1. Flowers should not be kept in the room of the client who is neutropenic. There are no special vases that are used with these clients that can protect them from infection.
2. **A neutropenic client should not have flowers in the room because the flowers may harbor *Aspergillus* or *Pseudomonas aeruginosa*. Neutropenic children are susceptible to infection. Precautions need to be taken so the child does not come in contact with any potential sources of infection. Fresh fruits and vegetables can also harbor molds and should be avoided. Telling the friend that the flowers are beautiful but that the child cannot have them is a tactful way not to offend the friend.**
3. Washing the vase will not change the reason for not having the flowers around the child.
4. This could scare the visitors and make them feel guilty that they might harm the child in some way.

TEST-TAKING HINT: Review neutropenic precautions; then by process of elimination determine that answers 1 and 3 are incorrect. Answer 4 is not a professional way of interacting with visitors.

34. 1. Inspecting the skin is a good measure to monitor for infection and should be done.
2. Mouth care is essential and should be done daily to help prevent infection. Chemotherapy puts the child at risk for mucositis.
3. Washing the hands is one of the most important measures to prevent infection.
4. **Monitoring the child's temperature and reporting it to the physician are important, but the temperature should not be taken rectally. The risk of injury to the mucous membranes is high. Rectal abscesses can occur in the damaged rectal tissue. The best method of taking the temperature is axillary, especially if the child has mouth sores.**

TEST-TAKING HINT: Review home-care instructions for children who have just received chemotherapy. These are measures to protect the child from infection and to monitor for infection.

35. 1. There is no need to have the client remain supine after a bone marrow aspiration is done.
2. The child can assume any position after a bone marrow aspiration.
3. The child usually receives conscious sedation during the procedure and will have nothing by mouth prior to the procedure. Oral fluids can be resumed after the procedure is completed.
4. **Children may experience minor discomfort after the procedure, and analgesics should be given as needed.**

TEST-TAKING HINT: Review the procedure for doing a bone marrow aspiration, and be aware of nursing care after the procedure. There should be no reason for the child to be in a specific position or to have fluids withheld after the procedure. Managing pain is always a priority need.

36. 1. Radiation should be done as part of therapy if there is metastasis.
2. Steroids are given as part of the treatment protocol but do not need to be given intravenously. Steroids do not pass through the blood brain barrier.
3. **Giving chemotherapy via spinal tap allows the drugs to get to the brain and helps prevent metastasis of the disease.**
4. Chemotherapy that is given intravenously will not pass through the blood brain barrier.

TEST-TAKING HINT: Chemotherapy does not pass through the blood brain barrier. Intrathecal chemotherapy needs to be done to protect the central nervous system from metastasis of the disease.

37. 1. It is better to provide high-protein nutritional supplements if the child can tolerate them.
2. It is better to provide high-caloric nutritional supplements.
3. Offering the child's favorite foods when the child is nauseated can create a later association with being sick; then the child may not want that food when not ill.
4. **Cool, clear liquids are better tolerated. Milk-based products cause secretions to be thick and can cause vomiting.**

TEST-TAKING HINT: **With nausea and vomiting, it is important to consider nutritional status. Answers 1 and 2 do not improve nutrition. Supportive nutritional supplements should be offered. Review measures to prevent nausea and provide nutrition.**

38. 1. **Using a wig is a good way for the child to find a way of keeping personal identity despite loss of hair.**
2. Just discussing the benefits of the therapy will not help the child with self-image.
3. Having the child play only with other children with cancer could make the child feel even worse because of the inability to interact with friends. The child needs to find acceptance as appearance begins to change.
4. Diverting the child's attention would be avoiding the truth and would not be dealing with the issues.

TEST-TAKING HINT: **Review the side effects on the body from the chemotherapy, and look at ways to help the child deal with body-image changes. Provide the child and family with accurate information of the side effects of the drugs, but also give the child ways to feel good.**

39. 1. The temperature should always be monitored, but the child has an exposure to chickenpox. The child needs to be protected from getting the disease as it can be life-threatening.
2. Chickenpox exposure is a real concern for a child who is immunocompromised, and action needs to be taken.
3. **The child should receive varicella zoster immune globulin within 96 hours of the exposure.**
4. Starting isolation at this time does not protect the child.

TEST-TAKING HINT: **Review protective precautions that should be utilized for**

immunocompromised children. **Chicken-pox can be deadly for these children.**

40. 1. **The calculated absolute neutrophil count is 400/mm³ (0.08 x 5000) and is neutropenic as it is less than 500/mm³.**
2. The absolute neutrophil count is incorrectly calculated. The child would not be neutropenic if the count were 5800/ mm³.
3. The absolute neutrophil count is incorrectly calculated. The child would not be neutropenic with a count of 4000/ mm³.
4. The absolute neutrophil count is incorrectly calculated. The child would not be neutropenic with a count of 800/mm³.

TEST-TAKING HINT: **To calculate the absolute neutrophil count, multiply the white blood cell count by the percentage of neutrophils ("polys," "segs," and "bands"). Precautions for infection should be used at all times with children who are immunosupressed, but greater precautions must be taken when the ANC is less than 500/mm³.**

41. 1. Antibiotics should be used only if the child has a bacterial infection.
2. **Hand-washing is the best method to prevent the spread of germs and protect the child from infection.**
3. All nurses should use the same techniques in caring for the child. Assigning the same nurses may not be possible.
4. Visitors should be screened for infection and communicable diseases, but visitors should not be limited to family members only.

TEST-TAKING HINT: **The first defense against infection is prevention. Strict hand-washing technique is a primary intervention to prevent the spread of infections. Review measures to protect the child from infection.**

42. 1. **Children with a normal or low white blood cell count who do not have non-T, non-B acute lymphoblastic leukemia, and who are CALLA-positive have a much better prognosis than those with high cell counts or other cell types.**
2. Race is not a factor in prognosis of leukemia.
3. The child should begin treatment as soon as diagnosed, but time in initiating treatment does not have an effect on prognosis.
4. A history of allergies has no connection to prognosis in acute lymphoblastic leukemia.

TEST-TAKING HINT: Review the important prognostic factors that affect long-term survival for children with acute lymphoblastic leukemia.

43. 1. **Allopurinol reduces serum uric acid. When there is lysis of cells from chemotherapy, there will be an increase in serum uric acid.**
    2. There is no specific medication that makes chemotherapy work better.
    3. Allopurinol is not an antiemetic.
    4. Allopurinol is not an analgesic.

TEST-TAKING HINT: Review the effects of the tumor lysis syndrome that occurs when chemotherapy is started with children with leukemia.

44. 1. Prednisone does not enhance protein metabolism.
    2. Prednisone may cause retention of sodium.
    3. There is no drug that increases absorption of chemotherapy.
    4. **Prednisone is used in many of the treatment protocols with leukemia because there is abnormal lymphocyte production.**

TEST-TAKING HINT: Prednisone is given in conjunction with chemotherapy. It helps modify the body's immune response.

45. 1. **All chemotherapy is immunosuppressive as most childhood cancers affect the immune system.**
    2. Not all chemotherapy drugs are alkylating agents.
    3. There is no replication of DNA with chemotherapy. Chemotherapy drugs such as the antimetabolites usually inhibit synthesis of DNA or RNA.
    4. There is no interruption of the cell cycle.

TEST-TAKING HINT: Review the function of each type of chemotherapy because the immune system is affected in childhood cancer.

46. 1. There is no immunity to recurrent cancers with remission of the leukemia.
    2. **The most devastating late effect of leukemia treatment is development of secondary malignancy.**
    3. After the child is in remission, the child may relapse, but there is no immunity to other malignancy.
    4. The child will not receive steroid treatment after completing therapy.

TEST-TAKING HINT: Review late effects of treatment of childhood cancer. This

should include chemotherapy as well as radiation treatments.

47. 1. Fever and pain may be some of the symptoms, but they can be from other forms of cancer. Joint pain is not a symptom of Hodgkin disease.
    2. Anorexia with weight loss can be a symptom of many other conditions.
    3. **Enlarged, painless, and movable lymph nodes in the cervical area are the most common presenting manifestations of Hodgkin disease.**
    4. Enlarged liver with jaundice is not a presenting symptom with Hodgkin disease.

TEST-TAKING HINT: Review the clinical manifestations of Hodgkin disease. Some of the manifestations are the same for many different cancers, so focus on the primary and most common manifestations.

48. 1. **A lymph node biopsy is done to confirm a histological diagnosis and staging of Hodgkin disease. The presence of Reed-Sternberg cells is characteristic of the disease.**
    2. Blast cells are usually seen with leukemia.
    3. A bone marrow aspiration is usually done to diagnose the type of leukemia.
    4. This test is done to diagnose neuroblastoma.

TEST-TAKING HINT: In reviewing Hodgkin disease, be aware of the specific cell identified to confirm diagnosis.

49. 1. **Long-term survival for all stages of Hodgkin disease is excellent. Early-stage disease can have a survival rate greater than 90%, with advanced stages having rates between 65% and 75%.**
    2. Hodgkin disease mostly affects adolescents.
    3. The treatment consists of chemotherapy and often radiation therapy and does not predict prognosis.
    4. Bone marrow transplant is not always necessary with the treatment of Hodgkin disease and will most likely worsen the prognosis.

TEST-TAKING HINT: Know the treatment and the prognosis of Hodgkin disease.

50. 1. It should not be necessary to give pain medication, as radiation therapy should not be painful.
    2. Neuropathy is not a normal side effect of radiation therapy.

3. The most common side effect is extensive malaise, which may be from damage to the thyroid gland, causing hypothyroidism.

4. No diet restriction is required for the radiation therapy. Continue with nutritional supplements as needed to maintain adequate nutrition.

TEST-TAKING HINT: Review the side effects of radiation therapy. Lack of energy may be difficult emotionally in adolescents, as they want to keep up with their peers.

51. 1. Palpating the abdomen of the child in whom a diagnosis of Wilms tumor is suspected should be avoided, because manipulation of the abdomen may cause seeding of the tumor.

2. Hematuria is a clinical manifestation.

3. Because the kidney is involved, hypertension should be assessed.

4. Height and weight are always important to obtain, as they can be used to calculate doses of medications and chemotherapy.

TEST-TAKING HINT: All of the assessment data are important, but the key phrase is "most important." Seeding of the tumor could spread cancerous cells.

52. 1. Chemotherapy is started after tumor removal, and radiation is done depending on stage and histological pattern.

2. Combination therapy of surgery and chemotherapy is the therapeutic management.

3. Combination therapy of surgery and chemotherapy is the primary therapeutic management. Radiation is done depending on clinical stage and histological pattern.

4. Radiation should be done after surgery and chemotherapy, depending on stage and histological pattern.

TEST-TAKING HINT: Staging and biopsy determine the treatment, but the child will always have the tumor and kidney removed, followed by chemotherapy.

53. 1. Prolonged bleeding indicates abnormalities of the clotting system.

2. Failure to thrive is a consequence of a present illness.

3. Fatigue and malaise result from decreases in red blood cells.

4. SCID is characterized by an absence of cell-mediated immunity, with the most common clinical manifestation being in-fection in children from age 3 months. These children do not usually recover from these infections.

TEST-TAKING HINT: Review the clinical manifestations of SCID, keeping in mind that the word "immunodeficiency" should indicate infection, which is the key to getting the correct answer.

54. 1. The clinical manifestations are different from those of Hodgkin disease, as the enlarged lymph nodes usually occur in the cervical area.

2. The clinical manifestations include symptoms of involvement. Rarely is a single sign or symptom diagnostic. Metastasis to the bone marrow or central nervous system may produce manifestations of leukemia.

3. The manifestations are not just limited to the abdomen, and NHL is not usually seen in young children.

4. There is not just lower extremity involvement with NHL.

TEST-TAKING HINT: Review the difference between Hodgkin disease and non-Hodgkin lymphoma.

55. 1. The clinical staging system used in Hodgkin disease is of little value in lymphoma. Other systems have been developed.

2. The use of aggressive combination chemotherapy has a major impact on the survival rates for children with a diagnosis of lymphoma. Because there is usually bone marrow involvement, there is a need for central nervous system prophylaxis.

3. Not all children receive a bone marrow transplant.

4. Usually there is a good prognosis for lymphoma with aggressive chemotherapy.

TEST-TAKING HINT: Be careful not to answer a question with a response that has the word "all" in it, because rarely will something always occur.

56. 1. Tumor involvement in the bone is usually osteosarcoma.

2. Tumors that are located in the kidney are most often a Wilms tumor.

3. Neuroblastoma tumors originate from embryonic neural crest cells that normally give rise to the adrenal medulla and the sympathetic nervous system. The majority of the tumors arise from the adrenal gland or from the

retroperitoneal sympathetic chain. Therefore, the primary site is within the abdomen.
4. In most tumors in children, there is liver involvement when there is metastasis to the liver.

TEST-TAKING HINT: Review the origin of neuroblastoma to determine the tumor sites.

57. 1. CMV infection is one common characteristic of human immunodeficiency virus infections, but it is not the most common.
2. Encephalitis is not a specific opportunistic infection noted in human immunodeficiency virus–infected children.
3. Meningitis is not a specific opportunistic infection noted in human immunodeficiency virus–infected children.
4. *Pneumocystis carinii* **pneumonia is the most common opportunistic infection that can occur in human immunodeficiency virus–infected children, and such children are treated prophylactically for this.**

TEST-TAKING HINT: Note the words "most common" in the question.

58. 1. The CD4 cell count indicates how well the immune system is working.
2. A Western blot test confirms the presence of human immunodeficiency virus antibodies.
3. An IgG level samples the immune system.
4. **Detection of human immunodeficiency virus in infants is confirmed by a p24 antigen assay, viral culture of human immunodeficiency virus, or polymerase chain reaction.**

TEST-TAKING HINT: Review the laboratory tests for HIV-infected clients. The important word in the question is "infant."

59. 1. Hepatitis B vaccine is administered according to the immunization schedule.
2. The varicella vaccine is avoided in the child who is human immunodeficiency virus–infected.
3. A Western blot test is not done and is not necessary.
4. **Immunizations against childhood illnesses are recommended for children exposed to or infected with human immunodeficiency virus. Pneumococcal and influenza vaccines are recommended.**

TEST-TAKING HINT: Review the immunization schedule, keeping in mind that human immunodeficiency virus–infected children should not receive live viruses.

60. 1. The child can attend day care. The risk of transmission remains the same at any age.
2. **The child can attend day care without any limitations but should not attend with a fever.**
3. There is no need to restrict the child's activity.
4. There is no law that requires notification of the child's condition.

TEST-TAKING HINT: Review the modes of transmission of human immunodeficiency virus infection in children. The day-care facility should practice universal precautions when caring for all its children.

Gastrointestinal Disorders

8

KEYWORDS

Anorectal malformation
Anterior fontanel
Appendectomy
Appendix
Bile
Biliary atresia
Bowel obstruction
Celiac disease
Cholestyramine
Cleft lip
Cleft palate
Congenital aganglionic megacolon
Constipation
Dehydration
Diarrhea
Electrolytes
Encopresis
Enema
Enterocolitis
Esophageal atresia
Esophagus
Fiber
Fistula
Fluid maintenance
Fundus
Gastroenteritis
Gastroesophageal reflux
Gastrostomy tube
Gluten
Hepatitis
Hirschsprung disease
Imperforate anus

Intestinal villi
Intussusception
Jaundice
Jejunal biopsy
Kasai procedure
Malabsorption
Malaise
Morphine
Necrotizing enterocolitis
Nissen fundoplication
Occult blood
Patient-controlled analgesia
Peristalsis
Peritonitis
Polyhydramnios
Prilosec
Pyloric stenosis
Reglan
Rotavirus
Rovsing sign
Short bowel syndrome
Stimulant laxative
Stoma
Stool
Stool softener
Sudden infant death syndrome
Tracheoesophageal fistula
Umbilical hernia
Vomiting
Yankauer suction
Zofran

ABBREVIATIONS

Gastroesophageal reflux (GER)
Gastrostomy tube (GT)
Nasogastric tube (NGT)
Necrotizing enterocolitis (NEC)
Nothing by mouth (NPO)
Patient-controlled analgesia (PCA)

Short bowel syndrome (SBS)
Sudden infant death syndrome (SIDS)

QUESTIONS

1. The nurse is teaching feeding techniques to new parents. The nurse emphasizes the importance of slowly warming the formula and testing the temperature prior to feeding the infant. The parent of a newborn asks, "Will my baby spit out the formula if it is too hot or too cold?" Select the nurse's best response.
   1. "Babies have a tendency to reject hot fluids but not cold fluids, which could result in abdominal discomfort."
   2. "Babies have a tendency to reject cold fluids but not hot fluids, which could result in esophageal burns."
   3. "Your baby would most likely spit out formula that was too hot, but your baby could swallow some of it, which could result in a burn."
   4. "Your baby is too young to be physically capable of spitting out fluids and will automatically swallow anything."

2. The mother of a newborn asks the nurse why she has to nurse so frequently. The nurse replies using which of the following principles?
   1. Formula tends to be more calorically dense, and formula-fed babies require fewer feedings than breastfed babies.
   2. The newborn's stomach capacity is small, and peristalsis is slow.
   3. The newborn's stomach capacity is small, and peristalsis is more rapid than in older children.
   4. Breastfed babies tend to take longer to complete a feeding than formula-fed babies.

3. A 2-month-old male is brought to the pediatric clinic. The infant has had vomiting and diarrhea for 24 hours. The infant's anterior fontanel is sunken. The child is irritable, and the nurse notes that the infant does not produce tears when he cries. Which of the following tasks will help confirm the diagnosis of dehydration?
   1. Urinalysis obtained by bagged specimen.
   2. Urinalysis obtained by sterile catheterization.
   3. Analysis of serum electrolytes.
   4. Analysis of cerebrospinal fluid.

4. A 4-month-old female is brought to the emergency department with severe dehydration. Her heart rate is 198, and her blood pressure is 68/38. The infant's anterior fontanel is sunken. The nurse notes that the infant does not cry when the intravenous line is inserted. The child's parents state that she has not "held anything down" in 18 hours. The nurse obtains a finger-stick blood sugar of 94. Which of the following would the nurse expect to do immediately?
   1. Administer a bolus of normal saline.
   2. Administer a bolus of $D_{10}W$.
   3. Administer a bolus of normal saline with 5% dextrose added to the solution.
   4. Offer the child an oral rehydrating solution such as Pedialyte.

5. The nurse is caring for a 2-year-old child who was admitted to the pediatric unit for moderate dehydration due to vomiting and diarrhea. The child is noted to be restless, with periods of irritability. The child is afebrile with a heart rate of 148 and a blood pressure of 90/42. Baseline laboratory tests reveal the following: Na 152, Cl 119, and glucose 115. The parents state that the child has not urinated in 12 hours. After establishing a saline lock, the nurse reviews the physician's orders. Which of the following orders should the nurse question?
   1. Administer a saline bolus of 10 mL/kg, which may repeat if child does not urinate.
   2. Recheck serum electrolytes in 12 hours.
   3. After the saline bolus, begin maintenance fluids of D5 ¼ NS with 10 mEq KCl/L.
   4. Give clear liquid diet as tolerated.

6. The nurse in the pediatric clinic receives a call from the parent of a 5-year-old and states that the child has been having diarrhea for 24 hours. The parent explains that the child vomited twice 2 hours ago and now claims to be thirsty. The parent asks what to offer the child because the child is refusing Pedialyte. Select the nurse's most appropriate response.
   1. "You can offer clear diet soda such as Sprite and ginger ale."
   2. "Pedialyte is really the best thing for your child, who, if thirsty enough, will eventually drink it."
   3. "Pedialyte is really the best thing for your child. Allow your child some choice in the way to take it. Try offering small amounts in a spoon, medicine cup, or syringe."
   4. "It really does not matter what your child drinks as long as it is kept down. Try offering small amounts of fluids in medicine cups."

7. The nurse is caring for a 9-month-old with diarrhea secondary to rotavirus. The child has not vomited and is mildly dehydrated. The nurse is sending the child home. Which of the following is likely to be included in the discharge teaching?
   1. Administer Immodium as needed.
   2. Administer Kaopectate as needed.
   3. Continue breastfeeding per routine.
   4. The infant may return to day care 24 hours after antibiotics have been started.

8. The nurse is working in the pediatric clinic and is seeing many children with diarrhea. Which of the following children can most likely be discharged without further evaluation?
   1. A 2-year-old who has had 24 hours of watery diarrhea that has changed to bloody diarrhea in the past 12 hours.
   2. A 10-year-old who has just returned from a Scout camping trip.
   3. A 2-year-old who had a relapse of one diarrhea episode after restarting a normal diet.
   4. A 6-year-old who has been having vomiting and diarrhea for 2 days and has decreased urine output.

9. The nurse receives a call from the parent of a 10-month-old who has vomited three times in the past 8 hours. The parent describes the baby as playful and wanting to drink. The parent asks the nurse what to give the child. Select the nurse's best response.
   1. "Replace the next feeding with regular water, and see if that is better tolerated."
   2. "Do not allow your baby to eat any solids; give half the normal formula feeding, and see if that is better tolerated."
   3. "Do not allow your baby to eat or drink anything for 24 hours to give the stomach a chance to rest."
   4. "Give your child a very small amount of Pedialyte. If vomiting continues, wait a half hour, and then give half of what you previously gave."

10. The parents of a 4-year-old ask the nurse how to manage their child's constipation.
Select the nurse's best response.
    1. "Add 2 ounces of apple or pear juice to the child's diet."
    2. "Be sure your child eats a lot of fresh fruit such as apples and bananas."
    3. "Encourage your child to drink more fluids."
    4. "Decrease bulky foods such as whole-grain breads and rice."

11. A 7-year-old is being seen in the pediatric clinic. The child is diagnosed with chronic
constipation that has been unresponsive to dietary and activity changes. Which of the
following pharmacological measures is most appropriate?
    1. Natural supplements and herbs.
    2. A stimulant laxative.
    3. A stool softener.
    4. Pharmacological measures are not used in pediatric constipation.

12. The nurse is reviewing the discharge instructions of a child diagnosed with
encopresis. Which of the following instructions should the nurse question?
    1. Limit the intake of milk.
    2. Encourage positive reinforcement for appropriate toileting habits.
    3. Obtain a complete dietary log.
    4. Follow up with a child psychologist or psychiatrist.

13. The nurse is caring for an infant diagnosed with Hirschsprung disease. The mother
states she is pregnant with a male and wants to know if her new baby will likely have
the disorder. Select the nurse's best response.
    1. "Genetics play a small role in Hirschsprung disease, so there is a chance the baby
will develop it as well."
    2. "There is no evidence to support a genetic link, so it is very unlikely the baby will
also have it."
    3. "It is rarely seen in boys, so it is not likely your new baby will have Hirschsprung
disease."
    4. "Hirschsprung disease is seen only in girls, so your new baby will not be at risk."

14. The nurse is caring for an infant newly diagnosed with Hirschsprung disease. Which
of the following does the nurse understand about this infant's condition?
    1. There is a lack of peristalsis in the large intestine and an accumulation of bowel
contents, leading to abdominal distention.
    2. There is excessive peristalsis throughout the intestine, resulting in abdominal
distention.
    3. There is a small-bowel obstruction leading to ribbon-like stools.
    4. There is inflammation throughout the large intestine, leading to accumulation of
intestinal contents and abdominal distention.

15. The nurse is caring for a 3-month-old male who is being evaluated for possible
Hirschsprung disease. His parents call the nurse and state that his diaper contains a
large amount of mucus and bloody diarrhea. The nurse notes that the infant is
irritable and his abdomen appears very distended. Which of the following should
be the nurse's next action?
    1. Reassure the parents that this is an expected finding and not uncommon.
    2. Call a code for a potential cardiac arrest, and stay with the infant.
    3. Immediately obtain all vital signs with a quick head-to-toe assessment.
    4. Obtain a stool sample for occult blood.

16. The nurse is caring for an 8-week-old male who has just been diagnosed with Hirschsprung disease. The parents ask what they should expect. Select the nurse's best response.
    1. "It is really an easy disease to manage. Most children are placed on stool softeners to help with constipation until the constipation resolves."
    2. "A permanent stool diversion, called a colostomy, will be placed by the surgeon to bypass the narrowed area."
    3. "Daily bowel irrigations will help your child maintain regular bowel habits."
    4. "Although your child will require surgery, there are different ways to manage the disease, depending on how much of your child's bowel is involved."

17. The nurse is caring for a 2-month-old infant diagnosed with GER. Which of the following should the nurse include in the plan of care to decrease the incidence of symptoms of GER?
    1. Place the infant in an infant seat immediately after feedings.
    2. Place the infant in the prone position immediately after feeding to decrease the risk of aspiration.
    3. Encourage the parents not to worry because most infants outgrow GER within the first year of life.
    4. Encourage the parents to hold the infant in an upright position for 30 minutes following a feeding.

18. The nurse is caring for a 6-week-old infant with cerebral palsy and GER. After two hospital admissions for aspiration, the child is scheduled for a Nissen fundoplication. The nurse knows that this procedure involves which of the following?
    1. The fundus of the stomach is wrapped around the inferior stomach, mimicking a lower esophageal sphincter.
    2. The fundus of the stomach is wrapped around the inferior esophagus, mimicking a cardiac sphincter.
    3. The fundus of the stomach is wrapped around the middle portion of the stomach, decreasing the capacity of the stomach.
    4. The fundus of the stomach is dilated, decreasing the likelihood of reflux.

19. The nurse is caring for a 4-month-old with GER. The infant is due to receive Reglan (metoclopramide). Based on the medication's mechanism of action, when should this medication be administered?
    1. Immediately before a feeding.
    2. 30 minutes after the feeding.
    3. 30 minutes before the feeding.
    4. At bedtime.

20. The nurse is administering Prilosec to a 3-month-old with GER. The child's parents ask the nurse how the medication works. Select the nurse's best response.
    1. "Prilosec is a proton pump inhibitor that is commonly used for reflux in infants."
    2. "Prilosec decreases stomach acid, so it will not be as irritating when your child spits up."
    3. "Prilosec helps food move through the stomach quicker, so there will be less chance for reflux."
    4. "Prilosec relaxes the pressure of the lower esophageal sphincter."

21. The nurse is caring for a 10-year-old who is being evaluated for possible appendicitis. The child has been complaining of nausea and sharp abdominal pain in the right lower quadrant. An abdominal ultrasound is scheduled, and a blood count has been obtained. The child vomits, finds the pain relieved, and calls the nurse. Which of the following should be the nurse's next action?
    1. Cancel the ultrasound, and obtain an order for oral Zofran.
    2. Cancel the ultrasound, and prepare to administer an intravenous bolus.
    3. Prepare for the probable discharge of the patient.
    4. Immediately notify the physician of the child's status.

22. The parents of a 6-year-old being evaluated for appendicitis tell the nurse the physician diagnosed their child as having a positive Rovsing sign. They ask the nurse what this means. Select the nurse's best response.
    1. "Your child's physician should answer that question."
    2. "A positive Rovsing sign means the child feels pain in the right side of the abdomen when the left side is palpated."
    3. "A positive Rovsing sign means pain is felt when the physician removes the hand from the abdomen."
    4. "A positive Rovsing sign means pain is felt in the right lower quadrant when the child coughs."

23. The nurse is caring for an 8-year-old who has just returned to the pediatric unit after an appendectomy for a ruptured appendix. Which of the following is the best position for the child?
    1. Semi-Fowler.
    2. Prone.
    3. Right side-lying.
    4. Left side-lying.

24. The nurse is about to receive a 4-year-old from the recovery room after an appendectomy for a non-ruptured appendix. The parents have not seen the child since the surgery and ask what to expect. Select the nurse's best response.
    1. "Your child will be very sleepy, have an intravenous line in the hand, and have a nasal tube to help drain the stomach. If your child needs pain medication, it will be given intravenously."
    2. "Your child will be very sleepy, have an intravenous line in the hand, and have white stockings to help prevent blood clots. If your child needs pain medication, we will give it intravenously or provide a liquid to swallow."
    3. "Your child will be wide awake and will have an intravenous line in the hand. If your child needs pain medication, we will give it intravenously or provide a liquid to swallow."
    4. "Your child will be very sleepy and will have an intravenous line in the hand. If your child needs pain medication, we will give it intravenously."

25. The nurse is caring for a 5-year-old who has just returned from having an appendectomy. Which of the following is the optimal way to manage pain?
    1. Intravenous morphine as needed.
    2. Liquid Tylenol with codeine as needed.
    3. Morphine administered through a PCA pump.
    4. Intramuscular morphine as needed.

26. The nurse is caring for a 3-year-old who had an appendectomy 2 days ago. When taking the child's temperature, the nurse notes that the child has a fever of 101.8°F (38.8°C). The nurse notes the child's breath sounds are slightly diminished in the right lower lobe. Which of the following actions is most appropriate for this patient?
    1. Teach the child how to use an incentive spirometer.
    2. Encourage the child to blow bubbles.
    3. Obtain an order for intravenous antibiotics.
    4. Obtain an order for acetaminophen.

27. The nurse is providing discharge instructions to the parents of a 10-year-old who had an appendectomy for a ruptured appendix 5 days ago. The nurse knows that further education is required when the child's parent states:
    1. "We will wait a few days before allowing our child to return to school."
    2. "We will wait 2 weeks before allowing our child to return to sports."
    3. "We will call the pediatrician's office if we notice any drainage around the wound."
    4. "We will encourage our child to go for walks every day."

28. The nurse is caring for a 6-year-old in the early stages of acute hepatitis. Which of the following manifestations should the nurse expect to find?
    1. Nausea, vomiting, and generalized malaise.
    2. Nausea, vomiting, generalized malaise, and pain in the left upper quadrant.
    3. Nausea, vomiting, generalized malaise, and yellowing of the skin and sclera.
    4. Yellowing of the skin and sclera without any other generalized complaints.

29. The nurse is caring for a 6-year-old with hepatitis. The child is hungry and wants to eat dinner. Which of the following foods should be offered?
    1. A tuna sandwich on whole wheat bread and a cup of skim milk.
    2. Clear liquids, such as broth, and Jell-O.
    3. A hamburger, French fries, and a diet soda.
    4. A peanut butter sandwich and a milkshake.

30. The nurse in the pediatric clinic is providing instructions to the parents of a 2-year-old child who has just been diagnosed with acute hepatitis. Which of the following would be an appropriate activity for the nurse to recommend?
    1. Riding a bike in an enclosed area such as a basement.
    2. Playing basketball.
    3. Playing video games in bed.
    4. Playing with puzzles in bed.

31. The nurse is caring for a 4-week-old infant with biliary atresia. Which of the following manifestations would the nurse expect to see?
    1. Abdominal distention, enlarged liver, enlarged spleen, clay-colored stool, and tea-colored urine.
    2. Abdominal distention, multiple bruises, bloody stools, and hematuria.
    3. Yellow sclera and skin tones, excessively oily skin, and prolonged bleeding times.
    4. No manifestations until the disease has progressed to the advanced stage.

32. The nurse is caring for an infant with biliary atresia. The parents ask why the child is receiving cholestyramine. Select the nurse's best response.
    1. To lower your child's cholesterol.
    2. To relieve your child's itching.
    3. To help your child gain weight.
    4. To help feedings be absorbed in a more efficient manner.

33. The nurse is caring for an infant with biliary atresia who is scheduled for a Kasai procedure. Which of the following is an accurate description of this surgery?
    1. A palliative procedure in which a bile duct is attached to a loop of bowel to assist with bile drainage.
    2. A curative procedure in which a connection is made between a bile duct and a loop of bowel to assist with bile drainage.
    3. A curative procedure in which a bile duct is banded to prevent bile leakage.
    4. A palliative procedure in which a bile duct is banded to prevent bile leakage.

34. The parents of a newborn diagnosed with a cleft lip and palate ask the nurse when their child's lip and palate will most likely be repaired. Select the nurse's best response.
    1. "The palate and the lip are usually repaired in the first few weeks of life so that the baby can grow and gain weight."
    2. "The palate and the lip are usually not repaired until the baby is approximately 6 months old so that the mouth has had enough time to grow."
    3. "The lip is repaired in the first few months of life, but the palate is not usually repaired until the child is 3 years old."
    4. "The lip is repaired in the first few weeks of life, but the palate is not usually repaired until the child is 18 months old."

35. The nurse is caring for a newborn with a cleft lip and palate. The mother states, "I will not be able to breastfeed my baby." Select the nurse's best response.
   1. "It sounds like you are feeling discouraged. Would you like to talk about it?"
   2. "Sometimes breastfeeding is still an option for babies with a cleft lip and palate. Would you like more information?"
   3. "Although breastfeeding is not an option, you have the option of pumping your milk and then feeding it to your baby with a special nipple."
   4. "We usually discourage breastfeeding babies with cleft lip and palate as it puts them at an increased risk for aspiration."

36. The nurse is caring for a 4-month-old who has just had an isolated cleft lip repaired. Select the best position for the child in the immediate postoperative period.
   1. Right side-lying.
   2. Left side-lying.
   3. Supine.
   4. Prone.

37. The nurse is caring for an 18-month-old infant whose cleft palate was repaired 12 hours ago. Which of the following should be included in the plan of care?
   1. Allow the infant to have familiar items of comfort such as a favorite stuffed animal and a pacifier.
   2. Once liquids have been tolerated, encourage a bland diet such as soup, Jell-O, and saltine crackers.
   3. Administer pain medication on a regular schedule, as opposed to an as-needed schedule.
   4. Use a Yankauer suction catheter on the infant's mouth to decrease the risk of aspiration of oral secretions.

38. The nurse is caring for a newborn with esophageal atresia. When reviewing the mother's history, the nurse would expect to find which of the following?
   1. A history of maternal polyhydramnios.
   2. A pregnancy that lasted more than 38 weeks.
   3. A history of poor nutrition during pregnancy.
   4. A history of alcohol consumption during pregnancy.

39. The nurse is in the room while a mother of a newborn is feeding her infant for the first time. The baby immediately begins coughing and choking. The nurse notes that the baby is extremely cyanotic. Which of the following should be the nurse's immediate action?
   1. Call the physician, and inform the physician of the situation.
   2. Have the mother stop feeding the infant, and observe to see if the choking episode resolves on its own.
   3. Immediately determine the infant's oxygen saturation, and have the mother stop feeding the infant.
   4. Take the infant from the mother, and administer blow-by oxygen while obtaining the infant's oxygen saturation.

40. The nurse is caring for a newborn who has just been diagnosed with tracheoesophageal atresia and is scheduled for surgery. Which of the following should the nurse expect to do in the preoperative period?
   1. Keep the child in a monitored crib, obtain frequent vital signs, and allow the parents to visit but not hold their infant.
   2. Administer intravenous fluids and antibiotics.
   3. Place the infant on 100% oxygen via a non-rebreather mask.
   4. Have the mother feed the infant slowly in a monitored area, stopping all feedings 4 to 6 hours before surgery.

41. The nurse is giving discharge instructions to the parents of a 1-month-old infant with tracheoesophageal atresia. The infant is being discharged with a GT. The nurse knows that the parents understand the discharge teaching when the mother states:
    1. "I will give my baby feedings through the GT but place liquid medications in the corner of the mouth to be absorbed."
    2. "I will flush the GT with 2 ounces of water after each feeding to prevent the GT from clogging."
    3. "I will clean the area around the GT with soap and water every day."
    4. "I will place petroleum jelly around the GT if any redness develops."

42. An expectant mother asks the nurse if her new baby will likely have an umbilical hernia. The nurse bases the response on which of the following?
    1. Umbilical hernias occur more often in large infants.
    2. Umbilical hernias occur more often in white infants than in African-American infants.
    3. Umbilical hernias occur twice as often in male infants.
    4. Umbilical hernias occur more often in premature infants.

43. The nurse is providing discharge teaching to the parents of an infant with an umbilical hernia. Which of the following should be included in the plan of care?
    1. If the hernia has not resolved on its own by the age of 12 months, surgery is generally recommended.
    2. If the hernia appears to be more swollen or tender, seek medical care immediately.
    3. To help the hernia resolve, place a pressure dressing over the area gently.
    4. If the hernia is repaired surgically, there is a strong likelihood that it will return.

44. The nurse is caring for an infant with pyloric stenosis. The parents ask if any future children will likely have pyloric stenosis. Select the nurse's best response.
    1. "You seem worried; would you like to discuss your concerns?"
    2. "It is very rare for a family to have more than one child with pyloric stenosis."
    3. "Pyloric stenosis can run in families. It is more common among males."
    4. "Although there can be a genetic link, it is very unusual for girls to have pyloric stenosis."

45. The nurse is caring for an 8-week-old infant being evaluated for pyloric stenosis. Which of the following statements made by the parents would be typical of a child with this diagnosis?
    1. "The baby is a very fussy eater and just does not want to eat."
    2. "The baby tends to have a very forceful vomiting episode approximately 30 minutes after most feedings."
    3. "The baby is always hungry."
    4. "The baby is happy in spite of getting really upset on spitting up."

46. The nurse is caring for a 7-week-old scheduled for a pyloromyotomy in 24 hours. Which of the following would the nurse expect to find in the plan of care?
    1. Keep infant NPO; begin intravenous fluids at maintenance.
    2. Keep infant NPO; begin intravenous fluids at maintenance; place NGT to low wall suction.
    3. Obtain serum electrolytes; keep infant NPO; do not attempt to pass NGT due to obstruction from pylorus.
    4. Offer infant small frequent feedings; keep NPO 6 to 8 hours before surgery.

47. The nurse receives a call from the mother of a 6-month-old who describes her child as sleepy and fussy. She states that her infant vomited once this morning and had two episodes of diarrhea. The last episode contained mucus and a small amount of blood. She asks the nurse what she should do. Select the nurse's best response.
    1. "Your infant will need to have some tests in the emergency room to determine if anything serious is going on."
    2. "Try feeding your infant in about 30 minutes; in the event of repeat vomiting, bring the infant to the emergency room for some tests and intravenous rehydration."
    3. "Many infants display these symptoms when they develop an allergy to the formula they are receiving; try switching to a soy-based formula."
    4. "Do not worry about the blood and mucus in the stool; it is not unusual for infants to have blood in their stools because their intestines are more sensitive."

48. The nurse is caring for a 5-month-old infant with a diagnosis of intussusception. The infant has periods of irritability during which the knees are brought to chest and the infant cries, alternating with periods of lethargy. Vital signs are stable and within age-appropriate limits. The physician elects to give an enema. The parents ask the purpose of is the enema. Select the nurse's most appropriate response.
    1. "The enema will confirm the diagnosis. If the test result is positive, your child will need to have surgery to correct the intussusception."
    2. "The enema will confirm the diagnosis. Although very unlikely, the enema may also help fix the intussusception so that your child will not immediately need surgery."
    3. "The enema will help confirm diagnosis and has a good chance of fixing the intussusception."
    4. "The enema will help confirm the diagnosis and may temporarily fix the intussusception. If the bowel returns to normal, there is a strong likelihood that the intussusception will recur."

49. A nurse working in an emergency room of a large pediatric hospital receives a transfer call from a reporting nurse at a local community hospital. The nurse will soon receive a 4-month-old who has been diagnosed with an intussusception. The infant is described as very lethargic with the following vital signs, T 101.8°F (38.7°C), HR 181, BP 68/38. The reporting nurse states the infant's abdomen is very rigid. Which of the following is the most appropriate action for the receiving nurse?
    1. Prepare to accompany the infant to a computed tomography scan to confirm the diagnosis.
    2. Prepare to accompany the infant to the radiology department for a reducing enema.
    3. Prepare to start a second intravenous line to administer fluids and antibiotics.
    4. Prepare to get the infant ready for immediate surgical correction.

50. The nurse is providing discharge instructions to the parents of an infant who has had surgery to open a low imperforate anus. The nurse knows that the discharge instructions have been understood when the child's parents say which of the following?
    1. "We will use an oral thermometer because we cannot use a rectal one."
    2. "We will call the physician if the stools change in consistency."
    3. "Our infant will never be toilet-trained."
    4. "We understand that it is not unusual for our infant's urine to contain stool."

51. The nurse is caring for a neonate with an anorectal malformation. The nurse notes that the infant has not passed any stool per rectum but that the infant's urine contains meconium. The nurse can make which of the following assumptions?
    1. The child likely has a low anorectal malformation.
    2. The child likely has a high anorectal malformation.
    3. The child will not need a colostomy.
    4. This malformation will be corrected with a nonoperative rectal pull-through.

52. The nurse is caring for a newborn with an anorectal malformation and has had a colostomy placed. The nurse knows that more education is needed when the infant's parent states which of the following?
    1. "I will make sure the stoma is red."
    2. "There should not be any discharge or irritation around the outside of the stoma."
    3. "I will keep a bag attached to avoid the contents of the small intestine coming in contact with the baby's skin."
    4. "As my baby grows, a pattern will develop over time, and there should be predictable bowel movements."

53. The parents of a child being evaluated for celiac disease ask the nurse why it is important to make dietary changes. Select the nurse's best response.
    1. "The body's response to gluten causes damage to the mucosal cells in the intestine, leading to absorption problems."
    2. "When the child with celiac disease consumes anything containing gluten, the body responds by creating specials cells called villi, which leads to more diarrhea."
    3. "The body's response to gluten causes the intestine to become more porous and hang on to more of the fat-soluble vitamins, leading to vitamin toxicity."
    4. "The body's response to gluten causes damage to the mucosal cells, leading to malabsorbtion of water and hard, constipated stools."

54. The nurse is caring for a 14-year-old with celiac disease. The nurse knows that the patient understands the diet instructions by ordering which of the following meals?
    1. Eggs, bacon, rye toast, and lactose-free milk.
    2. Pancakes, orange juice, and sausage links.
    3. Oat cereal, breakfast pastry, and nonfat skim milk.
    4. Cheese, banana slices, rice cakes, and whole milk.

55. The nurse is caring for a 3-year-old undergoing evaluation for celiac disease. Which of the following would the nurse expect to be included in the child's diagnostic workup?
    1. Obtain complete blood count and serum electrolytes.
    2. Obtain complete blood count and stool sample; keep child NPO.
    3. Obtain stool sample and prepare child for jejunal biopsy.
    4. Obtain complete blood count and serum electrolytes; monitor child's response to gluten-containing diet.

56. Which of the following manifestations suggests that an infant is developing NEC?
    1. The infant absorbs bolus orogastric feedings at a faster rate than previous feedings.
    2. The infant has bloody diarrhea.
    3. The infant has increased bowel sounds.
    4. The infant appears hungry right before a scheduled feeding.

57. The nurse is caring for a 1-month-old term infant who experienced an anoxic episode at birth. The health-care team suspects that the infant is developing NEC. Which of the following would the nurse expect to be included in the plan of care?
    1. Immediately remove the feeding NGT from the infant.
    2. Obtain vital signs every 4 hours.
    3. Prepare to administer antibiotics intravenously.
    4. Change feedings to half-strength and administer slowly via a feeding pump.

58. The nurse is conducting an in-service lecture on NEC to a group of colleagues. The nurse knows that she needs to provide more education when one of the participants states which of the following?
    1. "Encouraging the mother to pump her milk for the feedings helps prevent NEC."
    2. "Some sources state that the occurrence of NEC has increased because so many preterm infants are surviving."
    3. "When signs of sepsis appear, the infant will likely deteriorate quickly."
    4. "NEC occurs only in preemies and low-birth-weight infants."

59. The nurse is caring for an infant who has been diagnosed with SBS. The parents of the infant ask how the disease will affect their child. Select the nurse's best response.
    1. "Because your child has a shorter intestine than most, your child will likely experience constipation and will need to be placed on a bowel regimen."
    2. "Because your child has a shorter intestine than most, your child will not be able to absorb all the nutrients and vitamins in food and will need to get nutrients in alternative ways."
    3. "Unfortunately, most children with this diagnosis do not do very well."
    4. "The prognosis and course of the disease have changed because hyperalimentation is available.

60. The nurse is caring for a 3-month-old infant who has SBS and has been receiving TPN. The parents ask if their child will ever be able to eat. Select the nurse's best response.
    1. "Children with SBS are never able to eat and must receive all of their nutrition in intravenous form."
    2. "You will have to start feeding your child because children cannot be on TPN longer than 6 months."
    3. "We will start feeding your child soon so that the bowel continues to receive stimulation."
    4. "Your child will start receiving tube feedings soon but will never be able to eat by mouth."

61. Which of the following children may need extra fluids to prevent dehydration? Select all that apply.
    1. A 7-day-old receiving phototherapy.
    2. A 6-month-old with newly diagnosed pyloric stenosis.
    3. A 2-year-old with pneumonia.
    4. A 13-year-old who has just started her menses.
    5. A 2-year-old with full-thickness burns to the chest, back, and abdomen.

62. The nurse is interviewing the parents of a 6-year-old who has been experiencing constipation. Which of the following could be a causative factor? Select all that apply.
    1. Hypothyroidism.
    2. Muscular dystrophy.
    3. Myelomeningocele.
    4. Drinks a lot of milk.
    5. Active in sports.

1. 1. Swallowing is a reflex in neonates; infants younger than 6 weeks cannot voluntarily control swallowing.
2. Swallowing is a reflex in neonates; infants younger than 6 weeks cannot voluntarily control swallowing.
3. The infant is not capable of selectively rejecting fluid because swallowing is a reflex until 6 weeks.
4. **Swallowing is a reflex in infants younger than 6 weeks.**

TEST-TAKING HINT: Swallowing is a reflex that is present until the age of 6 weeks. The test taker should eliminate answers 1, 2, and 3 as they both suggest that the infant is capable of selectively rejecting fluids.

2. 1. The caloric content of breast milk and formula tends to be similar.
2. Peristalsis in infants is greater than in older children.
3. **The small-stomach capacity and rapid movement of fluid through the digestive system account for the need for small frequent feedings.**
4. Breastfed babies and formula-fed babies do not necessarily have a difference in feeding time.

TEST-TAKING HINT: The test taker should eliminate answers 1 and 4 because they both form generalizations that are not supported by current literature.

3. 1. The information obtained from a urinalysis of an infant is not as helpful as serum electrolytes. The infant has limited ability to concentrate urine, so the specific gravity is not usually affected.
2. The information obtained from a urinalysis of an infant is not as helpful as serum electrolytes. The infant has limited ability to concentrate urine, so the specific gravity is not usually affected. A urinalysis does not need to be obtained by catheterization.
3. **The analysis of serum electrolytes offers the most information and assists with the diagnosis of dehydration.**
4. Although critical in diagnosing meningitis, a lumber puncture and analysis of cerebrospinal fluid are not done to confirm dehydration.

TEST-TAKING HINT: Infants have limited ability to concentrate urine, so answers 1 and 2 can be eliminated immediately.

4. 1. **Dehydration is corrected with the administration of an isotonic solution, such as normal saline or lactated Ringer solution.**
2. Solutions containing dextrose should never be administered in bolus form because they may result in cerebral edema.
3. Solutions containing dextrose should never be administered in bolus form because they may result in cerebral edema.
4. Severe dehydration is not usually corrected with oral solutions; children with altered levels of consciousness should be kept NPO.

TEST-TAKING HINT: The test taker should immediately eliminate answers 2 and 3 as they both suggest administering glucose in bolus form, which is always contraindicated in the pediatric population. Answer 4 should be eliminated as the infant is severely dehydrated and not responding to painful stimulation, which is suggested by the lack of a cry on intravenous insertion.

5. 1. Fluid boluses of normal saline are administered according to the child's body weight. It is not unusual to have to repeat the bolus multiple times in order to see an improvement in the child's condition.
2. It is important to monitor serum electrolytes frequently in the dehydrated child.
3. **Potassium is contraindicated because the child has not yet urinated. Potassium is not added to the maintenance fluid until kidney function has been verified.**
4. The child with dehydration secondary to vomiting and diarrhea is placed on a clear liquid diet.

TEST-TAKING HINT: Be aware of the usual ways in which dehydration is treated. Answer 3 should be selected because the description states that the child has not urinated.

6. 1. When Pedialyte is not tolerated, it is usually recommended that clear sodas and juices be diluted. Diet beverages are not recommended because the sugar is needed to help the sodium be reabsorbed.
2. Pedialyte is the best choice. If the child is not encouraged to drink Pedialyte, the child may become severely dehydrated. Other ways to encourage oral rehydration need to be considered.

3. **Pedialyte is the first choice, as recommended by the American Academy of Pediatrics. Offering the child appropriate choices may allow the child to feel empowered and less likely to refuse the Pedialyte. Small, frequent amounts are usually better tolerated.**
4. Offering small amounts of liquids is important. The type of beverage does matter because many fluids may increase vomiting and diarrhea.

TEST-TAKING HINT: The test taker should eliminate answer 2 because it offers an ultimatum to a child. The child is likely to refuse the Pedialyte, worsening the state of dehydration.

7. 1. Immodium slows intestinal motility and allows overgrowth of organisms and should therefore be avoided.
2. Kaopectate slows intestinal motility and allows overgrowth of organisms and should therefore be avoided.
3. **Breastfeeding is usually well tolerated and helps prevent death of intestinal villi and malabsorption.**
4. Antibiotics are not effective in viruses. Children should not return to day care while they are still having diarrhea.

TEST-TAKING HINT: The test taker can eliminate answer 4 as antibiotics are not effective with viruses such as rotavirus. Answers 1 and 2 can be eliminated as antidiarrheal agents are not recommended in the pediatric population.

8. 1. Diarrhea containing blood needs further evaluation to determine the source of the blood and the child's blood counts and electrolyte balance.
2. Diarrhea following a camping trip needs further evaluation because it may be due to bacteria or parasites.
3. **It is common for children to have a relapse of diarrhea after resuming a regular diet.**
4. Children who have had vomiting and diarrhea for more than 2 days require evaluation to determine if IV rehydration and hospital admission are necessary.

TEST-TAKING HINT: The test taker should eliminate answers 1 and 4 because they describe children who may have altered electrolytes and blood counts due to prolonged diarrhea.

9. 1. Free water should not be given as it does not contain any electrolytes and can lead to critical electrolyte imbalances.

2. Formula should be avoided, and clear liquids such as Pedialyte should be offered.
3. Twenty-four hours are too long for the infant to remain NPO. The infant needs to drink a rehydration solution such as Pedialyte in order to avoid severe dehydration.
4. **Offering small amounts of clear liquids is usually well tolerated. The amount can be halved if the child vomits as long as the child does not appear to be dehydrated. The child in this scenario is described as playful and therefore does not appear to be at risk for dehydration.**

TEST-TAKING HINT: The test taker should eliminate answers 1 and 3 because they could cause harm to the infant.

10. 1. Two ounces of apple juice is most likely not a sufficient quantity to alter a 4-year-old child's bowel movements. It is appropriate for a young infant.
2. Although fresh fruits help decrease constipation, bananas tend to increase constipation.
3. **Increasing fluid consumption helps to decrease the hardness of the stool.**
4. Whole-grain bread is high in fiber and helps decrease constipation.

TEST-TAKING HINT: Answer 1 decreases constipation in the infant but not in the preschooler.

11. 1. Natural supplements and herbs are not recommended because the safety and efficacy are not standardized.
2. A stimulant laxative is not the drug of choice because it may increase abdominal discomfort and may lead to dependency.
3. **A stool softener is the drug of choice because it will lead to easier evacuation.**
4. Although diet and activity modification are tried first, medications are sometimes needed.

TEST-TAKING HINT: The test taker should eliminate answer 4 as it implies that medications are never given to the constipated child. In health care, there are very few cases of "never" and "always."

12. 1. Dairy products are limited as they can lead to constipation.
2. **Positive reinforcement is encouraged. The use of negative reinforcement is discouraged, however, as it may cause the child to attempt to be controlling by holding on to the stool.**

3. A complete dietary log should be kept to help correlate the foods that lead to constipation.
4. The child and family are encouraged to seek counseling, as there is often a psychological component to encopresis.

TEST-TAKING HINT: Recall the developmental needs of children and successful approaches to meet their needs.

13. 1. **There is a genetic component to Hirschsprung disease, so any future siblings are also at risk.**
2. There is a genetic component to Hirschsprung disease.
3. Hirschsprung disease is seen more commonly in males than females.
4. Hirschsprung disease is seen in both males and females but is more common in males.

TEST-TAKING HINT: The test taker can eliminate answers 3 and 4 as they are similar and therefore would not likely be the correct answer.

14. 1. **In Hirschsprung disease, a portion of the large intestine has an area lacking in ganglion cells. This results in a lack of peristalsis as well as an accumulation of bowel contents and abdominal distention.**
2. There is a lack of peristalsis at the aganglionic section of the bowel.
3. Hirschsprung disease does not include a small-bowel obstruction.
4. Hirschsprung disease does not present with inflammation throughout the large intestine.

TEST-TAKING HINT: The test taker should be familiar with the pathophysiology of Hirschsprung disease in order to select answer 1.

15. 1. All cases of bloody diarrhea need to be evaluated because this may be a sign of enterocolitis, which is a potentially fatal complication of Hirschsprung disease.
2. Although this is a potentially critical complication, calling a code is not necessary at this time as the infant is irritable and not unconscious.
3. **All vital signs need to be evaluated because the child with enterocolitis can quickly progress to a state of shock. A quick head-to-toe assessment will allow the nurse to evaluate the child's circulatory system.**
4. It is not a priority to test the stool for occult blood, as there is obvious blood in the sample.

TEST-TAKING HINT: The test taker should select answer 3 because there is not enough information to determine the status of the child. Obtaining vital signs will help the nurse to assess the situation.

16. 1. The constipation will not resolve with stool softeners. The affected bowel needs to be removed.
2. Most colostomies are not permanent. The large intestine is usually reattached, and the colostomy is taken down.
3. The child with Hirschsprung disease requires surgery to remove the aganglionic portion of the large intestine.
4. **The aganglionic portion needs to be removed. Although most children have a temporary colostomy placed, many infants are able to bypass the colostomy and have the bowel immediately reattached.**

TEST-TAKING HINT: The test taker should be led to answer 4 as it is the least restrictive of all answers and is the only one that states that the child will require surgery. All children with Hirschsprung disease are managed surgically.

17. 1. Placing the infant in an infant seat increases intra-abdominal pressure, placing the infant at increased risk for GER.
2. The prone position is not recommended as it may lead to sudden infant death syndrome.
3. Although most infants outgrow GER, providing the parents with this education will not help decrease the symptoms
4. **Keeping the infant in an upright position is the best way to decrease the symptoms of GER. The infant can also be placed in the supine position with the head of the crib elevated. A harness can be used to keep the child from sliding down.**

TEST-TAKING HINT: The test taker may be led to answers 3 and 4 as they are both correct. The question is looking for ways to decrease reflux. Although decreasing parental anxiety may help decrease reflux, the better answer is 4, as it more likely to be an effective management plan.

18. 1. The fundus is wrapped around the inferior esophagus, not the inferior stomach.
2. **The Nissen fundoplication involves wrapping the fundus of the stomach around the inferior esophagus, creating a lower esophageal sphincter or cardiac sphincter.**

3. The fundus is not wrapped around the middle portion of the stomach. There is no benefit to decreasing the stomach's capacity.
4. The fundus of the stomach is not dilated.

TEST-TAKING HINT: The test taker needs to be familiar with surgical options for GER disease.

19. 1. If Reglan is administered immediately before a feeding, the medication will not have enough time to take effect.
2. This medication should be administered prior to a feeding to be effective.
3. **Reglan increases gastric emptying and should be administered 30 minutes before a feeding.**
4. This medication should be administered prior to a feeding to be effective.

TEST-TAKING HINT: The test taker needs to be familiar with the administration of Reglan.

20. 1. Although this is an accurate description of the mechanism of action, it does not tell the parents how the medication functions.
2. **This accurate description gives the parents information that is clear and concise.**
3. Prilosec does not increase the rate of gastric emptying.
4. Prilosec does not relax the pressure of the lower esophageal sphincter.

TEST-TAKING HINT: The test taker should eliminate answers 1 and 4 because they do not communicate information in a manner that will be clear to many parents.

21. 1. The ultrasound should not be canceled but obtained emergently because the child probably has a perforated appendix. The child should be NPO because surgery is imminent.
2. The ultrasound should not be canceled but obtained emergently because the child probably has a perforated appendix.
3. The child will not be discharged due to most likely having a perforated appendix.
4. **The physician should be notified immediately, as a sudden change or loss of pain often indicates a perforated appendix.**

TEST-TAKING HINT: The test taker should eliminate answers 1 and 2 because there is no reason to cancel the ultrasound. The physician should always be notified of any changes in a patient's condition.

22. 1. This response is not helpful and dismisses the parent's concern.
2. **A positive Rovsing sign occurs when the left lower quadrant is palpated and pain is felt in the right lower quadrant.**
3. Pain that is felt when the hand is removed during palpation is called rebound tenderness.
4. Pain that is felt when the child coughs is called a positive cough sign.

TEST-TAKING HINT: The test taker should immediately eliminate answer 1 because it is not therapeutic and is dismissive.

23. 1. The semi-Fowler position does not provide the most comfort to the postoperative appendectomy child.
2. The prone position does not allow the nurse to visualize the incision easily and would probably be uncomfortable for the child.
3. **The right side-lying position promotes comfort and allows the peritoneal cavity to drain.**
4. The left side-lying position may not provide as much comfort and will not allow the peritoneal cavity to drain as freely as the right side-lying position.

TEST-TAKING HINT: The test taker should be led to answer 3 because lying on the same side as the abdominal incision is usually the most comfortable for the child.

24. 1. An NGT is not needed when an appendix has not ruptured.
2. Antiembolic stockings are not used in children this young, who will likely be moving the lower extremities and ambulating.
3. The child in the immediate postoperative period is usually not wide awake.
4. **In the immediate postoperative period, the child is usually sleepy but can be roused. The child usually has an intravenous line for hydration and pain medication.**

TEST-TAKING HINT: The test taker should eliminate answer 1 because NGTs are not used unless the appendix has ruptured. Answer 2 can also be eliminated because a 4-year-old who is post appendectomy is not at risk for blood clots.

25. 1. Intravenous morphine given as needed may cause the child to have periods of pain when the medication has worn off. The child may also be hesitant to ask for pain medication, fearing an invasive procedure.

2. Liquid Tylenol with codeine may not offer sufficient pain control in the immediate postoperative period.
3. **Morphine administered through a PCA pump offers the child control over managing pain. The PCA pump also has the benefit of offering a basal rate as well as an as-needed rate for optimal pain management.**
4. The intramuscular route should be avoided if less invasive routes are available. A 5-year-old fears invasive procedures and may deny pain to avoid receiving an injection.

TEST-TAKING HINT: The test taker needs to recall that PCA analgesia is very effective, even in young children.

26. 1. Many 3-year-olds have difficulty understanding how to use an incentive spirometer.
2. **Blowing bubbles is a developmentally appropriate way to help the preschooler take deep breaths and cough.**
3. In the early postoperative period, a fever is likely a respiratory issue and not a result of infection of the incision.
4. Although acetaminophen may be administered, encouraging the child to breathe deeply and cough will help prevent the fever from returning.

TEST-TAKING HINT: The test taker should be aware that a fever in the first few days after surgery is generally due to pulmonary complications, so that answer 3 can be eliminated. Remembering the developmental needs of the child, the test taker should select answer 2.

27. 1. The child should wait a few days to return to school to avoid being easily fatigued at first.
2. **The child should wait 6 weeks before returning to any strenuous activity.**
3. Any signs of infection should be reported to the primary care provider.
4. The child should be encouraged to walk every day because it will help the bowels return to normal and help the child regain stamina.

TEST-TAKING HINT: The test taker should note that the question is asking which of the answers indicate that more education is needed. Answer 2 should be selected because 2 weeks is too early to return to strenuous contact sports.

28. 1. **The early stages of acute hepatitis are referred to as the anicteric phase,**

during which the child usually complains of nausea, vomiting, and generalized malaise.
2. A tender enlarged liver is noted in the right upper quadrant.
3. The child does not appear jaundiced until the icteric phase.
4. The child does not appear jaundiced until the icteric phase. The child usually does not feel well during the early stages of acute hepatitis.

TEST-TAKING HINT: The test taker needs to be familiar with the manifestations of acute hepatitis. Knowing that the early stage is referred to as the anicteric phase, answers 3 and 4 can be eliminated.

29. 1. **A diet that is high in protein and carbohydrates helps maintain caloric intake and protein stores while preventing muscle wasting. A low-fat diet prevents abdominal distention.**
2. The child should be encouraged to consume a diet higher in protein.
3. The child should be encouraged to consume a low-fat diet.
4. The child should be encouraged to consume a low-fat diet.

TEST-TAKING HINT: The child with hepatitis is usually placed on a diet that is high in both protein and carbohydrates but low in fat.

30. 1. The child with acute hepatitis usually does not feel well, and activities should be limited to quiet, restful ones.
2. The child with acute hepatitis usually does not feel well, and activities should be limited to quiet, restful ones.
3. Video games are not developmentally appropriate for a 3-year-old
4. **Playing with puzzles is a developmentally appropriate activity for a 3-year-old on bedrest.**

TEST-TAKING HINT: The test taker should incorporate developmentally appropriate activities for the child in the early stages of acute hepatitis. Answers 1 and 2 can be eliminated as they are not activities that can be done while resting. Answer 4 should be selected because it is a better activity for a 3-year-old.

31. 1. **The infant with biliary atresia usually has an enlarged liver and spleen. The stools appear clay-colored due to the absence of bile pigments. The urine is tea-colored due to the excretion of bile salts.**

2. The urine typically contains bile salts, not blood. There is usually no blood noted in the stool.
3. The skin is usually dry and itchy, not oily.
4. Manifestations of biliary atresia usually appear by 3 weeks of life.

TEST-TAKING HINT: The test taker needs to be familiar with the manifestations of biliary atresia and should be led to select answer 1.

32. 1. Although cholestyramine is used to lower cholesterol, its primary purpose in the child with biliary atresia is to relieve pruritus.
    2. The primary reason cholestyramine is administered to the child with biliary atresia is to relieve pruritus.
    3. Cholestyramine is not administered to help the child gain weight.
    4. Cholestyramine does not assist with the absorption of feedings.

TEST-TAKING HINT: The test taker needs to consider the manifestations of the disease process when considering why medications are administered. The liver is unable to eliminate bile, which leads to intense pruritus.

33. **1. The Kasai procedure is a palliative procedure in which a bile duct is attached to a loop of bowel to assist with bile drainage.**
    2. The procedure is palliative, not curative because most children require a liver transplant after a few years.
    3. The Kasai procedure does not band a bile duct.
    4. The Kasai procedure does not band a bile duct.

TEST-TAKING HINT: The test taker should eliminate answers 2 and 3 as the majority of cases of biliary atresia require a liver transplant. The Kasai procedure is performed to give the child a few years to grow before requiring a transplant.

34. 1. The palate is not repaired until the child is approximately 18 months old to allow for growth. Waiting beyond 18 months may interfere with speech.
    2. The lip is usually repaired in the first few weeks of life, and the palate is usually repaired at approximately 18 months.
    3. The palate is repaired earlier than 3 years so that speech development is not impaired.
    4. The lip is repaired in the first few weeks of life, but the palate is not
    usually repaired until the child is 18 months old.

TEST-TAKING HINT: The test taker should consider the palate's involvement in the development of speech and therefore eliminate answer 3. The palate is usually given at least a year to grow sufficiently.

35. 1. Encouraging parents to express their feelings is important, but it is more appropriate to give the parents information on breastfeeding.
    2. Some mothers are able to breastfeed their infants who have a cleft lip and palate. The breast can help fill in the cleft and help the infant create suction.
    3. Breastfeeding is sometimes an option.
    4. Breastfeeding does not increase the risk of aspiration among infants with a cleft lip and palate.

TEST-TAKING HINT: The test taker should be led to select answer 2 because the breast can sometimes act to fill in the cleft.

36. 1. The infant may rub the face on the bedding if positioned on the side.
    2. The infant may rub the face on the bedding if positioned on the side.
    3. The supine position is preferred because there is decreased risk of the infant rubbing the suture line.
    4. The infant may rub the face on the bedding if positioned on the abdomen.

TEST-TAKING HINT: The test taker should be led to answer 3 because it is the only option in which the suture line is not at increased risk for injury.

37. 1. The child should not be allowed to use anything that creates suction in the mouth, such as pacifiers or straws.
    2. The child should not have anything hard in the mouth, such as crackers, cookies, or a spoon.
    3. Pain medication should be administered regularly to avoid crying, which places stress on the suture line.
    4. A Yankauer suction should not be used in the mouth because it creates suction and is a hard instrument that could irritate the suture line. The child should be positioned to allow secretions to drain out of the child's mouth. Suction should be used only in the event of an emergency.

TEST-TAKING HINT: The child who has had a cleft palate repair should have nothing in the mouth that could irritate the suture line. Answers 1, 2, and 4 can be eliminated.

38. **1. Maternal polyhydramnios is present because the infant cannot swallow and absorb the amniotic fluid in utero.**
2. Many mothers of infants with esophageal atresia deliver early due to the pressure of the unabsorbed amniotic fluid.
3. Although good nutrition is essential in every pregnancy, there is not a direct relationship between diet and esophageal atresia.
4. Although alcohol should not be consumed in any pregnancy, there is not a direct link between diet and esophageal atresia.

TEST-TAKING HINT: The test taker should select answer 1 because esophageal atresia prevents the infant from ingesting much, leading to increased amniotic fluid in utero.

39. 1. The infant's feeding should be stopped immediately and oxygen administered. The nurse should call for help but should not leave the infant while in distress.
2. The mother should stop feeding the infant, but oxygen should be applied while the infant is cyanotic. The infant should be placed on a monitor, and vital signs should be obtained.
3. Although obtaining oxygen saturations is extremely important, the infant is visually cyanotic, so the nurse should administer oxygen as a priority.
4. The infant should be taken from the mother and placed in the crib where the nurse can assess the baby. Oxygen should be administered immediately, and vital signs should be obtained.

TEST-TAKING HINT: The test taker should be led to answer 4 because the baby is cyanotic and needs oxygen.

40. 1. The infant should be monitored, and vital signs should be obtained frequently, but the parents should be encouraged to hold their baby.
2. Intravenous fluids are administered to prevent dehydration because the infant is NPO. Intravenous antibiotics are administered to prevent pneumonia because aspiration of secretions is likely.
3. The infant should receive only the amount of oxygen needed to keep saturations above 94%.
4. As soon as the diagnosis is made, the infant is made NPO immediately because the risk for aspiration is extremely high.

TEST-TAKING HINT: Infants with tracheoesophageal atresia are at great risk for
aspiration and subsequent pneumonia. With this knowledge, the test taker should eliminate answer 4 and select answer 2.

41. 1. Medications can be placed in the GT also.
2. Two ounces of water is too much water for an infant and could cause electrolyte imbalances. The tube can be flushed with 3 to 5 mL to prevent clogging.
3. The area around the GT should be cleaned with soap and water to prevent an infection.
4. If redness develops, the parents should call the physician because an infection could be present.

TEST-TAKING HINT: The test taker should immediately eliminate answer 1 because medications and feedings can be placed in the GT. The test taker should recall that 2 ounces of water after each feeding is a large amount (recalling that infants are typically fed at least every 4 hours).

42. 1. Umbilical hernias occur more often in low-birth-weight infants.
2. Umbilical hernias occur more often in African-American infants than in white infants.
3. Umbilical hernias affect males and females equally.
4. Umbilical hernias occur more often in premature infants.

TEST-TAKING HINT: The test taker needs to be familiar with the occurrence of umbilical hernias.

43. 1. Most umbilical hernias resolve spontaneously by age 2 to 3 years. Surgery is not usually recommended until the age of 3 because the hernia may resolve before that.
2. If the hernia appears larger, swollen, or tender, the intestine may be trapped, which is a surgical emergency.
3. A pressure dressing should never be placed over the hernia because it can cause irritation and does not help the hernia resolve.
4. If the hernia is corrected surgically, the recurrence rate is low.

TEST-TAKING HINT: The test taker should be led to select answer 2 because a change in the hernia indicates an incarcerated hernia, which is an emergency.

44. 1. This approach sounds like the nurse is avoiding the mother's question. It would be better to offer the information and then ask about her concerns.

2. It is not at all uncommon for a family to have multiple children with pyloric stenosis.

3. **Pyloric stenosis can run in families, and it is more common in males.**

4. Although pyloric stenosis occurs more often in males, it can occur in females, especially in siblings of a child with pyloric stenosis.

TEST-TAKING HINT: The test taker needs to be familiar with pyloric stenosis.

45. 1. Infants with pyloric stenosis tend to be perpetually hungry because most of their feedings do not get absorbed.
2. Infants with pyloric stenosis vomit immediately after a feeding, especially as the pylorus becomes more hypertrophied.
3. **Infants with pyloric stenosis are always hungry and often appear malnourished.**
4. Most infants with pyloric stenosis are irritable because they are hungry. Parents do not usually describe the vomiting episodes as "spitting up" because infants tend to have projectile vomiting.

TEST-TAKING HINT: Recall the dynamics of pyloric stenosis. Because feedings are not absorbed, the infant is irritable and hungry. The test taker can eliminate answers 1 and 4 and select answer 3.

46. 1. In addition to giving fluids intravenously and keeping the infant NPO, an NGT is placed to decompress the stomach.
2. **In addition to giving fluids intravenously and keeping the infant NPO, an NGT is placed to decompress the stomach.**
3. The pylorus is distal to the stomach, so an NGT is placed above the obstruction.
4. The infant is made NPO as soon as diagnosis is confirmed. Allowing the infant to feed perpetuates the vomiting and continued hypertrophy of the pylorus.

TEST-TAKING HINT: The test taker should consider the pathophysiology of pyloric stenosis and eliminate answers 1, 3, and 4.

47. 1. **The infant is displaying signs of intussusception. This is an emergency that needs to be evaluated to prevent ischemia and perforation.**
2. The mother should be told not to give the infant anything by mouth and bring the infant immediately to the emergency room.
3. Although similar symptoms may be seen among infants with allergies, a more serious illness must first be ruled out. It is

uncommon to see lethargy as a response to an allergy.

4. All bloody stools should be evaluated.

TEST-TAKING HINT: The child is described as lethargic and is having diarrhea and vomiting. This child needs to be seen to rule out an intussusception. At the very least, the mother should be told to bring the child to the emergency room because the described signs could also be seen in severe dehydration. The test taker should be led to select answer 1.

48. 1. The enema is used for confirmation of diagnosis and reduction. In most cases of intussusception in young children, an enema is successful in reducing the intussusception.
2. In most cases of intussusception in young children, an enema is successful in reducing the intussusception.
3. **In most cases of intussusception in young children, an enema is successful in reducing the intussusception.**
4. There is not a high likelihood that the intussusception will recur.

TEST-TAKING HINT: The test taker needs to be aware that intussusceptions in young children respond well to reduction by enema.

49. 1. The child has already been diagnosed and appears to have developed peritonitis, which is a surgical emergency.
2. Although reducing enemas have a high success rate among infants with intussusception, they are contraindicated in the presence of peritonitis.
3. Although a second intravenous line may be needed, the nurse's first priority is getting the child to the operating room.
4. **Intussusception with peritonitis is a surgical emergency, so preparing the infant for surgery is the nurse's top priority.**

TEST-TAKING HINT: The child has already been diagnosed and is displaying signs of shock and peritonitis. The nurse must act quickly and get the child the surgical attention needed to avoid disastrous consequences.

50. 1. Although a rectal thermometer should never be used in a child with an anorectal malformation, an oral thermometer should not be used in an infant or young child.
2. **A change in stool form is important to report because it could indicate stenosis of the rectum.**

3. The child with a low anorectal malformation should be capable of achieving bowel continence.
4. Any stool in the urine should be reported because it indicates a fistula is present.

TEST-TAKING HINT: The test taker should eliminate answer 3 as it contains the word "never." There are very few circumstances in health care in which "never" is the case.

51. 1. The child who has stool in the urine has a fistula connecting the rectum to the urinary tract, and the anorectal malformation cannot be low.
    2. **The presence of stool in the urine indicates that the anorectal malformation is high.**
    3. This child probably needs a colostomy.
    4. This malformation requires surgical correction.

TEST-TAKING HINT: The test taker needs to consider that stool is present in the urine, indicating a fistula is present and a more complex anorectal malformation exists, so answers 1 and 4 can be eliminated.

52. 1. The stoma should be red in color, indicating good perfusion.
    2. Discharge or irritation around the stoma could indicate the presence of an infection.
    3. **The colostomy contains stool from the large intestine; an ileostomy contains the very irritating stool from the small intestine.**
    4. Babies usually develop a pattern to their bowel habits as they grow.

TEST-TAKING HINT: Although it is important to keep a bag attached to the colostomy, the contents are not the irritating effluent of an ileostomy.

53. 1. **The inability to digest protein leads to an accumulation of an amino acid that is toxic to the mucosal cells and villi, leading to absorption problems.**
    2. Extra villi cells are not created. Instead, villi become damaged, leading to absorption problems.
    3. The intestine does not become more porous. There is difficulty with absorbing vitamins, leading to deficiencies, not toxicity.
    4. The child experiences diarrhea, not constipation.

TEST-TAKING HINT: The test taker needs to recall the pathophysiology of celiac disease in order to select answer 1. By

recalling that the child with celiac usually appears malnourished and experiences diarrhea, the test taker can eliminate answers 3 and 4.

54. 1. Rye toast contains gluten.
    2. Unless otherwise indicated, pancakes are made of flour, which contains gluten.
    3. Oat cereal contains gluten.
    4. **Cheese, banana slices, rice cakes, and whole milk do not contain gluten.**

TEST-TAKING HINT: The test taker needs to recall that children with celiac disease cannot tolerate gluten, which is found in wheat, barley, rye, and oats. Answers 1, 2, and 3 contain gluten.

55. 1. Although a blood count and serum electrolyte evaluation will likely be included in the child's evaluation, the diagnosis cannot be confirmed without a stool sample and jejuna biopsy.
    2. The child is not usually kept NPO but is monitored to assess the response to the gluten-free diet.
    3. **A stool sample for analysis of fat and a jejunal biopsy can confirm the diagnosis.**
    4. The child's response to a gluten-free diet is monitored.

TEST-TAKING HINT: The test taker should eliminate answers 1, 2, and 4 because they do not include preparing the child for a jejunal biopsy, which is the key to a definitive diagnosis of celiac disease.

56. 1. The feedings tend to take longer and often do not get absorbed before the next scheduled feeding.
    2. **Bloody diarrhea can indicate that the infant has NEC.**
    3. Bowel sounds tend to decrease, not increase.
    4. The infant does not appear hungry but irritable.

TEST-TAKING HINT: The test taker needs to be familiar with manifestations of NEC and be led to select answer 2.

57. 1. The feedings should immediately be stopped, but the NGT should be placed to allow decompression of the stomach.
    2. Vital signs should be obtained more frequently than every 4 hours because the infant is at high risk for peritonitis and sepsis.
    3. **Intravenous antibiotics are administered to prevent or treat sepsis.**
    4. Feedings are stopped immediately when a suspicion of NEC is present.

TEST-TAKING HINT: The test taker needs to consider the plan of care for an infant with NEC. This child is at risk for becoming critically ill, so feedings are stopped and vital signs are monitored very closely.

58. 1. It is thought that the breast milk contains macrophages that help fight infection, preventing NEC.
    2. Because NEC is seen primarily in preterm and low-birth-weight infants, their increased survival rate has lead to an increase in the occurrence of NEC.
    3. The infant's condition deteriorates rapidly when sepsis occurs, so early recognition and treatment are essential.
    4. **Although much more common in preterm and low-birth-weight infants, NEC is also seen in term infants as well.**

TEST-TAKING HINT: The test taker needs to be familiar with general concepts associated with NEC. Answer 4 contains the word "only," which is an absolute value that is rarely used in health care.

59. 1. Children with SBS experience diarrhea, not constipation.
    2. **Because the intestine is used for absorption, children with SBS usually need alternative forms of nutrition such as hyperalimentation.**
    3. Without knowing how much intestine is involved, the nurse cannot make this assumption about prognosis and should not share this information with the infant's parents.
    4. It is therapeutic to acknowledge the parents' concern. Without knowing the parents' knowledge base, this response may or may not be above the level of their comprehension.

TEST-TAKING HINT: The test taker should eliminate answer 1 as it is false. Answer 3 can also be eliminated because it makes a generalization that should not be made without knowing the details of the child's diagnosis.

60. 1. It is important for children with SBS to receive some feedings, either by tube or mouth, so that the intestine receives some stimulation.
    2. Although TPN can cause long-term challenges, there is not an absolute time limit.
    3. **It is important to begin feedings as soon as the bowel is healed so that it receives stimulation and does not atrophy.**

4. Feedings are provided by mouth or tube based on each child's needs.

TEST-TAKING HINT: The test taker could eliminate answers 1 and 4 as they contain the word "never," which is rarely used in health-care scenarios.

61. **1, 2, 3, 5.**
    1. **The lights in phototherapy increase insensible fluid loss, requiring the nurse to monitor fluid status closely.**
    2. **The infant with pyloric stenosis is likely to be dehydrated due to persistent vomiting.**
    3. **A 2-year-old with pneumonia may have increased insensible fluid loss due to tachypnea associated with respiratory illness. The nurse needs to monitor fluid status cautiously because fluid overload can result in increased respiratory distress.**
    4. An adolescent starting her menses is not at risk for dehydration.
    5. **The child with a burn experiences extensive extracellular fluid loss and is at great risk for dehydration. The younger child is at greater risk due to greater proportionate body surface area.**

TEST-TAKING HINT: The test taker needs to know that an infant needing phototherapy, an infant with persistent vomiting, a child with pneumonia, and a child with burns require more fluids because of the risk of dehydration.

62. **1, 2, 3, 4.**
    1. **Hypothyroidism can be a causative factor in constipation.**
    2. **Weakened abdominal muscles can be seen in muscular dystrophy and can lead to constipation.**
    3. **Myelomeningocele affects the innervation of the rectum and can lead to constipation.**
    4. **Excessive milk consumption can lead to constipation.**
    5. Activity tends to decrease constipation and increase regularity.

TEST-TAKING HINT: The test taker has to know which of these conditions can cause constipation.

Genitourinary Disorders

9

KEYWORDS

Albuminemia
Bladder exstrophy
Cryptorchidism
Dialysate
Disequilibrium syndrome
Enuresis
Epispadias
Glomerulonephritis
Hematuria
Hemodialysis

Hydronephrosis
Hypospadias
Inguinal hernia
Peritoneal dialysis
Phimosis
Proteinuria
Reticulocyte
Testicular torsion

ABBREVIATIONS

Acute renal failure (ARF)
Chronic renal failure (CRF)
Desmopressin acetate (DDAVP)
Hemolytic uremic syndrome (HUS)
Kilogram (kg)
Milliliter (mL)

Minimal change nephrotic syndrome
 (MCNS)
Urinary tract infection (UTI)
Vesicoureteral reflux (VUR)
Voiding cystourethrogram (VCUG)

QUESTIONS

1. The nurse is reviewing the basic anatomy and physiology of the genitourinary system.
   e The nurse knows that the bladder capacity of a 3-year-old could be estimated to be
   approximately how much?
   1. 1.5 oz.
   2. 3 oz.
   3. 4 oz.
   4. 5 oz.

2. The nurse is caring for a 4-year-old who weighs 15 kg. At the end of a 10-hour period, the nurse notes the urine output to be 150 mL. What action does the nurse take?
   1. The nurse notifies the physician because this urine output is too low.
   2. The nurse encourages the patient to increase oral intake in order to increase urine output.
   3. The nurse records the patient's urine output in the chart.
   4. The nurse administers isotonic fluid intravenously to help with the rehydration process.

3. A 3-year-old has a recurrent UTI. She had a UTI 3 months ago and was treated with an oral antibiotic. A follow-up urinalysis revealed results within normal range. The child has had no other problems until this visit. Choose the nurse's best response.
   1. The nurse should prepare for the following tests: urinalysis, urine culture, and VCUG.
   2. Signs and symptoms of renal failure should be evaluated.
   3. The nurse should prepare the child for likely admission to the pediatric unit.
   4. Send the child home on an antibiotic and instruct the parent to offer the child lots of fluids.

4. The nurse is instructing a group of girls and parents about the importance of preventing UTIs. Which of the following should the nurse teach?
   1. Avoiding constipation has no effect on the occurrence of UTIs.
   2. After urinating, always wipe from back to front to prevent fecal contamination.
   3. Hygiene is an important preventive measure and can be accomplished with frequent tub baths.
   4. Increasing fluids will help prevent and treat UTIs.

5. The nurse is working in a pediatric urgent care clinic. Which of the following patients can be discharged without the need for a urinalysis to evaluate for a UTI?
   1. A 4-month-old female who presents with a 2-day history of fussiness and poor appetite; her current vital signs include T 100.8°F (38.2°C) (axillary) and heart rate 120 beats per minute.
   2. An 8-year-old male who presents with a finger laceration; his mother states he had surgical reimplantation of his ureters 2 years ago.
   3. A 12-year-old female complaining of pain to her lower right back; she denies any burning or frequency at this time; she has an oral temperature of 101.5°F (38.6°C).
   4. A 4-year-old female who states "it hurts when I pee"; her parent states that she has been asking to urinate every 30 minutes; vital signs are within normal range.

6. An 8-month-old is being evaluated for a UTI. A urinalysis and urine culture are ordered. Which of the following is the best way to obtain the urine sample?
   1. Carefully cleanse the perineum from front to back, and apply a self-adhesive urine collection bag to the perineum.
   2. Insert an indwelling Foley catheter and begin antibiotic administration.
   3. Place a sterile cotton ball in the diaper, and immediately obtain the sample with a syringe after the first void.
   4. Using a straight catheter, obtain the sample, and immediately remove the catheter without waiting for the results of the urine sample.

7. On reviewing information about glomerulonephritis, the nurse knows that which of the following children is at risk for developing the disease?
   1. A 10-year-old recovering from viral pneumonia.
   2. A 6-year-old with new-onset type 1 diabetes.
   3. A 3-year-old who had impetigo 1 week ago.
   4. A 5-year-old with a history of five UTIs in the previous year.

8. The nurse is caring for a 7-year-old with glomerulonephritis. Which of the following combinations of signs is commonly associated with glomerulonephritis?
   1. Massive proteinuria, hematuria, decreased urinary output, and lethargy.
   2. Mild proteinuria, increased urinary output, and lethargy.
   3. Mild proteinuria, hematuria, decreased urinary output, and lethargy.
   4. Massive proteinuria, decreased urinary output, and hypotension.

9. The parents of a child with glomerulonephritis ask the nurse why the urine is such a funny color. What is the nurse's best response?
   1. "It is not uncommon for the urine to be discolored when children are receiving steroids and blood pressure medications."
   2. "There is blood in your child's urine that causes it to be tea-colored."
   3. "Your child's urine is very concentrated, so it appears to be discolored."
   4. "A ketogenic diet often causes the urine to be tea-colored."

10. The nurse is caring for a 7-year-old with glomerulonephritis. Which of the following findings requires immediate attention?
    1. The child sleeps most of the day and is very "cranky" when awake; blood pressure is 170/90.
    2. The child's urine output is 190 mL in an 8-hour period and is the color of Coca Cola.
    3. The child complains of a severe headache and photophobia.
    4. The child refuses breakfast and lunch and states that he "just is not hungry."

11. The parents of a child with glomerulonephritis ask how will they know that the condition is improving after they take their child home. What is the nurse's best response?
    1. "Your child's urine output will increase, and the urine will become less tea-colored."
    2. "Your child will rest more comfortably."
    3. "Your child's appetite will decrease."
    4. "Your child's laboratory test values will become more normal."

12. A 5-year-old is hospitalized with MCNS. The nurse obtains a history from the parents. Which statement by the parents is most consistent with MCNS?
    1. "Our child missed 2 days of school last week because of a really bad cold."
    2. "We went camping last week, and our child's legs were covered in bug bites."
    3. "Our child came home from school a week ago due to vomiting and stomach cramps."
    4. "Our child has a pet turtle but does not wash hands after playing with the turtle."

13. The nurse is teaching the family about MCNS and explains that the clinical manifestations are due to which of the following?
    1. Chemical changes in the composition of albumin.
    2. Increased permeability of the glomeruli.
    3. Obstruction of the capillaries of the glomeruli because of antibody-antigen complex formation.
    4. Loss of the kidney's ability to excrete waste and concentrate urine.

14. The parents of a child hospitalized with MCNS ask why the last blood test revealed elevated lipids. What is the nurse's best response?
    1. "If your child had just eaten a fatty meal, the lipids may have been falsely elevated."
    2. "It's not unusual to see elevated lipids in children because of the dietary habits of today."
    3. "Since your child is losing so much protein, the liver is stimulated and ends up making more lipids."
    4. "Your child's blood is very concentrated because of the edema, so the lipids are falsely elevated."

15. The nurse is caring for a 2-year-old hospitalized with MCNS. The edema has progressed from periorbital to generalized. The skin appears stretched, and areas of breakdown are noted over the bony prominences. The child has been receiving Lasix twice daily for several days. In order to reduce edema, which of the following does the nurse expect to be included in the treatment plan?
    1. An increase in the amount and frequency of Lasix.
    2. Addition of a second diuretic, such as mannitol.
    3. Administration of intravenous albumin.
    4. Elimination of all fluids and sodium from the child's diet.

16. A 3-year-old returns to the pediatric clinic after having had MCNS. His parents ask the nurse how to prevent the child from having it again. What is the nurse's best response?
    1. "It is very rare for a child to have a relapse after having fully recovered."
    2. "Unfortunately, many children have cycles of relapses, and there is very little that can be done to prevent it."
    3. "Your child is much less likely to get sick again if sodium is avoided in his diet."
    4. "Try to keep your child away from sick children because relapses have been associated with infectious illnesses."

17. The nurse is caring for a newborn male with hypospadias. His parents ask if circumcision is an option. Which is the nurse's best response?
    1. "Circumcision is a fading practice and is now contraindicated in most children."
    2. "Circumcision in children with hypospadias is recommended because it helps prevent infection."
    3. "Circumcision is an option, but it cannot be done at this time."
    4. "Circumcision can never be performed in a child with hypospadias."

18. A 6-week-old male is scheduled for a hypospadias and chordee repair. The parent tells the nurse, "I understand why the hypospadias repair is necessary, but do they have to fix the chordee as well?" What is the nurse's best response?
    1. "I understand your concern. Parents do not want their children to undergo extra surgery."
    2. "The chordee repair is done strictly for cosmetic reasons that may affect your son as he ages."
    3. "The repair is done to optimize his sexual function when he is older."
    4. "This is the best time to repair the chordee because he will be having surgery anyway."

19. A 13-month-old is being discharged following the repair of his epispadias. Which of the following statements made by the parents indicate that they understand the discharge teaching?
    1. "If a mucous plug forms in the urinary drainage tube, we will irrigate it gently to prevent a blockage."
    2. "If a mucous plug forms in the urinary drainage tube, we will allow it to pass on its own because this is a sign of healing."
    3. "We will make sure the dressing is loosely applied to increase the toddler's comfort."
    4. "If we notice any yellow drainage, we will know that everything is healing well."

20. A 2-year-old is admitted to the pediatric floor with a diagnosis of HUS. Which of the following would the nurse likely find in the child's history?
    1. The child has a history of frequent UTIs and possible VUR.
    2. The child and parents had vomiting and diarrhea, but the parents believe it was due to "probably something that they ate."
    3. The child was stung by a bee and experienced localized edema to the site for 3 days.
    4. The child had previously been healthy and did not show any signs of illness until this admission.

21. The nurse is reviewing the pathophysiology of HUS. The manifestations of the disease are due primarily to which of the following events?
    1. The swollen lining of the small blood vessels damages the red blood cells, which are then removed by the spleen, leading to anemia.
    2. There is a disturbance of the glomerular basement membrane, allowing large proteins to pass through.
    3. The red blood cell changes shape, causing it to obstruct microcirculation.
    4. There is a depression in the production of all formed elements of the blood.

22. A 16-month-old with HUS has had blood and urine samples sent to the laboratory. Which of the following results are most consistent with his HUS?
    1. Hematuria, massive proteinuria, elevated blood urea nitrogen, and creatinine.
    2. Hematuria, mild proteinuria, decreased blood urea nitrogen, and creatinine.
    3. Hematuria, mild proteinuria, increased blood urea nitrogen, and creatinine.
    4. Ketonuria, proteinuria, elevated blood urea nitrogen, and creatinine.

23. A 3-year-old is admitted to the pediatric unit with a diagnosis of HUS. The child is very pale and lethargic. Stools have progressed from watery to bloody diarrhea. Blood work indicates low hemoglobin and low hematocrit levels. The child has not had any urine output in 24 hours. The nurse expects which of the following to be added to the plan of care?
    1. Administration of blood products and initiation of dialysis.
    2. Administration of blood products and close observation of the child's hemodynamic status.
    3. Administration of blood products followed by diuretic therapy to force urinary output.
    4. Administration of clotting factors to diminish blood loss and continued monitoring of urinary output.

24. The nurse knows that which of the following need to be present to diagnose HUS?
    1. Increased red blood cells with a low reticulocyte count, increased platelet count, and renal failure.
    2. Decreased red blood cells with a high reticulocyte count, decreased platelet count, and renal failure.
    3. Increased red blood cells with a high reticulocyte count, increased platelet count, and renal failure.
    4. Decreased red blood cells with a low reticulocyte count, decreased platelet count, and renal failure.

25. A 5-year-old is being discharged from the hospital following the diagnosis of HUS. The child has been free of diarrhea for 1 week, and renal function has returned. The parent asks the nurse when the child can return to school. What is the nurse's best response?
    1. "Immediately, as your child is no longer contagious."
    2. "It would be best to keep your child home for a few more weeks because the immune system is weak, and there could be a relapse of HUS."
    3. "Your child will be contagious for approximately another 10 days, so it is best to not allow a return just yet."
    4. "It would be best to keep your child home to monitor urinary output."

26. A newborn is diagnosed with bladder exstrophy that includes a malformed pelvis. Which of the following is a priority of care?
    1. Change the diaper frequently and assess for skin breakdown.
    2. Keep the exposed bladder open in a warm and dry environment to avoid any heat loss.
    3. Immediately administer a dextrose-containing solution intravenously to avoid any possibility of hypoglycemia.
    4. Cluster all care to allow the child to sleep, grow, and gain strength for the upcoming surgical repair.

27. Which of the following medications would most likely be included in the postoperative care of a child with repair of bladder exstrophy?
    1. Lasix.
    2. Mannitol.
    3. Meperidine.
    4. Oxybutynin.

28. The nurse is providing discharge instructions to the parents of an infant born with bladder exstrophy who had a continent urinary reservoir placed. Which of the following statements should be included?
    1. "Allowing your child to sleep on the abdomen will provide comfort during the immediate postoperative period."
    2. "As your child grows, be cautious around playgrounds because the surface could be a health hazard."
    3. "As your child grows, be sure to encourage many different foods because it is not likely that food allergies will develop."
    4. "In order to encourage your child's development, keep the environment stimulating by having brightly colored things around, such as balloons."

29. The nurse understands that the clinical manifestations in hydronephrosis are due to which of the following?
    1. A structural abnormality in the urinary system causes urine to back up and can cause pressure and cell death.
    2. A structural abnormality causes urine to flow too freely through the urinary system, leading to fluid and electrolyte imbalances.
    3. Decreased production of urine in one or both kidneys, resulting in an electrolyte imbalance.
    4. Urine with an abnormal electrolyte balance and concentration leads to increased blood pressure and subsequent increased glomerular filtration rate.

30. A 20-month-old is admitted with hydronephrosis. The nurse notes which of the following findings?
    1. Increased blood pressure, metabolic alkalosis, polydipsia, and polyuria.
    2. Increased blood pressure, metabolic acidosis, and bacterial growth in the urine.
    3. Increased blood pressure, metabolic alkalosis, and bacterial growth in the urine.
    4. Increased blood pressure, metabolic acidosis, polydipsia, polyuria, and bacterial growth in the urine.

31. A 16-month-old is admitted to the pediatric unit with a diagnosis of hydronephrosis. Which of the following should be included in the plan of care?
    1. Intake and output as well as vital signs should be strictly monitored.
    2. Fluids and sodium in the diet should be limited.
    3. Steroids should be administered as ordered.
    4. The child's contact with other people should be limited to avoid infection.

32. The nurse in a diabetic clinic sees a 10-year-old who is a new diabetic and has had trouble maintaining blood glucose levels within normal limits. The patient's parent states the child has had several daytime "accidents." The nurse knows that this is referred to as which of the following?
    1. Primary enuresis.
    2. Secondary enuresis.
    3. Diurnal enuresis.
    4. Nocturnal enuresis.

33. At a well-child health screening, the parent of a 7-year-old voices concern over the child's continued bed-wetting at night. The parent, on going to bed, has tried getting the child up at 11:30 p.m., but the child still wakes up wet. What is the nurse's best response about what the parent should do next?
    1. "There is a medication called DDAVP that decreases the volume of the urine. The physician thinks that will work for your child."
    2. "When your child wakes up wet, be very firm, and indicate how displeased you are. Have your child change the sheets to see how much work is involved."
    3. "Limit fluids in the evening, and start a reward system in which your child can choose a reward after a certain number of dry nights."
    4. "Bed-wetting alarms are readily available, and most children do very well with them."

34. The nurse receives a call from the parent of a 15-year-old male. The son woke up complaining of intense pain and swelling to the scrotal area. He has vomited twice and is also complaining of abdominal pain. Which of the following should the nurse suggest?
    1. Encourage him to drink clear liquids until the vomiting subsides; if he gets worse, bring him to the emergency room.
    2. Bring him to the pediatrician's office for evaluation.
    3. Bring him to the emergency room immediately.
    4. Encourage him to rest; apply ice to the scrotal area, and go to the emergency room if the pain does not improve.

35. The nurse knows that which of the following causes the symptoms seen in testicular torsion?
    1. Twisting of the spermatic cord interrupts the blood supply.
    2. Swelling of the scrotal sac leads to testicular displacement.
    3. Unmanaged undescended testes cause testicular displacement.
    4. Microthrombi formation in the vessels of the spermatic cord causes interruption of the blood supply.

36. The day surgery nurse knows that the parent of a 13-year-old male understands postoperative teaching for a repair of testicular torsion by saying which the following?
    1. "We will encourage him to rest for a few days, but he can return to football practice in a week."
    2. "We will keep him in bed for 4 days and let him gradually increase his activity after that."
    3. "We will seek therapy as he ages because he is now infertile."
    4. "We will make sure he knows how to do testicular self-examination on a monthly basis."

37. The nurse is caring for a 3-week-old female diagnosed with an inguinal hernia. The nurse knows that which of the following protruding into the groin most likely caused the inguinal hernia?
    1. Bowel.
    2. Fallopian tube.
    3. Large thrombus formation.
    4. Muscle tissue.

38. The parents of a 6-week-old male ask the nurse if there is a difference between an inguinal hernia and a hydrocele. What is the nurse's best response?
    1. "The terms are used interchangeably and mean the same thing."
    2. "The symptoms are similar, but an inguinal hernia occurs when tissue protrudes into the groin, whereas a hydrocele is a fluid-filled mass in the groin."
    3. "A hydrocele is the term used when an inguinal hernia occurs in females."
    4. "A hydrocele presents in a manner similar to that of an inguinal hernia but causes increased concern because it is often malignant."

39. The nurse is speaking to the parents of an infant with an inguinal hernia. The nurse knows the parents understand the teaching when they say which of the following?
    1. "There are no risks associated with waiting to have the hernia reduced; surgery is done for cosmetic reasons."
    2. "It is normal to see the bulge in the baby's groin decrease with a bowel movement."
    3. "We will wait for surgery until the baby is older because narcotics for pain control will be required for several days."
    4. "It is normal for the bulge in the baby's groin to look smaller when the baby is asleep."

40. The nurse is working in the emergency department when an infant with a diagnosis of incarcerated hernia is brought in. The nurse would expect to hear the parents report a history of which of the following?
    1. Acute onset of pain, abdominal distention, and a mass that cannot be reduced.
    2. Gradual onset of pain, abdominal distention, and a mass that cannot be reduced.
    3. Acute onset of pain, abdominal distention, and a mass that is easily reduced.
    4. Gradual onset of pain, abdominal distention, and a mass that is easily reduced.

41. The parent of a 3-year-old is shocked to hear the diagnosis of Wilms tumor and says, "How could I have missed a lump this big?" What is the nurse's best response?
    1. "Do not be hard on yourself. It's easy to overlook something that has probably been growing for months when we see our children on a regular basis."
    2. "I understand you must be very upset. Your child would have had a better prognosis had you caught it earlier."
    3. "It really takes a trained professional to recognize something like this."
    4. "Do not blame yourself. This mass grows so fast that it was probably not noticeable a few days ago."

42. The nurse is caring for a 4-year-old child with a Wilms tumor. Which of the following would the nurse expect to find on assessment?
    1. Decreased blood pressure, increased temperature, and a firm mass located in one flank area.
    2. Increased blood pressure, temperature within normal limits, and a firm mass located in one flank area.
    3. Increased blood pressure, temperature within normal limits, and a firm mass located on one side or the other of the midline of the abdomen.
    4. Decreased blood pressure, temperature within normal limits, and a firm mass located on one side or the other of the midline of the abdomen.

43. The nurse is caring for a child who has just been diagnosed with a Wilms tumor. The child is scheduled for a magnetic resonance imaging of the lungs. The parents ask the nurse the reason for this test as a Wilms tumor involves the kidney, not the lung. What is the nurse's best response?
    1. "I'm not sure why your child is going for this test. I will check and get back to you."
    2. "It sounds like we made a mistake. I will check and get back to you."
    3. "The test is done to check to see if the disease has spread to the lungs."
    4. "We want to check the lungs to make sure your child is healthy enough to tolerate surgery."

44. The parents overhear the health-care team refer to their child's disease as in stage III. The parents ask the nurse what this means. The nurse responds, knowing which of the following?
    1. The tumor is confined to the abdomen, but it has spread to the lymph nodes or peritoneal area; the prognosis is poor.
    2. The tumor is confined to the abdomen, but it has spread to the lymph nodes or peritoneal area; the prognosis is still very good.
    3. The tumor has been found in three other organs beyond the peritoneal area; the prognosis is poor.
    4. The tumor has spread to other organs beyond the peritoneal area; the prognosis is poor.

45. The nurse is caring for a child due for surgery on a Wilms tumor. The nurse knows that the child's procedure will consist of which of the following?
    1. Only the affected kidney will be removed.
    2. Both the affected kidney and the other kidney will be removed in case of recurrence.
    3. The mass will be removed from the affected kidney.
    4. The mass will be removed from the affected kidney, and a biopsy of the tissue of the unaffected kidney will be done.

46. The nurse anticipates that the child who has had a kidney removed will have a high level of pain and will require invasive and noninvasive measures for pain relief. The nurse anticipates that the child will have pain because of which of the following?
    1. The kidney is removed laparoscopically, and there will be residual pain from accumulated air in the abdomen.
    2. There is a postoperative shift of fluids and organs in the abdominal cavity, leading to increased discomfort.
    3. The chemotherapy makes the child more sensitive to pain.
    4. The radiation therapy makes the child more sensitive to pain.

47. The parents of a 7-year-old tell the nurse they do not understand the difference between CRF and ARF. What is the nurse's best response?
    1. "There really is not much a difference because the terms are used interchangeably."
    2. "Most children experience ARF. It is highly unusual for a child to experience CRF.
    3. CRF tends to occur suddenly and is irreversible.
    4. ARF is often reversible, whereas CRF results in permanent deterioration of kidney function.

48. The nurse is caring for a 9-year-old in the pediatric intensive care unit. The patient had a tonsillectomy 6 days ago and was seen in the emergency room 4 hours ago due to postoperative hemorrhage. The patient's parent noted that her child was "swallowing a lot and finally began vomiting large amounts of blood." The child's vital signs are as follows: T 99.5° F (37.5°C), HR 124, BP 84/48, and RR 26. The nurse knows that this patient is at risk for which type of renal failure?
    1. CRF due to advanced disease process.
    2. Prerenal failure due to dehydration.
    3. Primary kidney damage due to a lack of urine flowing through the system.
    4. Postrenal failure due to a hypotensive state.

49. The nurse is caring for an 11-year-old diagnosed with ARF. The patient complains of "not feeling well," having "butterflies in the chest," and arms and legs "feeling like Jell-O." The nurse places the child on a cardiac monitor and notes that the QRS complex is wider than before and that an occasional premature ventricular contraction is seen. The nurse would expect to administer which of the following?
    1. An isotonic saline solution with 20 mEq KCl/L.
    2. Sodium bicarbonate via slow intravenous push.
    3. Calcium gluconate via slow intravenous push.
    4. Oral potassium supplements.

50. The nurse is caring for a 10-kg toddler who is diagnosed with ARF. The toddler has a 24-hour urine output of 110 mL and is afebrile. After calculating daily fluid maintenance, which of the following would the nurse expect the toddler's daily allotment of fluids to be?
    1. 1000 mL of oral and intravenous fluids.
    2. 2000 mL of oral and intravenous fluids.
    3. 350 mL of oral and intravenous fluids.
    4. Sips of clear fluids and ice chips only.

51. The nurse is caring for a 1-year-old diagnosed with ARF. The patient's parent calls the nurse to the bedside and says "My child's eyes cannot open." Edema is noted throughout the child's body, and the liver is enlarged. The child's urine output is less than 0.5 mL/kg/hr, and vital signs are as follows: HR 146, BP 176/92, and RR 42. The child is noted to have nasal flaring and retractions with inspiration. The lung sounds are coarse throughout. Despite receiving oral Kayexalate, the child's serum potassium continues to rise. Which of the following treatments will provide the most benefit to the patient?
    1. Additional rectal Kayexalate.
    2. Intravenous furosemide.
    3. Endotracheal intubation and ventilatory assistance.
    4. Placement of a Tenckhoff catheter for peritoneal dialysis.

52. The parent of a child diagnosed with ARF asks the nurse why peritoneal dialysis was selected instead of hemodialysis. What is the nurse's best response?
    1. "Hemodialysis is not used in the pediatric population."
    2. "Peritoneal dialysis has no complications, so it is a treatment used without hesitation."
    3. "Peritoneal dialysis removes fluid at a slower rate than hemodialysis, so many complications are avoided."
    4. "Peritoneal dialysis is much more efficient than hemodialysis."

53. The nurse is caring for a 12-year-old receiving peritoneal dialysis. The nurse notes the return to be cloudy, and the child is complaining of abdominal pain. The child's parents ask what the next step will likely be. What is the nurse's best response?
    1. "We will probably place antibiotics in the dialysis fluid before the next dwell time."
    2. "Many children experience cloudy returns. We do not usually worry about it."
    3. "We will probably give your child some oral antibiotics just to make sure nothing else develops."
    4. "The abdominal pain is likely due to the fluid going in too slowly. We will increase the rate of administration with the next fill."

54. The nurse is working in the pediatric intensive care unit, caring for a child receiving peritoneal dialysis. The nurse notes that the child has not been having adequate volume in the return. The child is currently edematous and hypertensive. The nurse would anticipate the physician to do which of the following?
    1. Increase the glucose concentration of the dialysate.
    2. Decrease the glucose concentration of the dialysate.
    3. Administer antihypertensives and diuretics but not change the dialysate concentration.
    4. Decrease the dwell time of the dialysate.

55. The nurse is working in a hemodialysis center for children. During hemodialysis, the nurse notes that a 10-year-old becomes confused and restless. The child complains of a headache and nausea and has generalized muscle twitching. The nurse knows that this situation is called disequilibrium syndrome and may be prevented by which of the following?
    1. Slowing the rate of solute removal during dialysis.
    2. Ensuring the patient is warm during dialysis.
    3. Administering antibiotics before dialysis.
    4. Obtaining an accurate weight the night before dialysis.

56. The nurse is caring for a 9-year-old diagnosed with CRF. The child's blood pressure has been consistently elevated. The nurse knows that chronic hypertension in the child who has CRF is due to which of the following?
    1. Retention of sodium and water.
    2. Obstruction of the urinary system.
    3. Accumulation of waste products in the body.
    4. Generalized metabolic alkalosis.

57. The nurse knows that the child with CRF is at risk for spontaneous fractures because of an electrolyte imbalance. Which of the following best describes the imbalance that occurs?
    1. Decreased serum phosphorus and calcium levels.
    2. Depletion of phosphorus and calcium stores from the bones.
    3. Change in the structure of the bones, causing calcium to remain in the bones.
    4. Nutritional needs are poorly met, leading to a decrease in many electrolytes such as calcium and phosphorus.

58. The nurse on the pediatric unit is verifying that the patients have received the correct lunches. She knows that the child with CRF needs to receive which of the following diets?
    1. A diet high in calories, protein, and all minerals and electrolytes.
    2. A diet with high calories but low protein and minerals.
    3. A diet high in calories, protein, and calcium and low in potassium and phosphorus.
    4. A diet high in calories, protein, phosphorus, and calcium and low in potassium and sodium.

59. The nurse is caring for a 7-year-old who received a kidney transplant 1 week ago. The child complains to the nurse about abdominal pain, and the parents note that the child has been very irritable. The nurse notes a 10% weight gain and elevated blood urea nitrogen and creatinine levels. The nurse asks the parents if the child has been taking which of the following medications?
    1. Codeine tablets.
    2. Furosemide.
    3. MiraLAX powder.
    4. Corticosteroids.

60. A 10-year-old with renal failure is scheduled to undergo renal transplantation. The nurse knows that this treatment option is which of the following?
    1. A curative procedure that will free the patient from any more treatment modalities.
    2. An ideal treatment option for families with a history of dialysis noncompliance.
    3. A treatment option that will free the patient from dialysis.
    4. A treatment option that is very new to the pediatric population.

61. The parents of a 3-year-old are concerned that the child is having "more accidents" during the day. Which of the following questions would be appropriate for the nurse to ask in order to obtain more information? Select all that apply.
    1. "Has there been a stressful event in the child's life, such as the birth of a sibling?"
    2. "Has anyone else in the family had problems with accidents?"
    3. "Does your child seem to be drinking more than usual?"
    4. "Is your child more irritable, and does your child seem to be in pain when urinating?"
    5. "Is your child having difficulties sharing at preschool?"

62. Which of the following is true of a Wilms tumor? Select all that apply.
    1. It is also referred to as neuroblastoma.
    2. It can occur at any age but is seen most often between the ages of 2 and 5 years.
    3. It can occur on its own or can be associated with many congenital anomalies.
    4. It is a slow-growing tumor.
    5. It is associated with a very poor prognosis.

ANSWERS AND RATIONALES

1. 1. The capacity of the bladder can be estimated by adding 2 to the child's age in years.
   2. The capacity of the bladder can be estimated by adding 2 to the child's age in years.
   3. The capacity of the bladder can be estimated by adding 2 to the child's age in years.
   4. **The capacity of the bladder can be estimated by adding 2 to the child's age in years.**

   TEST-TAKING HINT: **The test taker can eliminate answer 1 because 1.5 oz represents a very small bladder capacity.**

2. 1. This urine output is within the expected range of 0.5–1 mL/kg/hr and is therefore not too low.
   2. This urine output is within the expected range of 0 .5–1 mL/kg/hr and is therefore not too low.
   3. **Recording the patient's urine output in the chart is the appropriate action because the urine output is within the expected range of 0.5–1 mL/kg/hr.**
   4. This urine output is within the expected range of 0.5–1 mL/kg/hr and is therefore not too low.

   TEST-TAKING HINT: **The test taker can eliminate answers 1, 2, and 4 because they address strategies for caring for a dehydrated child.**

3. 1. **Urinalysis and urine culture are routinely used to diagnose UTIs. VCUG is used to determine the extent of urinary tract involvement when the child has a second UTI within 1 year.**
   2. There are no data to suggest that renal failure should be evaluated.
   3. A UTI is usually treated with oral antibiotics at home, not routinely requiring admission to the hospital.
   4. A second UTI requires more extensive evaluation and diagnostic testing.

   TEST-TAKING HINT: **The test taker can eliminate answer 2 because it is the only answer that does not address the UTI. Answer 1 is the best choice because it will provide more data about the cause of the child's recurrent UTIs.**

4. 1. The increased pressure associated with evacuating the hardened stool can result in the backflow of urine into the bladder, leading to infection.
   2. To prevent infection, a female child should wipe from front to back.

3. Tub baths are not recommended because they may cause irritation of the urethra, leading to infection.
   4. **Increasing fluids will help flush the bladder of any organism, encouraging urination and preventing stasis of urine.**

   TEST-TAKING HINT: **The test taker can eliminate answers 1, 2, and 3 because they do not provide accurate information.**

5. 1. Irritability and lack of appetite can indicate a UTI. Signs of infection, such as fever and increased heart rate, should be evaluated to determine whether an infection exists.
   2. **Although this child has had a history of urinary infections, the child is currently not displaying any signs and therefore does not need a urinalysis at this time.**
   3. Pain to the lower right back can indicate infection of the upper urinary tract. Although the child currently denies any burning or frequency, the child currently has a fever coupled with flank pain, which needs evaluation.
   4. Frequency and urgency are classic signs of a UTI.

   TEST-TAKING HINT: **The test taker should be led to answer 2 because it states that the child is not currently having any manifestations of a UTI.**

6. 1. A sample obtained from a urine bag would contain microorganisms from the skin, causing contamination of the sample.
   2. There is no need to leave the catheter in because it serves as a portal for infection. Antibiotics are not administered through a Foley catheter.
   3. The cotton ball would not remain sterile and would therefore contaminate the urine sample.
   4. **An in-and-out catheterization is the best way to obtain a urine culture in a child who is not yet toilet-trained.**

   TEST-TAKING HINT: **The test taker can eliminate answers 1 and 3 because they both lead to a contaminated sample.**

7. 1. Glomerulonephritis can be caused by a streptococcal infection. This organism is commonly associated with respiratory and skin infections.
   2. Type 1 diabetes is not a cause of glomerulonephritis.
   3. **Impetigo is a skin infection caused by the streptococcal organism that is commonly associated with glomerulonephritis.**

4. Frequent UTIs have not been associated with glomerulonephritis.

TEST-TAKING HINT: The test taker may be distracted by answer 1 because streptococcal infections are associated with glomerulonephritis. However, answer 1 states that the illness is viral, so that answer is not a correct choice.

8. 1. Unlike nephrotic syndrome, protein is lost in mild-to-moderate amounts.
2. Urinary output is decreased in the patient with glomerulonephritis.
3. **Mild-to-moderate proteinuria, hematuria, decreased urinary output, and lethargy are common findings in glomerulonephritis.**
4. Hypertension, not hypotension, is a common finding in glomerulonephritis.

TEST-TAKING HINT: The test taker should eliminate answers 1 and 4 because glomerulonephritis does not cause massive proteinuria. Answer 2 can be eliminated because increased urine output is not associated with glomerulonephritis.

9. 1. Steroids and antihypertensives do not cause urine to change color.
2. **Blood in the child's urine causes it to be tea-colored.**
3. The tea color of the urine is due to hematuria, not concentration.
4. The child with glomerulonephritis is not on a ketogenic diet. The ketogenic diet does not cause the urine to change color.

TEST-TAKING HINT: The test taker can immediately eliminate answer 4 because the child is not placed on a ketogenic diet.

10. 1. Children with glomerulonephritis usually have an elevated blood pressure and tend to rest most of the day.
2. The urine output is often decreased, and the color is often tea-colored due to hematuria.
3. **A severe headache and photophobia can be signs of encephalopathy due to hypertension, and the child needs immediate attention.**
4. Anorexia is often seen with glomerulonephritis.

TEST-TAKING HINT: The test taker should eliminate answers 1, 2, and 4 because they are manifestations of glomerulonephritis.

11. 1. **When glomerulonephritis is improving, urine output increases, and the urine becomes less tea-colored. These are**

signs that can be monitored at home by the child's parents.
2. As glomerulonephritis improves, the child should have more energy and rest less.
3. The child's appetite should increase as the condition improves.
4. Although the laboratory test values will normalize, this is not something that will be readily apparent to the family at home.

TEST-TAKING HINT: The test taker should be led to answer 1 because the manifestations represent improvement in the disease process that can be easily recognized by the parents.

12. 1. **An upper respiratory infection often precedes MCNS by a few days.**
2. Bug bites are not typically associated with MCNS.
3. Vomiting and abdominal cramping are not typically associated with MCNS.
4. Pet turtles often carry salmonella, which can cause vomiting and diarrhea but not MCNS.

TEST-TAKING HINT: The test taker should be led to answer 1 because MCNS is most often associated with upper respiratory infections.

13. 1. Albumin does not undergo any chemical changes in MCNS.
2. **Increased permeability of the glomeruli in MCNS allows large substances such as protein to pass through and be excreted in the urine.**
3. Obstruction of the capillaries of the glomeruli due to the formation of antibody-antigen complexes occurs in glomerulonephritis.
4. Loss of the kidneys' ability to excrete waste and concentrate urine occurs in renal failure.

TEST-TAKING HINT: The test taker should recognize the pathophysiology of MCNS.

14. 1. In MCNS, the lipids are truly elevated. Lipoprotein production is increased because of the increased stimulation of the liver hypoalbuminemia.
2. The elevated lipids are unrelated to the child's dietary habits.
3. **In MCNS, the lipids are truly elevated. Lipoprotein production is increased because of the increased stimulation of the liver hypoalbuminemia.**
4. The lipids are not falsely elevated.

TEST-TAKING HINT: The test taker can eliminate answers 1 and 2 because they do not represent changes associated with a disease process.

15. 1. The dosage of the diuretic may be adjusted, but other medications such as albumin are likely to be used.
2. Mannitol is not usually used in the treatment of MCNS.
3. **In cases of severe edema, albumin is used to help return the fluid to the bloodstream from the subcutaneous tissue.**
4. Although sodium and fluids are restricted in the severely edematous child, they are not eliminated completely.

TEST-TAKING HINT: The test taker can eliminate answer 2 because mannitol is used to treat edema of the central nervous system.

16. 1. It is not unusual for a child to experience relapses.
2. Many children do experience relapses, but exposure to infectious illnesses has been linked to relapses.
3. There is no correlation between the consumption of sodium and nephrotic syndrome.
4. **Exposure to infectious illness has been linked to the relapse of nephrotic syndrome.**

TEST-TAKING HINT: The test taker can eliminate answers 1 and 2 because relapses are common and can be prevented.

17. 1. Although routine circumcision is no longer recommended by the American Academy of Pediatrics, it is not contraindicated in most children.
2. It is not recommended that circumcision of children with hypospadias be done immediately because the foreskin may be needed later for repair of the defect.
3. **It is usually recommended that circumcision be delayed in the child with hypospadias because the foreskin may be needed for repair of the defect.**
4. Circumcision can usually be performed in the child with hypospadias when the defect is corrected.

TEST-TAKING HINT: The test taker can eliminate answer 4 because "never" is infrequently the case in health care.

18. 1. This response is empathetic. It does not, however, answer the parent's concern, whereas a simple explanation would immediately do so.
2. Although a cosmetic component exists, straightening the penis is important for future sexual function.
3. **Releasing the chordee surgically is necessary for future sexual function.**
4. Although the two surgeries are usually done simultaneously, each has its own importance and necessity.

TEST-TAKING HINT: The test taker should be led to answer 3 because it provides the parents with a simple, accurate explanation.

19. 1. **Any mucous plugs should be removed by irrigation to prevent blockage of the urinary drainage system.**
2. The mucous plug should be removed by irrigation because it could cause a blockage of the urinary drainage system.
3. The dressing is usually a compression type of dressing that helps decrease edema.
4. Foul-smelling yellow drainage is often a sign of infection that needs to be evaluated.

TEST-TAKING HINT: The test taker can eliminate answer 2 and 4 because they have potential to cause injury to the child.

20. 1. Frequent UTIs and VUR do not lead to HUS.
2. **HUS is often preceded by diarrhea that may be caused by _E. coli_ present in undercooked meat.**
3. Insect stings are not associated with HUS.
4. HUS is usually preceded by diarrhea.

TEST-TAKING HINT: The test taker can eliminate answer 1 because there is no correlation between UTIs and HUS.

21. 1. **The swollen lining of the small blood vessels damages the red blood cells, which are then removed by the spleen.**
2. The increased permeability of the basement membrane occurs in MCNS.
3. The red blood cell changing shape is typical of sickle cell anemia.
4. The depression of all formed elements of the blood occurs in aplastic anemia.

TEST-TAKING HINT: The question requires familiarity with the pathophysiology of HUS.

22. 1. Protein is not lost in massive amounts in HUS.
2. BUN and creatinine are usually increased in HUS.
3. **Hematuria, mild proteinuria, increased BUN, and creatinine are all present in HUS.**
4. Ketonuria is not present in HUS.

TEST-TAKING HINT: The test taker can eliminate answer 4 because ketonuria is not associated with HUS.

23. 1. **Blood products are given to control the anemia. Because the child is symptomatic, dialysis is the treatment of choice.**
    2. Blood products are administered to control anemia. Because the child is symptomatic, dialysis is the treatment of choice.
    3. Diuretics are given to prevent fluid overload, but they cannot cause the child in renal failure to produce urine.
    4. Clotting factors are not used in HUS. The nurse would expect the plan to include dialysis, because the child is no longer producing urine.

TEST-TAKING HINT: The test taker can eliminate answer 3 because diuretics will not cause a child in renal failure to produce urine.

24. 1. The triad in HUS includes decreased red blood cells (with a high reticulocyte count as the body attempts to produce more red blood cells), decreased platelet count, and renal failure.
    2. **The triad in HUS includes decreased red blood cells (with a high reticulocyte count as the body attempts to produce more red blood cells), decreased platelet count, and renal failure.**
    3. The triad in HUS includes decreased red blood cells (with a high reticulocyte count as the body attempts to produce more red blood cells), decreased platelet count, and renal failure.
    4. The triad in HUS includes decreased red blood cells (with a high reticulocyte count as the body attempts to produce more red blood cells), decreased platelet count, and renal failure.

TEST-TAKING HINT: The test taker can eliminate answers 1 and 3 because platelets are not increased in HUS.

25. 1. Children with HUS are considered contagious for up to 17 days after the resolution of diarrhea and should be placed on contact isolation.
    2. Once the child recovers from HUS, there is usually no relapse.
    3. **Children with HUS are considered contagious for up to 17 days after the resolution of diarrhea and should be placed on contact isolation.**

4. Once free of diarrhea for approximately 17 days, the child is considered not to be contagious and should be encouraged to return to developmentally appropriate activities as tolerated.

TEST-TAKING HINT: The test taker can eliminate answer 1 because the child is still considered contagious.

26. 1. **Preventing infection from stool contamination and skin breakdown is the top priority of care.**
    2. The bladder should be covered with a moist dressing and not kept open where it can be exposed to pathogens or subject to irritation from drying.
    3. A child should never receive an intravenous bolus of dextrose because it can lead to cerebral edema.
    4. Although the child should be encouraged to rest, it is important to change the diaper immediately to prevent fecal contamination and subsequent infection.

TEST-TAKING HINT: The test taker can eliminate answers 2 and 3 because they have potential to cause harm to the infant.

27. 1. Lasix is a loop diuretic that is not routinely used in the care of the child with a repair of bladder exstrophy.
    2. Mannitol is an osmotic diuretic that is not routinely used in the care of the child with a repair of bladder exstrophy.
    3. Meperidine is a narcotic that is not a first-line drug for pain management after a bladder reconstruction.
    4. **Oxybutynin is used to control bladder spasms.**

TEST-TAKING HINT: The test taker can eliminate answer 2 because mannitol is a diuretic that is used for central nervous system edema.

28. 1. The infant should not be allowed to sleep on the abdomen because the prone position has been associated with sudden infant death syndrome.
    2. **Many children with urological malformations are prone to latex allergies. The surfaces of playgrounds are often made of rubber, which contains latex.**
    3. Many children with urological malformations are prone to latex allergies. Foods such as bananas can cause a latex allergy.
    4. Although children need a stimulating environment, balloons are dangerous because many contain latex and can also be a choking hazard.

TEST-TAKING HINT: The test taker can eliminate answer 1 because infants should be placed to sleep on their backs to prevent sudden infant death syndrome.

29. 1. **Hydronephrosis is due to a structural abnormality in the urinary system, causing urine to back up, leading to pressure and potential cell death.**
2. Hydronephrosis is due to pressure created by an obstruction, causing urine to back up. There is no free flow of urine.
3. A decreased production of urine does not lead to hydronephrosis.
4. Hydronephrosis is not caused by abnormalities in the urine.

TEST-TAKING HINT: This question requires familiarity with the pathophysiology of hydronephrosis.

30. 1. The blood pressure is increased as the body attempts to compensate for the decreased glomerular filtration rate. Polydipsia and polyuria occur as the kidney's ability to concentrate urine decreases. Metabolic acidosis occurs, not alkalosis.
2. The blood pressure is increased, not decreased, because the body attempts to compensate for the decreased glomerular filtration rate. Metabolic acidosis occurs because there is a reduction in hydrogen ion secretion from the distal nephron. There is bacterial growth in the urine due to the urinary stasis caused by the obstruction.
3. The blood pressure is increased as the body attempts to compensate for the decreased glomerular filtration rate. Metabolic acidosis, not alkalosis, occurs because there is a reduction in hydrogen ion secretion from the distal nephron. There is bacterial growth in the urine due to the urinary stasis caused by the obstruction.
4. **The blood pressure is increased as the body attempts to compensate for the decreased glomerular filtration rate. Metabolic acidosis is caused by a reduction in hydrogen ion secretion from the distal nephron. Polydipsia and polyuria occur as the kidney's ability to concentrate urine decreases. There is bacterial growth in the urine due to the urinary stasis caused by the obstruction.**

TEST-TAKING HINT: The test taker can eliminate answers 1 and 3 because hydronephrosis does not lead to metabolic alkalosis.

31. 1. **Fluid status is monitored to ensure adequate urinary output. Assessing blood pressure monitors kidney function.**
2. Fluid and sodium restriction are not required in hydronephrosis.
3. Steroids are not routinely used in the treatment of hydronephrosis.
4. Limiting the child's exposure to other people does not help prevent UTIs.

TEST-TAKING HINT: The test taker can eliminate answer 2 because fluids and sodium are not eliminated from the child's diet.

32. 1. Primary enuresis refers to urinary incontinence in a child who has never had voluntary bladder control.
2. **Secondary enuresis refers to urinary incontinence in a child who previously had bladder control.**
3. Diurnal enuresis refers to daytime urinary incontinence.
4. Nocturnal enuresis refers to nighttime urinary incontinence.

TEST-TAKING HINT: The test taker should be led to answer 2 because a disease process causes the child's enuresis.

33. 1. Although DDAVP is used for enuresis, it is not the first treatment chosen. Behavior modification and positive reinforcement are usually tried first.
2. Having the child help with changing the bed is a good idea. The child should be approached in a positive manner, however, not a punitive one, so as not to threaten self-esteem.
3. **Limiting the child's fluids in the evening will help decrease the nocturnal urge to void. Providing positive reinforcement and allowing the child to choose a reward will increase the child's sense of control.**
4. Enuresis alarms are readily available, but behavior modification and positive reinforcement are usually tried first.

TEST-TAKING HINT: The test taker can eliminate answer 2 because negative reinforcement is not recommended and is not helpful.

34. 1. The child is having symptoms of testicular torsion, which is a surgical emergency and needs immediate attention. The child should not wait to go to the emergency room and should be told not to drink anything in anticipation of surgery.
2. Testicular torsion is a surgical emergency, and time should not be wasted at the pediatrician's office when the child needs surgery.

3. **The child is having symptoms of testicular torsion, which is a surgical emergency and needs immediate attention.**
4. The child should be brought to the emergency room immediately because testicular torsion is a surgical emergency. Ice and scrotal support can be used for relief of discomfort, but bringing the child to the emergency room is the priority.

TEST-TAKING HINT: The test taker should be led to answer 3 because testicular torsion is a surgical emergency.

35. 1. **Testicular torsion is caused by an interruption of the blood supply due to twisting of the spermatic cord.**
2. Swelling of the scrotal sac occurs because of testicular torsion; it is not a cause of testicular torsion.
3. Unmanaged undescended testes may be a risk factor but not a cause of testicular torsion.
4. Microthrombi formation in the vessels of the spermatic cord does not occur in testicular torsion.

TEST-TAKING HINT: This question depends on familiarity with the pathophysiology of testicular torsion.

36. 1. Lifting and strenuous activity should be avoided for 2 to 4 weeks.
2. The child should not be placed on bedrest and should be encouraged to gradually increase activity while resting as necessary.
3. Most cases of testicular torsion involve only one testis, so most children do not become infertile.
4. **The child and family should be taught the importance of testicular self-examination.**

TEST-TAKING HINT: The test taker can eliminate answer 1 because this activity could place the postoperative child at risk for injury.

37. 1. Bowel is the most common tissue to protrude into the groin in males.
2. **Fallopian tube or an ovary is the most common tissue to protrude into the groin in females.**
3. Large thrombus formation does not commonly protrude into the groin.
4. Muscle tissue does not commonly protrude into the groin.

TEST-TAKING HINT: The test taker should be led to answer 2 because the question specifically states that the child is a female.

38. 1. The terms are not used interchangeably. Inguinal hernia refers to protrusion of abdominal tissue into the groin, and a hydrocele refers to a fluid-filled mass in the scrotum.
2. **The symptoms are similar, but an inguinal hernia occurs when tissue protrudes into the groin, and a hydrocele is a fluid-filled mass in the groin.**
3. A hydrocele does not occur in females.
4. A hydrocele is not associated with an increased risk of malignancy.

TEST-TAKING HINT: This question depends on knowledge of the definitions of inguinal hernia and hydrocele.

39. 1. Surgery is usually done at an early age to avoid incarceration, in which the hernia causes impaired circulation to the surrounding tissue.
2. The hernia tends to look larger when the child strains or has a bowel movement.
3. The surgery is usually done on an outpatient basis, and narcotics are not usually needed.
4. **The hernia often appears smaller when the child is asleep.**

TEST-TAKING HINT: The test taker can eliminate answer 1 because there are risks associated with waiting for the repair, and surgery is not done solely for cosmetic reasons.

40. 1. **Signs of an incarcerated hernia include an acute onset of pain, abdominal distention, and a mass that cannot be reduced. Other signs are bloody stools, edema of the scrotum, and a history of poor feeding.**
2. The pain is not gradual but is acute in onset.
3. The mass is not easily reduced.
4. The mass is not easily reduced, and the child experiences acute, not gradual, onset of pain.

TEST-TAKING HINT: The test taker can eliminate answers 2 and 4 because the onset of pain is not gradual.

41. 1. Wilms tumor grows very rapidly and doubles in size in fewer than 2 weeks.
2. This response places blame on the parent. Wilms tumor has a very good prognosis, even when first diagnosed at a more advanced stage.
3. This response is condescending and does not acknowledge the parent as the person who knows the child best.

4. The tumor is fast-growing and could very easily not have been evident a few days earlier.

TEST-TAKING HINT: The test taker can eliminate answer 2 because the nurse should never cause the parent to feel guilt and responsibility over any diagnosis.

42. 1. The blood pressure may be increased if there is renal damage. The mass will be located on one side or the other of the midline of the abdomen. There is no reason for the child's temperature to be affected.
    2. The blood pressure may be increased if there is renal damage. The mass will be located on one side or the other of the midline of the abdomen. There is no reason for the child's temperature to be affected.
    3. The blood pressure may be increased if there is renal damage. The mass will be located on one side or the other of the midline of the abdomen. There is no reason for the child's temperature to be affected.
    4. The blood pressure may be increased if there is renal damage. The mass is located on one side or the other of the midline of the abdomen. There is no reason for the child's temperature to be affected.

TEST-TAKING HINT: The test taker can eliminate answers 1 and 2 because the mass is felt in the abdomen, not the back.

43. 1. When the nurse is unsure of the answer, it is best to check and get back to the parents. The nurse should be aware that tests of other organs are often performed to evaluate for the presence of metastases.
    2. The test is ordered to check for metastasis to the lungs.
    3. The test is done to see if the disease has spread to the lungs.
    4. A chest x-ray, not a magnetic resonance image, is ordered routinely to evaluate the health of the lungs prior to surgery.

TEST-TAKING HINT: The test taker should be led to answer 3 because further testing evaluates metastasis to other organs.

44. 1. The tumor is confined to the abdomen but has spread to the lymph nodes or peritoneal area. The prognosis is still very good.
    2. The tumor is confined to the abdomen but has spread to the lymph nodes or peritoneal area. The prognosis is still very good.
    3. Stage III does not indicate that the tumor has spread to three other organs.

4. The tumor has not spread to other organs beyond the peritoneal area. This would represent stage IV, but with aggressive treatment the child would still have a good prognosis.

TEST-TAKING HINT: The test taker should be led to answer 2 because this represents stage III.

45. **1. The treatment of a Wilms tumor involves removal of the affected kidney.**
    2. Removal of the unaffected kidney is not necessary and is not done.
    3. The entire kidney is removed.
    4. A biopsy of the tissue of the unaffected kidney is not necessary and is not obtained.

TEST-TAKING HINT: The test taker should eliminate answers 3 and 4 because the entire kidney is removed, not only the mass.

46. 1. A large incision is used because the kidney is not removed laparoscopically at this time.
    2. There is a postoperative shift of fluids and organs in the abdominal cavity, leading to increased discomfort.
    3. The increased pain is due to shifting of fluid and organs.
    4. The increased pain is due to shifting of fluid and organs.

TEST-TAKING HINT: The test taker should eliminate answer 1 because the kidney is not removed laparoscopically.

47. 1. Both disease processes are characterized by the kidney's inability to excrete waste. CRF occurs gradually and is irreversible, whereas ARF occurs suddenly and may be reversible.
    2. Children can experience CRF and ARF.
    3. CRF is irreversible, and it tends to occur gradually.
    4. ARF is often reversible, whereas CRF results in permanent deterioration of kidney function.

TEST-TAKING HINT: The test taker should eliminate answer 1 because the terms "acute" and "chronic" are not used interchangeably.

48. 1. CRF occurs gradually.
    2. Examples of causes of prerenal failure include dehydration and hemorrhage.
    3. Primary kidney failure occurs when the kidney experiences a direct injury. Examples include HUS and glomerulonephritis.
    4. Postrenal failure occurs when there is an obstruction to urinary flow. Hypotension does not cause postrenal failure.

TEST-TAKING HINT: **The test taker should eliminate answer 1 because there is no evidence of a chronic disease process.**

49. 1. The patient is demonstrating signs of hyperkalemia; therefore, intravenous potassium would be contraindicated.
    2. Sodium bicarbonate would be administered when metabolic acidosis is present.
    3. **Calcium gluconate is the drug of choice for cardiac irritability secondary to hyperkalemia.**
    4. The patient is demonstrating signs of hyperkalemia; therefore, oral potassium supplements would be contraindicated.

    TEST-TAKING HINT: **The test taker should eliminate answer 1 because the patient is already showing signs of increased potassium levels.**

50. 1. 1000 mL represents the daily fluid requirement in a healthy child.
    2. 2000 mL is double the fluid requirement of a healthy child and is contraindicated in a child in the oliguric phase of ARF.
    3. **350 mL is approximately a third of the daily fluid requirement and is recommended for the child in the oliguric phase of ARF. If the child were febrile, the fluid intake would be increased.**
    4. Sips of clear fluids and ice chips would not replace the insensible losses. All oral intake needs to be measured and accurately recorded because "sips" can be very subjective.

    TEST-TAKING HINT: **The question specifies that the child is afebrile; therefore, the test taker can eliminate answers 1 and 2 because extra fluid is not required.**

51. 1. Although the child will likely receive additional Kayexalate, the child's condition will likely not improve without dialysis.
    2. Although the child will likely receive intravenous furosemide, the child's condition will likely not improve without dialysis.
    3. Endotracheal intubation and ventilatory assistance may be required, but ultimately the child will need dialysis.
    4. **Placement of a Tenckhoff catheter for peritoneal dialysis is needed when the child's condition deteriorates despite medical treatment.**

    TEST-TAKING HINT: **The test taker should be led to answer 4 because dialysis is the treatment required to reverse the existing clinical manifestations.**

52. 1. Hemodialysis is used in the pediatric population.
    2. Peritoneal dialysis has many complications, such as peritonitis.
    3. **Peritoneal dialysis removes fluid at a slower rate that is more easily controlled than that of hemodialysis.**
    4. Hemodialysis is much more efficient than peritoneal dialysis.

    TEST-TAKING HINT: **The test taker should eliminate answer 2 because very few treatments are without complications.**

53. 1. **Cloudy returns and abdominal pain are signs of peritonitis and are usually treated with the administration of antibiotics in the dialysis fluid.**
    2. Cloudy returns and abdominal pain are signs of peritonitis and need to be treated.
    3. Cloudy returns and abdominal pain are signs of peritonitis and are usually treated with the administration of antibiotics in the dialysis fluid.
    4. Cloudy returns and abdominal pain are signs of peritonitis. In addition to peritonitis, abdominal pain can be caused by the rapid infusion of dialysis fluid.

    TEST-TAKING HINT: **The test taker can eliminate answer 2 because pain would be increased if the rate of administration were increased.**

54. 1. **Increasing the concentration of glucose will pull more fluid into the return.**
    2. Decreasing the concentration of glucose will pull less fluid into the return.
    3. Antihypertensives and diuretics may be administered, but changing the concentration of glucose in the dialysate will help regulate the fluid balance.
    4. Increasing the dwell time would help pull more fluid into the return. Decreasing the dwell time would pull less fluid into the return.

    TEST-TAKING HINT: **The test taker should eliminate answers 2 and 4 because they decrease the amount of return.**

55. 1. **The child is experiencing signs of disequilibrium syndrome, which is caused by free water shifting from intravascular spaces and can be prevented by slowing the rate of dialysis.**
    2. The patient's temperature is not a causative factor in disequilibrium syndrome.
    3. Antibiotics are used to prevent peritonitis, not disequilibrium syndrome.

4. The child's weight should be obtained immediately prior to dialysis.

TEST-TAKING HINT: The test taker should eliminate answers 2 and 3 because they are not associated with disequilibrium syndrome.

56. 1. **The retention of sodium and water leads to hypertension.**
2. The obstruction of the urinary system can lead to renal failure but is not a direct cause of hypertension.
3. The accumulation of waste products leads to metabolic acidosis.
4. In CRF, the body experiences a state of metabolic acidosis, not alkalosis.

TEST-TAKING HINT: The test taker should eliminate answer 4 because metabolic alkalosis is not associated with CRF.

57. 1. The kidneys are unable to excrete phosphorus, so phosphorus levels increase, and calcium levels fall.
2. **The calcium and phosphorus levels are drawn from the bones in response to low calcium levels.**
3. The calcium is drawn from the bones in response to low serum calcium levels.
4. Although the child may not be consuming enough calcium, dietary deficiency is not the primary cause of hypocalcemia.

TEST-TAKING HINT: The test taker should eliminate answer 4 because dietary imbalances are not the primary cause of hypocalcemia in renal failure.

58. 1. The child's diet should be high in calories and protein, but not all minerals and electrolytes should be high. Sodium, potassium, and phosphorus should be restricted.
2. The child with CRF needs a diet high in protein.
3. **The child with CRF needs a diet high in calories, protein, and calcium and low in potassium and phosphorus.**
4. Phosphorus should be restricted because the kidneys are unable to excrete phosphorus.

TEST-TAKING HINT: The test taker should eliminate answer 2 because it is important for the child to have a diet high in protein.

59. 1. The child is demonstrating signs of rejection. Although pain control is always important, antirejection medications are of utmost importance.
2. Furosemide may be given to reduce edema, but antirejection medications are the most important for this child.

3. MiraLAX powder will help with constipation, but it will not help prevent rejection.
4. **Corticosteroids are considered to be part of the antirejection regimen that is essential after a kidney transplant.**

TEST-TAKING HINT: The test taker should be led to answer 4 because it is the only listed answer that is part of an antirejection regimen.

60. 1. There are extensive post-transplant care requirements.
2. This treatment option is not ideal for families with a history of noncompliance because there is extensive post-transplant care associated with the receipt of a kidney.
3. **Renal transplantation frees the patient from dialysis.**
4. Renal transplantation is not new to the pediatric population.

TEST-TAKING HINT: The test taker should eliminate answer 1 because transplantation is a treatment, not a cure.

61. 1, 2, 3, 4.
1. **Stressors such as the birth of a sibling can lead to incontinence in a child who previously had bladder control.**
2. **A pattern of enuresis can often be seen in families.**
3. **Increased thirst and incontinence can be associated with diabetes.**
4. **Irritability and incontinence can be associated with UTIs.**
5. Preschool-age children do not habitually share, so this information would not help the nurse in gathering more information on enuresis.

TEST-TAKING HINT: The test taker should be able to eliminate answer 5 by knowing lack of sharing is not unusual in preschoolers.

62. 2, 3.
1. It is referred to as a nephroblastoma, not a neuroblastoma.
2. **It can occur at any age but is seen most often between the ages of 2 and 5 years.**
3. **It can occur on its own or can be associated with many congenital anomalies.**
4. It is a tumor that grows very quickly.
5. It is associated with a very good prognosis.

TEST-TAKING HINT: The test taker would have to know about Wilms tumor to answer the question.

Endocrinology Pediatric Review Questions

10

KEYWORDS

Adrenal gland
Gonadotropin
Hyperthyroidism
Hypothyroidism
Myxedema

Pancreas
Pituitary gland
Type I diabetes
Type II diabetes

ABBREVIATIONS

Adrenocorticotropic hormone (ACTH)
Antidiuretic hormone (ADH)
Chronic renal failure (CRF)
Diabetes insipidus (DI)
Diabetes mellitus (DM)
Emergency department (ED)
Health-care professional (HCP)
Insulin-like growth factor-1 (IGF-1)

Insulin-like growth factor binding
  protein-3 (IGFBP-3)
Intravenous (IV)
Syndrome of inappropriate antidiuretic
  hormone (SIADH)
Thyrocalcitonin (TC)
Thyroid hormone (TH)
Thyroid-stimulating hormone (TSH)

QUESTIONS

1. At the 6-month follow-up visit for an 8-year-old who is being evaluated for short stature, the nurse again measures and plots the child's height on the growth chart. Which explanation should the nurse give the child and family?
   1. "We want to make sure you were measured accurately the last two visits."
   2. "We need to calculate how tall you will be when you grow to adult height."
   3. "We need to see how many inches you have grown since your last visit."
   4. "We need to know your height so that a dosage of medication can be calculated for you."

2. What key information should be explained to the family of a 3-year-old who has short stature and abnormal laboratory test results?
   1. Due to the diurnal rhythm of the body, growth hormone levels are elevated following the onset of sleep.
   2. Exercise can stimulate growth hormone secretion.
   3. The initial screening tests need to be repeated for accuracy.
   4. Growth hormone levels in children are so low that stimulation testing must be done.

3. A 6-year-old white girl comes with her mother for evaluation of her acne, breast buds, axillary hair, and body odor. What information should the nurse explain to them?
   1. This is a typical age for girls to go into puberty.
   2. Encourage the girl to dress and act appropriately for her chronological age.
   3. She should be on birth control as she is fertile.
   4. She may be short if her epiphyses close early.

4. The nurse is working on the pediatric floor, caring for an infant who is very fussy and has a diagnosis of DI. Which parameter should the nurse monitor while the infant is on fluid restrictions?
   1. Oral intake.
   2. Urine output.
   3. Appearance of the mucous membranes.
   4. Pulse and temperature.

5. A 12-year-old comes to the clinic with a diagnosis of Graves disease. What information should the nurse discuss with the child?
   1. Suggest weight loss.
   2. Encourage attending school.
   3. Emphasize that the disease will go into remission.
   4. Encourage the child to take responsibility for daily medications.

6. The school nurse notices that a 14-year-old who used to be an excellent student and very active in sports is losing weight and acting very nervous. The teen was recently checked by the primary care provider, who noted the teen had a very low level of TSH. The nurse recognizes that the teen has which condition?
   1. Hashimoto thyroid disease.
   2. Graves disease.
   3. Hypothyroidism.
   4. Juvenile autoimmune thyroiditis.

7. A newborn develops tetany and a seizure just prior to discharge from the nursery. The newborn is diagnosed with hypocalcemia secondary to hypoparathyroidism and is started on calcium and vitamin D. Which information would be most important for the nurse to teach the parents?
   1. They should observe the baby for signs of tetany and seizures.
   2. They should observe for weakness, nausea, vomiting, and diarrhea, all signs of vitamin D toxicity.
   3. They should administer the calcium and vitamin D daily as prescribed.
   4. They should call the clinic if they have any questions about care of the newborn.

8. A teen who was hospitalized for CRF develops symptoms of polyuria, polydipsia, and bone pain. What body mineral might be causing these symptoms?
   1. Elevated calcium.
   2. Low phosphorus.
   3. Low vitamin D.
   4. High aluminum hydroxide.

9. The family of a young child has been told the child has DI. What information should the nurse emphasize to the family?
   1. One caregiver needs to learn to give the injections of vasopressin (Pitressin).
   2. Children should wear MedicAlert tags if they are over 5 years old.
   3. DI is different from DM.
   4. Over time, the child may grow out of the need for medication.

10. A nurse is working with a child who has had a bone age evaluation. Which explanation of the test should the nurse give?
    1. "The bone age will give you a diagnosis of your child's short stature."
    2. "If the bone age is delayed, the child will continue to grow taller."
    3. "The x-ray of the bones is compared with that of the age-appropriate, standardized bone age."
    4. "If the bone age is not delayed, no further treatment is needed."

11. You are caring for a school-aged child with myxedematous skin changes. The HCP wants information about the child's appearance. Which descriptive terms should you use to describe your observations of the child's skin?
    1. The skin is oily and scaly.
    2. The skin has pale, thickened patches.
    3. The eyes are sunken, and the hair is thickened.
    4. The eyes are puffy, the hair is sparse, and the skin is dry.

12. A child is brought to the ED with what is presumed to be acute adrenocortical insufficiency. Which of the following should the nurse do first?
    1. Insert an IV line to administer fluids and cortisol.
    2. Prepare for admission to the intensive care unit.
    3. Indicate the likelihood of a slow recovery.
    4. Discuss the likelihood of the child's imminent death.

13. The nurse is working with a school-aged child with a diagnosis of Addison disease (chronic adrenocortical insufficiency). The child takes oral cortisol supplements and has to get monthly injections of desoxycorticosterone acetate injections. What teaching should be done at each visit for the injections?
    1. "Keep an extra month's supply of all medications on hand at all times."
    2. "Wear a MedicAlert bracelet at all times"
    3. "The drug has a bitter taste."
    4. "Weight gain is inevitable."

14. The nurse is instructing a family on the side effects of cortisone. What aspects of administering the medication should the nurse emphasize?
    1. Weight gain and dietary management.
    2. Bitterness of the taste of the medication.
    3. Excitability and sleepiness resulting from the medication.
    4. Taking the medication with food to decrease gastric irritation.

15. An infant is born with ambiguous genitalia. Genetic testing and an ultrasound are ordered. The infant has a large clitoris, but there is no vaginal orifice. The labia appear to be sac-like darkened tissue. No testes are located. What suggestion should the nurse offer the family?
    1. Take the baby home, and wait until the gender is determined to name "it."
    2. Because the parents wanted a boy, give the baby a boy's name.
    3. Give the baby a neutral name that fits either a boy or a girl.
    4. Call the infant "baby" until they know the gender.

16. A baby has hypertension as a result of partial 21-hydroxylase deficiency. The parents asks the nurse to clarify why the baby is being sent home on cortisone. Which of the following is the nurse's best response about cortisone?
    1. Increases the utilization of fatty acids for energy.
    2. Depresses the secretion of ACTH.
    3. Stimulates the adrenal glands.
    4. Increases the response to inflammation.

17. A school-aged child is diagnosed with bilateral pheochromocytomas. The nurse recalls that the tumor, benign in most children, arises from the adrenal medulla. Which clinical manifestations should the nurse check for in this child?
    1. Hypertension, headache, and decreased gastrointestinal activity.
    2. Hypoglycemia, lethargy, and increased gastrointestinal activity.
    3. Bradycardia, diarrhea, and weight gain.
    4. Hypotension, constipation, and anuria.

18. A teen comes into the clinic with complaints of having been under a lot of stress recently. The teen is being treated for Addison disease and is taking cortisol and aldosterone orally. Today, the teen shows symptoms of muscle weakness, fatigue, salt craving, and dehydration. What should the nurse discuss with the patient regarding the medications?
    1. The dosage may need to be decreased in times of stress.
    2. The dosage may need to be increased in times of stress.
    3. The aldosterone should be stopped, and the cortisol should be increased.
    4. The cortisol may need to be given IV to raise its level.

19. A 6-year-old is diagnosed with growth hormone deficiency. A prescription is written for a dose of 0.025 mg/kg of somatotropin subcutaneously three times weekly. The child weighs 27 kg (59.4 lb). What dose of medication should the nurse administer three times weekly?
    1. 1 mg.
    2. 0.5 mg.
    3. 0.675 mg.
    4. 2 mg.

20. The medication for the child in the previous problem comes in a vial of 5 mg of somatropin (rDNA) and is mixed with a diluent of 5 mL. There is 5 mL of solution in each vial. What amount of the solution should the nurse draw up to give the appropriate dose each time?
    1. 1 mL.
    2. 0.5 mL.
    3. 0.675 mL.
    4. 2 mL.

21. A 7-year-old is diagnosed with central precocious puberty. The child has to receive a monthly intramuscular injection of leuprolide acetate (Lupron). The child has great fears of pain and needles and requires considerable stress reduction techniques each time an injection is due. What could the nurse suggest that might help manage the pain?
    1. Apply a eutectic mixture of local anesthetics (EMLA) of lidocaine and prilocaine to the site at least 60 minutes before the injection.
    2. Have extra help on hand to help hold the child down.
    3. Apply cold to the area prior to injection.
    4. Identify a reward to bribe the child to behave during the injection.

22. A child weighs 21 kg. The parent asks for the weight in pounds. Which is the correct equivalent?
    1. Approximately 50 lb.
    2. 42 lb.
    3. 60 lb.
    4. 46 lb, 3 oz.

23. Two parents bring their teen to the clinic with a tender, enlarged right breast. The nurse explains that which hormone(s) secreted by the anterior pituitary influence(s) this process?
    1. Thyrotropin.
    2. Gonadotropin.
    3. Oxytocin.
    4. Somatotropin.

24. A toddler is admitted to the pediatric floor for hypopituitarism following removal of a craniopharyngioma. The toddler has polyuria, polydipsia, and dehydration. What area of the brain was most affected by the surgery?
    1. Posterior pituitary.
    2. Anterior pituitary.
    3. Autonomic nervous system.
    4. Sympathetic nervous system.

25. Which of the following hormones does the anterior pituitary secrete? Select all that apply.
    1. Thyroxine.
    2. Luteinizing hormone.
    3. Prolactin (luteotropic hormone).
    4. ACTH.
    5. Epinephrine.
    6. Cortisol.

26. The adrenal cortex secretes sex hormones. Identify which hormones would result in male feminization of a young child. Select all that apply.
    1. Estrogen.
    2. Testosterone.
    3. Progesterone.
    4. Cortisol.
    5. Androgens.

27. A child comes into the clinic and is suspected to have Cushing syndrome. Which test(s) could be utilized to determine cortisol levels in this patient? Select all that apply.
    1. Fasting blood glucose.
    2. Thyroid panel (TSH, T3, T4).
    3. 24-hour urine for 17-hydroxycorticoids.
    4. Radiographic studies of the bones.
    5. Cortisone suppression test.
    6. Urine culture.
    7. Complete blood count.

28. A teen comes into the clinic with anxiety. Over the last 2 weeks, the teen has had some muscle twitching and has a positive Chvostek sign. Which explanation could the nurse provide to the parent about a Chvostek sign?
    1. It is a facial muscle spasm elicited by tapping the facial nerve.
    2. Muscle pain occurs when touched.
    3. The sign occurs because of increased intracranial pressure.
    4. The sign is a result of a vitamin D overdose.

29. A school-aged girl is working on a school project on glands and asks the clinic nurse to explain the function of the thymus gland. Which answer is correct?
    1. It produces hormones that help with digestion.
    2. It is a gland that disappears by the time a baby is born.
    3. A major function is to stimulate the pituitary to act as the master gland.
    4. The gland helps with immunity in fetal life and early childhood.

30. A parent with a toddler who has ambiguous genitalia asks the nurse how long before the child identifies his or her gender? Which is the best answer?
    1. "A child does not know his or her gender until he or she is a teen."
    2. "A child knows his or her gender by the age of 18 to 30 months."
    3. "A child knows from the time of birth what his or her gender is."
    4. "A child of 4 to 6 years is beginning to learn his or her gender."

31. The percentile of weight-for-age for an 8-kg boy who is 9 months old is ____ ?

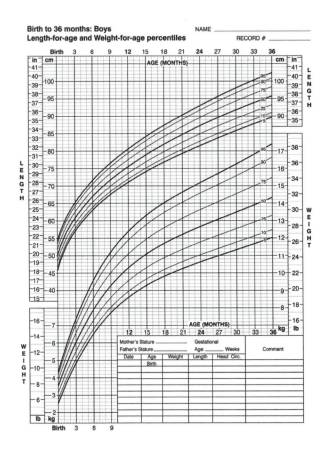

Birth to 36 months: Boys
Length-for-age and Weight-for-age percentiles

NAME _____

RECORD # _____

32. The nurse is working in the well-child clinic, and a new patient is brought in for a visit. The parent brings the record along with the 21-month-old child. The records show a birth weight of 8 lb; the 6-month weight was 16 lb; the 12-month weight was 18 lb; and the 15-month weight was 19 lb. With the record showing that the toddler's weight-for-age has been decreasing on the growth chart, the nurse should do what initially?
1. Omit plotting the previous weight-for-age on the new growth chart.
2. Point out the growth chart to the new HCP.
3. Consider the toddler a child with failure to thrive.
4. Weigh the child, and plot on a new growth chart.

33. The thyroid gland secretes two types of hormones, TH and TC. Mark TH or TC in the correct spaces below.
1. _____ This hormone regulates the metabolic rate of all cells.
2. _____ This hormone regulates body heat production.
3. _____ This hormone affects milk production during lactation and menstrual flow.
4. _____ This hormone maintains calcium metabolism.
5. _____ This hormone maintains appetite and secretion of gastrointestinal substances.
6. _____ This hormone increases gluconeogenesis and utilization of glucose.

34. A child with adrenal insufficiency is sick with the flu. The parent calls the office and wants to know what to do. What is the first thing the nurse should advise this parent?
1. Withhold all medications, and bring the child to the office.
2. Encourage the child to drink water and juices.
3. Give the child a dose of cortisol, and bring the child to the office.
4. Let the child rest; the child will be better in the morning.

35. A toddler is being evaluated for SIADH. The nurse should observe the child for which symptoms? Select all that apply.
   1. Dehydration.
   2. Fluid retention.
   3. Hyponatremia.
   4. Hypoglycemia.
   5. Myxedema.

36. What should the parent of a child with DI be taught about administering desmopressin acetate nasal spray? Select all that apply.
   1. The use of the flexible nasal tube.
   2. Nasal congestion causes this route to be ineffective.
   3. The medication should be administered every 48 hours.
   4. The medication should be administered every 8 to 12 hours.
   5. Overmedication results in signs of SIADH.
   6. Nasal sprays do not always work as well as injections.

37. A school-aged child comes in with a sore throat and fever. The child was recently diagnosed with Graves disease and is taking propylthiouracil. What concerns should the nurse have about this child?
   1. The child must not be taking her medication.
   2. The child may have leukopenia.
   3. The child needs to start an antibiotic.
   4. The child is participating in sports before she is euthyroid.

38. An 8-year-old with type I DM is complaining of a headache and dizziness and is visibly perspiring. The nurse caring for the child should do which of the following?
   1. Administer glucagon intramuscularly.
   2. Offer the child 8 oz of milk.
   3. Administer rapid-acting insulin (lispro).
   4. Offer the child 8 oz of water or calorie-free liquid.

39. The nurse is caring for a 10-year-old post parathyroidectomy. Discharge teaching should include which of the following?
   1. How to administer injectable growth hormone.
   2. The importance of supplemental calcium in the diet.
   3. The importance of increasing folic acid in the diet.
   4. How to administer subcutaneous insulin.

40. The nurse is teaching the family about caring for their 7-year-old, who has been diagnosed with type I DM. What information should the nurse provide about type I DM?
   1. Best managed through diet, exercise, and oral medication.
   2. Can be prevented by proper nutrition and activity.
   3. Characterized mainly by insulin resistance.
   4. Characterized mainly by insulin deficiency.

41. The most appropriate nursing diagnosis for a patient with type I DM is which of the following?
   1. Risk for infection related to reduced body defenses.
   2. Impaired urinary elimination (enuresis).
   3. Risk for injury related to medical treatment.
   4. Anticipatory grieving.

42. The nurse caring for a patient with type I DM is teaching how to self-administer insulin. The proper injection technique is which of the following?
   1. Position the needle with the bevel facing downward before injection.
   2. Spread the skin prior to intramuscular injection.
   3. Aspirate for blood return prior to injection.
   4. Elevate the subcutaneous tissue before injection.

43. The nurse is caring for a child who complains of constant hunger, constant thirst, frequent urination, and recent weight loss without dieting. The nurse can expect that care for this child will include which of the following?
    1. Limiting daily fluid intake.
    2. Weight management consulting.
    3. Strict intake and output monitoring.
    4. Frequent blood glucose testing.

44. The nurse is obtaining the medical history of an 11-year-old diagnosed with hypopituitarism. An important question for the nurse to ask the parents is which of the following?
    1. "Is the child receiving vasopressin intramuscularly or subcutaneously?"
    2. "What time of day do you administer growth hormone?"
    3. "Does your child have any concerns about being taller than the peer group?"
    4. "How often is your child testing blood glucose?"

45. The nurse is caring for a patient with a diagnosis of hyperthyroidism. An important nursing intervention is which of the following?
    1. Encourage an increase in physical activity.
    2. Do preoperative teaching for thyroidectomy.
    3. Promote opportunities for periods of rest.
    4. Do dietary planning to increase caloric intake.

46. A 13-year-old with type II DM asks the nurse, "Why do I need to have this hemoglobin A_{1c} test?" The nurse's response is based on which of the following?
    1. To determine how balanced the child's diet has been.
    2. To make sure the child is not anemic.
    3. To determine how controlled the child's blood sugar has been.
    4. To make sure the child's blood ketone level is normal.

47. The nurse caring for a 14-year-old girl with DI understands which of the following about this disorder?
    1. DI is treated on a short-term basis with hormone replacement therapy.
    2. DI may cause anorexia if proper meal planning is not addressed.
    3. DI is treated with vasopressin on a lifelong basis.
    4. DI requires strict fluid limitation until it resolves.

48. A 7-year-old is tested for DI. Twenty-four hours after his fluid restriction has begun, the nurse notes that his urine continues to be clear and pale, with a low specific gravity. The most likely reason for this is which of the following?
    1. Twenty-four hours is too early to evaluate effects of fluid restriction.
    2. The urine should be concentrated, and it is unlikely the child has DI.
    3. The child may have been sneaking fluids and needs closer observation.
    4. In DI, fluid restriction does not cause urine concentration.

49. The nurse has completed discharge teaching of the family of a 10-year-old diagnosed with DI. Which of the following statements best demonstrates the family's correct understanding of DI?
    1. "My child's disease was probably brought on by a bad diet and little exercise."
    2. "My father is a diabetic, and that may be why my child has it."
    3. "My child will need to check blood sugar several times a day."
    4. "My child will have to use the bathroom more often than other children."

50. The nurse is interviewing the parent of a 9-year-old girl. The parent expresses concern because the daughter already has pubic hair and is starting to develop breasts. Which of the following statements would be most appropriate?
    1. "Your daughter should get her period in approximately 6 months."
    2. "Your daughter is developing early and should be evaluated for precocious puberty."
    3. "Your daughter is experiencing body changes that are appropriate for her age."
    4. "Your daughter will need further testing to determine the underlying cause."

51. The nurse is taking care of a 10-year-old patient diagnosed with Graves disease. The nurse could expect this patient to have recently had which of the following?
    1. Weight gain, excessive thirst, and excessive hunger.
    2. Weight loss, difficulty sleeping, and heat sensitivity.
    3. Weight gain, lethargy, and goiter.
    4. Weight loss, poor skin turgor, and constipation.

52. A 12-year-old with type II DM presents with a fever and a 2-day history of vomiting. The nurse obtaining the history observes that the child's breath has a fruity odor and breathing that is deep and rapid. The nurse should do which of the following?
    1. Offer the child 8 oz of clear non-caloric fluid.
    2. Test the child's urine for ketones.
    3. Prepare the child for an IV infusion.
    4. Offer the child 25 g of carbohydrates.

53. A student has an insulin-to-carbohydrate ratio of 1:10. The school nurse understands which of the following?
    1. The student administers 10 U of regular insulin for every carbohydrate consumed.
    2. The student is trying to limit carbohydrate intake to 10 g per 24 hours.
    3. The student administers 1 U of regular insulin for every 10 carbohydrates consumed.
    4. The student plans to eat 10 g of carbohydrate for every gram of fat or protein.

54. A student takes metformin (Glucophage) three times a day. The nurse expects this student has which of the following?
    1. Type I DM.
    2. Gastrointestinal reflux.
    3. Inflammatory bowel disease.
    4. Type II DM.

55. Adolescents with diabetes have problems with low self-esteem. The nurse knows the most likely reason for this is which of the following?
    1. Managing diabetes decreases independence.
    2. Managing diabetes complicates perceived ability to "fit in."
    3. Obesity complicates perceived ability to "fit in."
    4. Hormonal changes are exacerbated by fluctuations in insulin levels.

56. The school nurse is talking to a 14-year-old about managing type I DM. Which of the following statements indicates the student's understanding of the disease?
    1. "It really does not matter what type of carbohydrate I eat as long as I take the right amount of insulin."
    2. "I should probably have a snack right after gym class."
    3. "I need to cut back on my carbohydrate intake and increase my lean protein intake."
    4. "Losing weight will probably help me decrease my need for insulin."

57. The nurse is assigned to care for a newborn with goiter. The nurse's primary concern is which of the following?
    1. Reassuring the parents that the condition is only temporary and will be treated with medication.
    2. Maintaining a patent airway and preparing for emergency ventilation.
    3. Preparing the infant for surgery and initiating preoperative teaching with the parents.
    4. Obtaining a detailed history, particularly of medications taken during the mother's pregnancy.

58. A 13-year-old is being seen for an annual physical examination. The child has lost 10 lb despite reports of excellent appetite. Appearance is normal, except for slightly protruding eyeballs, and the parents report the child has had difficulty sleeping lately. The nurse should do which of the following?
    1. Prepare the family for a neurology consult.
    2. Explain the need for an ophthalmology consult.
    3. Discuss the plan for thyroid function tests.
    4. Explain the plan for an 8-hour fasting blood glucose test.

59. A 12-year-old with hyperthyroidism is being treated with standard antithyroid drug therapy. A parent calls the office stating that the child has a sore throat and fever. The nurse's best response is which of the following?
    1. "Bring your child to the office or emergency room immediately."
    2. "Slight fever and sore throat are normal side effects of the medication."
    3. "Give your child the appropriate dose of ibuprofen, and call back if symptoms worsen."
    4. "Give your child at least 8 oz of clear fluids, and call back if symptoms worsen."

Answer the following three questions with reference to the following figure.

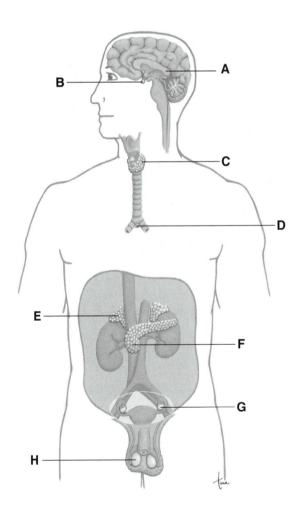

60. Hypofunction of which endocrine gland might cause type II DM?

_____

61. Hyperfunction of which endocrine gland might cause Cushing syndrome?

_____

62. Exophthalmic goiter is caused by hyperfunction of which endocrine gland?

_____

1. 1. One would not be able to determine if measuring was incorrect at a previous visit.
2. Expected adult height can be determined using a formula that takes into account the parents' height and can be calculated at any visit.
3. **Height velocity is the most important aspect of a growth evaluation and can demonstrate deceleration in growth if it is present.**
4. The dose of growth hormone replacement medication is based on weight.

TEST-TAKING HINT: The key point is the third visit. The HCP is interested in height velocity over time. The need for multiple measurements ensures that there is a measurable growth delay.

2. 1. Growth hormone levels elevate during sleep but cannot be used to determine a definitive diagnosis.
2. Exercise increases growth hormone secretion but cannot be used for definitive diagnosis.
3. Screening tests assist in determining in which direction further studies should be done.
4. **The need for additional testing requires explanation. The abnormal IGF-1 and insulin-like growth factor binding protein require a definitive diagnosis when the levels are either abnormally high or low. Very young children do not secrete adequate levels of growth hormone to measure accurately and thus require challenge/stimulation testing.**

TEST-TAKING HINT: The test taker should know that definitive diagnosis requires that more specific testing be done.

3. 1. Although girls in the United States mature earlier than in previous decades, the lowest age at which puberty is considered normal is 7 years for white girls and 6 years for African American girls.
2. **Dressing and acting appropriately for her chronological age should be encouraged for the well-being of the child.**
3. Although she is fertile if she is pubescent, it is not developmentally necessary to consider the use of birth control at this time.
4. The estrogen that is produced during puberty does assist in the closure of the epiphyseal plates. With proper medication management, however, the estrogen will be suppressed, and she will continue to grow.

TEST-TAKING HINT: White girls sometimes enter puberty as early as 7 years of age. This is rare, however, and the extent of her pubertal development should prompt concern.

4. 1. Although monitoring fluid intake is necessary, the child is on fluid restriction, and the amount of intake will be prescribed.
2. **It is crucial to monitor and record urine output. The infant with DI has hyposecretion of ADH, and fluid restriction has little effect on urine formation. This infant is at risk for dehydration and for fluid and electrolyte imbalances.**
3. It is a basic part of assessing the infant with fluid restriction to monitor skin turgor and the appearance of the mucous membranes, but they are not an absolute determination of overall well-being.
4. It is a basic part of assessing the infant to check pulse and temperature (the infant can become very hyperthermic), but neither would be an absolute indicator of well-being.

TEST-TAKING HINT: DI results from pituitary dysfunction. The posterior pituitary targets the renal tubules and acts on the distal and collecting tubules to make them permeable to water, thus increasing resorption and decreasing excretion of urine.

5. 1. Children with Graves disease have voracious appetites and lose weight.
2. Encouraging school and continuation of typical activities is better in terms of long-term management. Gym class and after-school sports should be restricted until the child is euthyroid.
3. Graves disease may go into remission after 2 or 3 years; there are some children, however, for whom it does not.
4. **Because the child is 12 years old, encouraging responsibility for health care is important. The child still needs family involvement and ongoing supervision but should not be completely dependent on family for care.**

TEST-TAKING HINT: The age of the patient is the key to answering the question.

6. 1. Hashimoto thyroiditis is a term that refers to hypothyroid disease. Laboratory tests would reveal a high TSH level.
2. **Graves disease is hyperthyroidism and presents with low TSH levels, weight loss, and excessive nervousness.**

3. Hypothyroidism is accompanied by a high TSH level.
4. Juvenile autoimmune thyroiditis is a term referring to hypothyroid disease. Laboratory tests would reveal a high TSH level.

TEST-TAKING HINT: The clues to the answer are the low TSH level and the child's symptoms.

7. 1. The baby has hypocalcemia and is being treated for this condition by the team. This should be reviewed with the family.
   2. **Vitamin D toxicity is a serious consequence of therapy and should be the top priority in teaching.**
   3. Reminding the family to give the medication as prescribed is helpful and should be a basic part of discharge care, but it is not the most important information.
   4. Giving the family the phone number for calling the clinic is part of basic care for discharge to home, but it is not the most important information.

TEST-TAKING HINT: Going over the side effects and risks of vitamin D treatment educates the family about what to watch for when giving the new medications.

8. 1. **The most common causes of secondary hyperparathyroidism are chronic renal disease and anomalies of the urinary tract. Blood studies indicate very high levels of calcium because the kidney is unable to process it.**
   2. Renal impairment causes phosphorus levels to become very high, and patients in renal failure are often put on low-phosphorus diets to control the levels.
   3. Massive doses of vitamin D are utilized to help improve the calcium levels in the bloodstream. Vitamin D toxicity has symptoms of weakness, vomiting, and diarrhea.
   4. Aluminum hydroxide keeps phosphorus mobilized so it can be excreted.

TEST-TAKING HINT: CRF is caused by the kidney's inability to process waste and excess minerals. Review which substances in excess cause which symptoms.

9. 1. Training two caretakers in the administration of the vasopressin reinforces the importance of the need to give the medication and ensures that medication can be given when the primary caretaker is unable to administer it. For someone on long-term injectable medication, two people need to know how to administer it for the above reason.

2. Children should wear MedicAlert tags as soon as they are diagnosed.
3. **Explaining that DI is different from DM is crucial to the parents' understanding of the management of the disease. DI is a rare condition that affects the posterior pituitary gland, whereas DM is a more common condition that affects the pancreas.**
4. Children with DI do not grow out of their condition and will require close medical management and medications for the rest of their lives.

TEST-TAKING HINT: The term "diabetes" is associated with DM. As DI is an uncommon condition that is treated differently, families may easily confuse it with the more common condition DM.

10. 1. Bone age is a method of assessing skeletal maturity and does not give a diagnosis.
    2. The child with a delayed bone age may continue to grow. In many children with a delayed bone age, medication is required to help them continue to grow.
    3. **The bone age is a method of evaluating the epiphyseal growth centers of the bone using standardized, age-appropriate tables.**
    4. A bone age that is not delayed in a child of short stature is more concerning than if the growth were delayed. This means that further testing and evaluation are needed if the growth delay is to be reversed.

TEST-TAKING HINT: Explaining a bone age film clarifies for the family why the test is needed.

11. 1. Oily skin is not associated with a low serum thyroxine level. It is more consistent with hyperthyroidism.
    2. Pale, thickened patches of skin are not associated with hypothyroidism.
    3. Sunken eyes and thickened hair are not associated with hypothyroidism, in which the hair is more often thin.
    4. **Myxedema, associated with low serum thyroxine and raised thyrotropin levels, is characteristic of hypothyroid dysfunction and presents with swelling or puffiness of the limbs and face, sparse hair, and very dry skin. These signs may be accompanied by slowness of movements and mental dullness.**

TEST-TAKING HINT: Describing various assessments is integral to charting accurately. Myxedema is a term used to describe hypothyroid skin.

12. 1. **Initially, in the ED, the child will be given an IV line, vital signs will be taken frequently, and seizure precautions will be taken.**
2. The child will be sent to the intensive care unit after being stabilized.
3. When children start to recover from an adrenocortical crisis, their progress is often very rapid, within 24 hours.
4. The child will present with headache, nausea and vomiting, high fever, high blood pressure, weakness, and abdominal pain. With prompt diagnosis and the institution of cortisol and fluids, a good recovery is likely.

TEST-TAKING HINT: The question is asking for a procedure that needs explaining while in the ED.

13. 1. **Keeping an extra month's supply of all medications, along with a prefilled syringe of hydrocortisone, will enable the family to treat an impending adrenal crisis before it gets severe.**
2. Wearing a MedicAlert bracelet is advantageous and can be periodically mentioned to the family.
3. Patients will know the medication has a bitter taste if they are taking the medication.
4. Weight gain will occur over time, but with good diet and adequate exercise this can be controlled.

TEST-TAKING HINT: Steroids are essential to life, so it is important to remind the family to have extra medication on hand at all times.

14. 1. Weight gain can and should be controllable with appropriate eating habits and adequate exercise.
2. The patient will quickly figure out that the medication tastes bitter and that the taste needs to be masked.
3. Anorexia and depression can result from taking steroids.
4. **Cortisone should be taken with food to decrease gastric irritation.**

TEST-TAKING HINT: Administration of cortisone can cause serious gastric irritation. The nurse should teach the family to anticipate this problem and ensure that the medicine is taken with food.

15. 1. The baby should not be discharged from the hospital without a name, and never call the infant "it."
2. The fact that the baby is a girl may be difficult for the family to accept, but the gender should be determined before discharge.
3. **Selecting a gender-neutral name enables the family and child to gradually accept and adjust to the baby's medical condition and sex.**
4. Calling the infant "baby" is akin to using the word "it."

TEST-TAKING HINT: The family needs to be given some positive way to cope with the fact that the infant's gender is in question.

16. 1. Cortisone increases the mobilization and utilization of fatty acids for energy, but it does not influence the hypertension.
2. **Cortisone suppresses the ACTH being secreted by the pituitary. Because very little, if any, cortisol is produced by the adrenal glands, the ACTH acts to increase cardiac activity and constrict the blood vessels, leading to hypertension.**
3. The adrenal glands synthesize and secrete cortisol.
4. Cortisone suppresses lymphocytes, eosinophils, and basophils, resulting in a decreased inflammatory and allergic response.

TEST-TAKING HINT: Regulation of hormonal secretions is based on negative feedback. The 21-hydroxylase deficiency is causing the adrenal gland to secrete too little cortisol. The pituitary is producing excess ACTH, trying to increase the adrenal secretion of cortisol, and causing the hypertension.

17. 1. **A pheochromocytoma is a rare tumor of the adrenal glands that secretes excess catecholamines, which are a group of amines secreted in the body that act as neurotransmitters. Examples include epinephrine, norepinephrine, and dopamine. Hypertension, headache, and decreased gastric motility are common with pheochromocytoma.**
2. A pheochromocytoma is a rare tumor of the adrenal glands that secretes excess catecholamines such as epinephrine, norepinephrine, and dopamine. Hypoglycemia and lethargy are not typical of pheochromocytoma. The excess catecholamines cause increased, not decreased, gastric motility.
3. A pheochromocytoma is a rare tumor of the adrenal glands that secretes excess catecholamines such as epinephrine, norepinephrine, and dopamine. Bradycardia, diarrhea, and weight gain are not typical of pheochromocytoma.

4. A pheochromocytoma is a rare tumor of the adrenal glands that secretes excess catecholamines such as epinephrine, norepinephrine, and dopamine. These excess catecholamines cause hypertension, not hypotension. Although they can cause decreased gastrointestinal activity, anuria is not typical of pheochromocytoma.

TEST-TAKING HINT: The tumor arises from the adrenal medulla. The adrenal medulla secretes epinephrine and norepinephrine. Symptoms are those of excess hormones from the adrenal medulla.

18. 1. Addison disease is another term for chronic adrenocortical insufficiency. Medications that replace normal glucocorticoids need to be increased, not decreased, in times of stress.
    2. **Because the adrenal glands are not producing enough glucocorticoids, the dosage of both the cortisol and aldosterone must be increased and sometimes tripled in times of stress.**
    3. Addison disease is another term for chronic adrenocortical insufficiency. Both medications need to be continued.
    4. Addison disease is another term for chronic adrenocortical insufficiency. Oral medications should be increased in times of stress.

TEST-TAKING HINT: The adrenal gland is not able to produce enough hormone, especially during times of stress.

19. 1. Determine the dosage of medication by multiplying 27 kg by the medication prescribed at 0.025 mg/kg. The total dosage needed is 0.675 mg.
    2. Determine the dosage of medication by multiplying 27 kg by the medication prescribed at 0.025 mg/kg. The total dosage needed is 0.675 mg.
    3. **Determine the dosage of medication by multiplying 27 kg by the medication prescribed at 0.025 mg/kg. The total dosage needed is 0.675 mg.**
    4. Determine the dosage of medication by multiplying 27 kg by the medication prescribed at 0.025 mg/kg. The total dosage needed is 0.675 mg.

TEST-TAKING HINT: Multiplying the milligrams per kilogram of weight by the patient's kilograms of weight yields the total milligrams dosage ordered.

20. 1. Determine the amount of solution by setting up an equation of 5 mg/5 mL as 0.675 mg:X.

2. Determine the amount of solution by setting up an equation of 5 mg/5 mL as 0.675 mg:X.
3. **Determine the amount of solution by setting up an equation of 5 mg/5 mL as 0.675 mg:X.**
4. Determine the amount of solution by setting up an equation of 5 mg/5 mL as 0.675 mg:X.

TEST-TAKING HINT: The medication is mixed as 1 mg per each mL. Give 0.675 mL of the solution three times weekly.

21. 1. **EMLA cream works well for skin and cutaneous pain. Having the child assist in putting on the EMLA patch involves the child in the pain-relieving process.**
    2. Because this is a monthly injection, it would not be appropriate to hold the child down forcefully, as this creates greater fear and anxiety.
    3. Apply ice to the opposite side of the body.
    4. Bribing children teaches them that the more they cry and fuss, the more they are rewarded.

TEST-TAKING HINT: Developing a trusting relationship with the child by allowing the child to help apply the EMLA cream gives the child some control in relieving the pain.

22. 1. 2.2 kg = 1 lb. Multiplying the kilograms by 2.2 yields 46.2 lb.
    2. 2.2 kg = 1 lb. Multiplying the kilograms by 2.2 yields 46.2 lb.
    3. 2.2 kg = 1 lb. Multiplying the kilograms by 2.2 yields 46. 2 lb.
    4. **2.2 kg = 1 lb. Multiplying the kilograms by 2.2 yields 46.2 lb.**

TEST-TAKING HINT: Parents frequently ask for "lay" terms of medical data. Knowing that there are 2.2 kg in each pound enables determination of this number.

23. 1. Thyrotropin and somatotropin are secreted by the anterior pituitary but do not directly influence breast development.
    2. **Oxytocin is secreted by the posterior pituitary but does target the uterus and production of milk from the breasts.**
    3. The gonadotropins stimulate the gonads to mature and produce sex hormones.
    4. Thyrotropin and somatotropin are secreted by the anterior pituitary but do not directly influence breast development.

TEST-TAKING HINT: The anterior pituitary is responsible for stimulating and inhibiting the secretions from the various target organs.

24. 1. **The posterior pituitary is responsible for the secretion of ADH and control of the renal tubules. The symptoms are those of DI.**
2. The anterior pituitary functions as the master gland for growth, sexual function, and skin but does not directly influence the urinary system.
3. The autonomic nervous system is not directly responsible for polyuria, polydipsia, and dehydration.
4. The sympathetic nervous system is not directly responsible for polyuria, polydipsia, and dehydration.

TEST-TAKING HINT: The symptoms are classic for posterior pituitary dysfunction.

25. 1. Thyroxine is secreted by the thyroid gland.
2. **Luteinizing hormone, prolactin, and ACTH are secreted by the anterior pituitary.**
3. **Luteinizing hormone, prolactin, and ACTH are secreted by the anterior pituitary.**
4. **Luteinizing hormone, prolactin, and ACTH are secreted by the anterior pituitary.**
5. Epinephrine is secreted by the adrenal medulla.
6. Cortisol is secreted by the adrenal cortex.

TEST-TAKING HINT: The pituitary is the master gland and is responsible for stimulating and inhibiting target glands. The thyroid and the adrenal glands are target glands.

26. 1. **Estrogen and progesterone are hormones secreted by the adrenal cortex that in excess would cause feminization of a young male child.**
2. Testosterone is secreted by the testes and does not result in feminization.
3. **Estrogen and progesterone are hormones secreted by the adrenal cortex that in excess would cause feminization.**
4. Cortisol is a glucocorticoid that is secreted by the adrenal cortex but does not result in feminization.
5. Androgens are secreted by the adrenal cortex but would cause masculinization of the child.

TEST-TAKING HINT: The sex hormones influence the development of the reproductive organs and secondary sexual characteristics. Male feminization is a result of hypofunction of primarily the male sex hormones.

27. 1. A fasting blood glucose is helpful in determining the child's overall health but does not demonstrate excess cortisol production by the body.
2. A thyroid panel is helpful in determining the child's overall health but does not demonstrate excess cortisol production by the body.
3. **A 24-hour urine for 17-hydroxycorticoids or a cortisone suppression test is used for diagnosing overproduction of cortisol by the body.**
4. Radiographic bone studies are helpful in determining the child's overall health but do not demonstrate excess cortisol production by the body.
5. **A 24-hour urine for 17-hydroxycorticoids or a cortisone suppression test is used for diagnosing overproduction of cortisol by the body.**
6. A urine culture is helpful in determining the child's overall health but does not demonstrate excess cortisol production by the body.
7. A complete blood count is helpful in determining the child's overall health but does not demonstrate excess cortisol production by the body.

TEST-TAKING HINT: Cortisol levels can be measured with urine-specific testing.

28. 1. **Chvostek sign is a facial muscle spasm elicited by tapping on the facial nerve in the region of the parotid gland, indicates heightened neuromuscular activity, and leads the nurse to suspect hypoparathyroidism.**
2. Chvostek sign is a facial muscle spasm elicited by tapping on the facial nerve in the region of the parotid gland, indicates heightened neuromuscular activity, and leads the nurse to suspect hypoparathyroidism.
3. Chvostek sign is a facial muscle spasm elicited by tapping on the facial nerve in the region of the parotid gland, indicates heightened neuromuscular activity, and leads the nurse to suspect hypoparathyroidism.
4. Chvostek sign is a facial muscle spasm elicited by tapping on the facial nerve in the region of the parotid gland, indicates heightened neuromuscular activity, and leads the nurse to suspect hypoparathyroidism.

TEST-TAKING HINT: The patient has had twitching for the last 2 weeks, and the nurse will want to see if the twitching can be elicited. If so, then the nurse would strongly suspect the child has hypothyroidism.

29. 1. The glands that line the gastrointestinal tract contain cells that produce hormones that control and coordinate secretion of digestive enzymes.
    2. The thymus gland is well developed in infancy, attains its greatest size at puberty and then is changed into fatty tissue.
    3. The pituitary gland is the master gland for the body.
    4. The thymus acts to provide immunity to the very young body.

TEST-TAKING HINT: The girl wants information about how the body develops immunity.

30. 1. Teens know their gender and may try on the roles of the opposite gender.
    2. Children 18 months to 30 months learn their gender from examining and touching their body parts and learning roles that are either male or female.
    3. Newborns do not identify with one gender or the other.
    4. By 4 to 6 years of age, children have a clear understanding of their gender and the male or female roles that they are assigned.

TEST-TAKING HINT: Erikson's stages of psychosexual development define a 2-year-old as in the "autonomy vs. shame and doubt" stage. The 2-year-old explores the body and is given specific behaviors that indicate the gender.

31. 10th percentile. The child would be in the 10th percentile in comparison with other boys the same age.

TEST-TAKING HINT: Mark the age of the child on the horizontal axis and find the weight on the vertical axis; the weight-for-age percentile is where the two lines intersect.

32. 1. The data from the previous primary care provider are important for comparison purposes.
    2. The provider should be made aware of the decelerating weight for age. This pictorial information can then be reviewed with the parent.
    3. Failure to thrive is a diagnosis that can be organic, nonorganic, or idiopathic.

Labeling a patient as having failure to thrive prior to the assessment is inappropriate.
    4. Weighing toddlers can be a challenge, because they are very active. The new weight should be obtained with only a diaper on the child. It should be recorded along with the previous provider's weights.

TEST-TAKING HINT: Working with professionals takes teamwork and allows the patient and family to feel as though they have selected a well-run practice.

33. 1. TH; the main physiological effect of TH is to regulate the basal metabolic rate and thereby control the process of growth and tissue differentiation.
    2. TH; the main physiological effect of TH is to regulate the basal metabolic rate and thereby control the process of growth and tissue differentiation.
    3. TC; the main effects that TC causes are related to maintenance of blood calcium levels by decreasing calcium concentration in the blood.
    4. TC; the main effects that TC causes are related to maintenance of blood calcium levels by decreasing calcium concentration in the blood.
    5. TH; the main physiological effect of TH is to regulate the basal metabolic rate and thereby control the process of growth and tissue differentiation.
    6. TH; the main physiological effect of TH is to regulate the basal metabolic rate and thereby control the process of growth and tissue differentiation.

TEST-TAKING HINT: TH is involved in many activities, and TC functions primarily to maintain calcium balance.

34. 1. The family should administer the reserve hydrocortisone injection intramuscularly immediately and then bring the child to the office.
    2. When children with adrenal insufficiency get the flu or are ill, the situation can be life-threatening. The family should administer the reserve hydrocortisone injection intramuscularly and then bring the child to the office.
    3. When children with adrenal insufficiency get the flu or are ill, the situation can be life-threatening. The family should administer the reserve hydrocortisone injection intramuscularly and then bring the child to the office. There is no harm in giving extra hydrocortisone.

4. When children with adrenal insufficiency get the flu or are ill, the situation can be life-threatening.

TEST-TAKING HINT: Because this child cannot produce cortisol, the levels fall and cause abdominal pain, nausea, and vomiting. The child needs additional cortisol to recover.

35. 1. Dehydration is not a feature of SIADH.
    2. **ADH assists the body in retaining fluids and subsequently decreases serum osmolarity while the urine osmolarity rises. When serum sodium levels are decreased below 120 mEq/L, the child becomes symptomatic.**
    3. **ADH assists the body in retaining fluids and subsequently decreases serum osmolarity while the urine osmolarity rises. When serum sodium levels are decreased below 120 mEq/L, the child becomes symptomatic.**
    4. Hypoglycemia is not a feature of SIADH.
    5. Myxedema is not a feature of SIADH.

TEST-TAKING HINT: The posterior pituitary is responsible for secretion of ADH. SIADH is oversecretion of ADH.

36. 1. **Administering desmopressin acetate per nasal spray is a means of providing the necessary medication in a steady state, if it is given using the flexible nasal tube every 8 to 12 hours. This decreases nasal irritation.**
    2. **If the child becomes ill with rhinorrhea, the nasal spray will need to be administered via the buccal mucosa or rectum or the medication changed to tablets.**
    3. Administering desmopressin acetate per nasal spray is a means of providing the necessary medication in a steady state, if it is given using the flexible nasal tube every 8 to 12 hours.
    4. **Administering desmopressin acetate per nasal spray is a means of providing the necessary medication in a steady state, if it is given using the flexible nasal tube every 8 to 12 hours.**
    5. **Side effects of the DDAVP are those of SIADH.**
    6. Administering desmopressin acetate per nasal spray is a means of providing the necessary medication in a steady state, if it is given using the flexible nasal tube every 8 to 12 hours.

TEST-TAKING HINT: Administering medication necessitates the parent be instructed in the technique, side effects, and what to do if the medication cannot be administered for some reason.

37. 1. Propylthiouracil is used to suppress thyroid function. One of the grave complications of the medication is leukopenia.
    2. **Propylthiouracil is used to suppress thyroid function. One of the grave complications of the medication is leukopenia.**
    3. Propylthiouracil is used to suppress thyroid function. One of the grave complications of the medication is leukopenia.
    4. Propylthiouracil is used to suppress thyroid function. One of the grave complications of the medication is leukopenia.

TEST-TAKING HINT: Side effects of a medication need to be assessed quickly. During the first few weeks of therapy there is a risk of blood dyscrasias. The propylthiouracil prevents the conversion of iodine to its usable form.

38. 1. Glucagon is given only for severe hypoglycemia. The child's symptoms are those of mild hypoglycemia.
    2. **Milk is best to give for mild hypoglycemia, which would present with the symptoms described.**
    3. Insulin is appropriate for elevated blood glucose, but the symptoms listed are those of hypoglycemia, not hyperglycemia. It is important for the test taker to be able to distinguish between the two.
    4. Water is appropriate for mild hyperglycemia, but the symptoms listed are those of hypoglycemia.

TEST-TAKING HINT: The test taker should first determine hyper- or hypoglycemia, which should permit elimination of two choices, then choose the best answer. When describing symptoms of a diabetic patient, look for ways to determine either hypoglycemia or hyperglycemia.

39. 1. Growth hormone is appropriate if the patient had panhypopituitarism.
    2. **Parathyroid is responsible for calcium reabsorption; therefore, supplemental calcium in the diet is the important point to be discussed in patient teaching.**
    3. Folic acid is another dietary supplement and a distraction.
    4. Information about insulin injection is appropriate for DM, not parathyroid disorder.

TEST-TAKING HINT: The test taker needs to know the function of the parathyroid glands.

40. 1. Type II DM is best managed by diet, exercise, and oral medication.
    2. Type II DM can best be prevented via diet and activity; type I DM is not preventable.
    3. Though insulin resistance can be one of the factors in type I DM, it is not the primary factor.
    4. **Individuals with type I DM do not produce insulin. If one does not produce insulin, type I DM is the diagnosis.**

TEST-TAKING HINT: The test taker should know the difference between type I and type II DM.

41. 1. **Risk for infection is a correct nursing diagnosis. Understanding DM is understanding the effect it has on peripheral circulation and impairment of defense mechanisms.**
    2. Although many children with type I DM present with enuresis, impaired urinary elimination is not the best response.
    3. Treatment includes injections, but this is not a risk for injury.
    4. Type I DM, although lifelong, is not a terminal illness and can be well managed, so grieving is not an appropriate diagnosis.

TEST-TAKING HINT: The test taker needs to understand diabetes to choose correctly.

42. 1. Correct needle position is with the bevel facing upward.
    2. Injection is subcutaneous, so tissue is not spread, as it would be for intramuscular injection.
    3. Aspiration for blood is no longer recommended for subcutaneous injections.
    4. **Skin tissue is elevated to prevent injection into the muscle when giving a subcutaneous injection. Insulin is only given subcutaneously.**

TEST-TAKING HINT: The test taker must understand that insulin is only given subcutaneously. The test taker can eliminate answers 2 and 3 by knowing how to give an intramuscular injection.

43. 1. Limiting fluids is appropriate for a child presenting with the symptoms of DI.
    2. Weight loss without the other presenting symptoms might be indicative of a need for a weight/nutrition consult.
    3. Strict intake and output monitoring is included in the care of a child with DI.

4. **Frequent blood glucose testing is included in the care of a child with type I DM. The symptoms described in the question are characteristic of a child just prior to the diagnosis of type I DM.**

TEST-TAKING HINT: In a question that lists symptoms, it is important to determine the diagnosis. In this case, the test taker can anticipate type I DM and know that frequent glucose monitoring is part of the plan of care.

44. 1. Vasopressin is a medication used to treat the uncontrolled diuresis associated with DI.
    2. **Growth hormone is used to treat a child with hypopituitarism.**
    3. Hypopituitarism promotes short, not tall, stature.
    4. Although hypoglycemia might be a factor when a child is undergoing diagnostic testing for hypopituitarism, blood sugar testing is not part of the treatment plan.

TEST-TAKING HINT: When presented with a question like this, the test taker must first consider the diagnosis and the clinical manifestations. Knowing that this diagnosis is considered primarily when a child presents with short stature and slowed growth curve, answer 2 is most appropriate.

45. 1. A child with hyperthyroidism displays increased activity.
    2. Thyroidectomy is not the first choice for treating hyperthyroidism, although it is considered if other treatments fail.
    3. **Because increased activity is characteristic of hyperthyroidism, providing opportunity for rest is a recommended nursing intervention.**
    4. Weight loss despite increased appetite and intake might be a symptom of hyperthyroidism. Just increasing calories is not the best option, because the cause and treatment of the thyroid's hyperactivity needs to be addressed.

TEST-TAKING HINT: The test taker needs to know the signs and symptoms of hyperthyroidism to determine appropriate nursing interventions.

46. 1. Balanced diet, although important, does not determine hemoglobin A_{1c}.
    2. Anemia would be a correct choice if the question asked about hemoglobin, not hemoglobin A_{1c}.
    3. **Hemoglobin A_{1c}, or glycosylated hemoglobin, reflects average blood glucose levels over 2 to 3 months. Frequent high blood glucose levels**

would result in a higher hemoglobin A_{1c}, suggesting that blood glucose needs to be in better control.

4. Presence of ketones in the blood, although associated with the absence of insulin and with high blood glucose levels, is not directly correlated with hemoglobin A_{1c}.

TEST-TAKING HINT: The test taker needs to know the purpose of the hemoglobin A_{1c} test.

47. 1. DI is caused by undersecretion of ADH (vasopressin). Replacement therapy with vasopressin is a long-term option, however, not a short-term one.
2. DI is not to be confused with DM, for which dietary planning is a large part of management.
3. **Vasopressin is the treatment of choice. It is important for patients and parents to understand that DI is a lifelong disease.**
4. Although a sign of DI is excessive urination, fluid replacement is needed, not restriction. Fluid restriction is only part of the diagnostic phase.

TEST-TAKING HINT: The test taker needs to understand the long-term implications of the diagnosis.

48. 1. Within 24 hours of fluid restriction, the urine becomes concentrated in a healthy child.
2. Because the urine is not concentrated, the child is likely to have DI.
3. Children should be carefully observed to make sure they are not sneaking fluids; however, the assumption that this child has been doing so should not be made.
4. **Children with DI cannot concentrate urine.**

TEST-TAKING HINT: Understanding that DI causes uncontrolled diuresis, the test taker should choose answer 4. Answers 1 and 3 assume that there is something wrong with the diagnostic procedure and would be less likely to be correct. Answer 2 is the opposite of 4.

49. 1. The primary causes of DI are idiopathic, organic, and brain trauma, unlike the causes for type II DM, for which diet and exercise are major factors.
2. DI does not have a hereditary factor.
3. Blood sugar monitoring is important with DM, not DI.
4. **Despite the use of vasopressin to treat the symptoms of DI, breakthrough urination is likely.**

TEST-TAKING HINT: The test taker needs to understand the difference between DI and DM.

50. 1. Menarche usually occurs within 2 years after the start of breast development.
2. Age 9 is the average age of thelarche (breast bud development), which is followed shortly by the appearance of pubic hair.
3. **The changes described in the question are normal for a healthy 9-year-old female.**
4. No further testing is required.

TEST-TAKING HINT: Understanding that the question describes a set of normal changes, the test taker could eliminate answers 2 and 4. Because the parent in the question is expressing concern, the most appropriate answer from the remaining two is the one offering reassurance, answer 3.

51. 1. Graves disease causes hyperthyroidism. Gradual weight loss, not weight gain, is a sign.
2. **Weight loss, increased activity, and heat intolerance can be expected when the thyroid gland is hyperfunctional.**
3. Weight gain as a symptom makes this answer incorrect.
4. Constipation and dry skin with poor turgor are more likely in a patient with hypothyroidism.

TEST-TAKING HINT: The test taker needs to know the presenting signs and symptoms of Graves disease.

52. 1. The fruity odor is that of acetone. The patient is exhibiting signs of ketoacidosis. The history of vomiting and the Kussmaul breathing preclude oral rehydration.
2. Although it is likely that ketones would be present, the child is in a life-threatening situation. Checking urine is not necessary.
3. **This patient needs fluid and electrolyte therapy to restore tissue perfusion prior to beginning IV insulin therapy.**
4. The patient is hyperglycemic, not hypoglycemic.

TEST-TAKING HINT: The patient's history of vomiting should clue the test taker to disregard choices for food or fluids by mouth, answers 1 and 4. Answer 2 might be possible, as the urine would test positive for ketones, but the deep and rapid breathing should help the test taker choose answer 3.

53. 1. 10 U of regular insulin is a very high dose; a carbohydrate ratio refers to the amount of carbohydrates allowed per unit of regular insulin. This dose would be appropriate if the child were planning a meal of 100 g of carbohydrates.
2. Limiting carbohydrate intake is not a factor in managing type I DM.
3. **An insulin-to-carbohydrate ratio refers to the amount of insulin given per gram of carbohydrate. A ratio of 1:5 means 1 U for every 5 carbohydrates.**
4. The ratio is insulin to carbohydrate, not carbohydrate to fat or protein.

TEST-TAKING HINT: The test taker needs to understand the insulin-to-carbohydrate ratio.

54. 1. Type I DM is managed with insulin, not oral agents.
2. Metoclopramide, not metformin, can be used to treat reflux.
3. Methylprednisolone (Medrol) can be used to treat inflammatory bowel disease.
4. **Metformin is commonly used to manage type II DM.**

TEST-TAKING HINT: Even being unfamiliar with the name metformin, the test taker might guess that Glucophage would have something to do with destruction or digestion of glucose, thereby being able to correctly eliminate answers 2 and 3.

55. 1. Managing DM increases rather than decreases independence.
2. **Because the desire to fit in is so strong in adolescence, the need to manage one's diabetes can compromise the patient's perception of ability to do so. For example, an adolescent with type I DM has to plan meals and snacks, test blood sugar, limit choices of when and what to eat, and always be concerned with the immediate health consequences of actions as simple as eating. The fact that these limitations can negatively affect self-esteem is an essential concept for the nurse caring for adolescents with diabetes to understand.**
3. Obesity is not necessarily associated with type I DM.
4. Hormone changes in adolescence often result in increasing insulin demands; however, increased insulin need not correlate with low self-esteem.

TEST-TAKING HINT: The test taker needs to understand normal development in the
adolescent and that fitting in is extremely important.

56. 1. **This is true. A carbohydrate is a carbohydrate, and insulin dosing is based on blood sugar level and carbohydrates to be eaten.**
2. Snacks should be ingested before planned exercise rather than after.
3. Nutritional needs of children with DM do not differ from those without DM.
4. Weight loss is likely a factor in managing type II DM; type I DM is often preceded by dramatic weight loss. The nutritional needs of children with type I DM are essentially the same as those not affected.

TEST-TAKING HINT: The test taker needs to understand the basics of DM and how it is managed. Insulin and carbohydrates have to complement each other for good control.

57. 1. Goiter in a newborn can be life-threatening and is usually treated by surgical removal or partial removal of the thyroid.
2. **Goiter in a newborn can cause tracheal compression, and positioning to help relieve pressure (i.e., neck hyperextension) is essential. Emergency precautions for ventilation and possible tracheostomy are also instituted.**
3. Although preparation for surgery might be necessary, the most important intervention is protecting the infant's airway.
4. Certain medications (antithyroid drugs) taken by the mother could predispose the infant to developing a goiter. Although the history is important, it is not the first priority for the nurse caring for this patient.

TEST-TAKING HINT: The test taker, if unsure of the correct response, should choose the one pertaining to the ABCs: airway, breathing, and cardiac status.

58. 1. The patient exhibits signs of Graves disease, the primary cause of hyperthyroidism in children. A neurology consultation is not indicated.
2. Despite the exophthalmos, an eye consultation is not indicated.
3. **Diagnostic evaluation for hyperthyroidism is based on thyroid function tests. It is expected in this case that T4 and T3 levels would be elevated, as the thyroid gland is overfunctioning.**
4. Fasting blood glucose is used to help evaluate for other endocrine disorders, such as Cushing syndrome and DM.

TEST-TAKING HINT: One of the first nursing considerations is identifying children with hyperthyroidism.

59. 1. **A complication of antithyroid drug therapy is leukopenia. Fever and sore throat, therefore, need to be evaluated immediately. This is an essential component of discharge teaching for patients with Graves disease.**
    2. Because of the above explanation, this response is not appropriate.
    3. This is a tempting choice for the test taker, as fever and sore throat appear to be fairly benign symptoms. Because the question includes information regarding Graves disease and medication therapy, however, the test taker should eliminate this answer.
    4. It is most likely that medication, not fluid status, contributes to the child's symptoms.

TEST-TAKING HINT: The test taker needs to be familiar with adverse effects of all medications administered or that the family is taught about.

60. F

61. E

62. C

11

Neuromuscular or Muscular Disorders

KEYWORDS

Atrophy (wasting or decrease in size of muscles)

Congenital (present at birth)

Contracture (shortening of muscle or scar tissue, resulting in deformity)

Dystrophy (disorder where muscles weaken and atrophy)

ABBREVIATIONS

Cerebral palsy (CP)

Cranial nerve (CN)

Guillain-Barré syndrome (GBS)

Magnetic resonance imaging (MRI)

QUESTIONS

1. An adolescent presents with sudden-onset unilateral facial weakness. The teen has drooping of one side of the mouth, is unable to close the eye on the affected side, has no other symptoms, and otherwise feels well. The nurse could summarize the condition by which of the following?
   1. The prognosis is poor.
   2. This may be a stroke.
   3. It is a fifth CN palsy.
   4. This is paralysis of the facial nerve.

2. The nurse is performing an admission assessment on a 9-year-old who has just been diagnosed with systemic lupus erythematosus. Which assessment findings should the nurse expect?
   1. Headaches and nausea.
   2. Fever, malaise, and weight loss.
   3. A papular rash covering the trunk and face.
   4. Abdominal pain and dysuria.

3. The parents of a preschooler diagnosed with muscular dystrophy are asking questions about the course of their child's disease. The nurse should tell them which of the following?
   1. Muscular dystrophies are disorders associated with progressive degeneration of muscles, resulting in relentless and increasing weakness.
   2. The weakness that the child is currently experiencing will probably not increase.
   3. The child will be able to function normally and require no special accommodations.
   4. The extent of degeneration depends on performing daily physical therapy.

4. The nurse is teaching the parents of a child with Duchenne (pseudohypertrophic) muscular dystrophy. The nurse should tell them that some of the progressive complications include which of the following?
   1. Dry skin and hair, hirsutism, protruding tongue, and mental retardation.
   2. Anorexia, gingival hyperplasia, and dry skin and hair.
   3. Contractures, obesity, and pulmonary infections.
   4. Trembling, frequent loss of consciousness, and slurred speech.

5. The Gower sign for assessing Duchenne muscular dystrophy can be elicited by having a patient do which of the following?
   1. Close the eyes and touch the nose with alternating index fingers.
   2. Hop on one foot and then the other.
   3. Bend from the waist to touch the toes.
   4. Walk like a duck and rise from a squatting position.

6. A 5-year-old has been diagnosed with pseudohypertrophic muscular dystrophy. Which of the following nursing interventions would be appropriate?
   1. Discuss with the parents the potential need for respiratory support.
   2. Explain that this disease is easily treated with medication.
   3. Suggest exercises that will limit the use of muscles and prevent fatigue.
   4. Assist the parents in finding a nursing facility for future care.

7. The nurse is discussing nutrition with the parents of a child with Duchenne muscular dystrophy. The nurse tells the parents that which of the following foods would be best for their child?
   1. High-carbohydrate, high-protein foods.
   2. No special food combinations.
   3. Extra protein to help strengthen muscles.
   4. Low-calorie foods to prevent weight gain.

8. Which of the following will help a school-aged child with muscular dystrophy stay active longer?
   1. Normal activities, such as swimming.
   2. Using a treadmill every day.
   3. Several periods of rest every day.
   4. Using a wheelchair on getting tired.

9. The mother of a child with Duchenne muscular dystrophy asks the nurse who in the family should have genetic screening. Who should the nurse say must be tested? Select all that apply.
   1. The mother and father.
   2. The sister.
   3. The brother.
   4. The aunts and all female cousins.
   5. The uncles and all male cousins.

10. The nurse is teaching family members of a child newly diagnosed with muscular dystrophy about early signs. The nurse knows that teaching was successful when a parent states that which of the following signs may indicate the condition early?
    1. Increased muscle strength.
    2. Difficulty climbing stairs.
    3. High fevers and tiredness.
    4. Respiratory infections and obesity.

11. The nurse is caring for a school-aged child with Duchenne muscular dystrophy in the elementary school. Which of the following would be an appropriate nursing diagnosis?
    1. Anticipatory grieving.
    2. Anxiety reduction.
    3. Increased pain.
    4. Activity intolerance.

12. The nurse knows that teaching has been successful when the parent of a child with muscle weakness states that the diagnostic test for muscular dystrophy is which of the following?
    1. Electromyelogram.
    2. Nerve conduction velocity.
    3. Muscle biopsy.
    4. Creatine kinase level.

13. Spinal cord injuries are frequently misdiagnosed in children because of a phenomenon called spinal cord injury without radiographic abnormality. This occurs because of which of the following?
    1. Children can suffer momentary severe subluxation and trauma to the spinal cord.
    2. The immature spinal column in children does not allow for quality films.
    3. Children are more prone to spinal cord injuries because of their size.
    4. Children are unable to quantify pain and do not report symptoms appropriately.

14. The nurse is preparing to receive a child in the emergency room. Radio report given by Emergency Medical Service indicates a possible spinal cord injury. The nurse should be prepared for a child with which of the following?
    1. Severe pain.
    2. Elevated temperature.
    3. Respiratory depression.
    4. Increased intracranial pressure.

15. Concerning a child with post-traumatic spinal cord injury, the nurse knows teaching has been successful when the parent states that which of the following can cause autonomic dysreflexia?
    1. Exposure to cold temperatures.
    2. Distended bowel or bladder.
    3. Bradycardia.
    4. Headache.

16. The nurse receives a call from the local Emergency Medical Services stating that an ambulance is arriving with an 8-month-old with a decreased level of consciousness. When assessing the neurological status of an 8-month-old, the nurse should check for which of the following?
    1. Clarity of speech.
    2. Interaction with staff.
    3. Developmental delay.
    4. Ability to follow instructions.

17. The nurse is admitting a child with a spinal cord injury. A plan of care should be based on the fact that a patient suffering from complete spinal cord injury will experience which of the following symptoms?
    1. Loss of motor and sensory function below the level of the injury.
    2. Loss of interest in normal activities.
    3. Have extreme pain below the level of the injury.
    4. Loss of some function, with sparing of function below the level of the injury.

18. The nurse is planning care for a patient with a T12 spinal cord injury. Which life-long complications should the patient and family know about? Select all that apply.
    1. Skin integrity.
    2. Incontinence.
    3. Loss of large and small motor activity.
    4. Loss of voice.
    5. Flaccid paralysis.

19. After spinal cord surgery, a patient suddenly complains of a severe headache. What should be the nurse's first action?
    1. Check the blood pressure.
    2. Check for a full bladder.
    3. Ask if pain is present somewhere else.
    4. Ask if other symptoms are present.

20. A nurse working in the neuro-intensive care unit has a patient with a spinal cord injury at T4. The patient suddenly becomes dangerously hypertensive and brady-cardic. Which of the following interventions is appropriate in this situation?
    1. Call the neurosurgeon immediately, as this sounds like sudden intracranial hypertension.
    2. Check to be certain that the patient's bladder is not distended.
    3. Administer Hyperstat to treat the blood pressure.
    4. Administer atropine for bradycardia.

21. A nurse is receiving an infant with myelomeningocele from an outside hospital. Which of the following priority items should be placed at the newborn's bedside?
    1. A bottle of normal saline.
    2. A rectal thermometer.
    3. Extra blankets.
    4. A blood pressure cuff.

22. The nurse is caring for an infant with myelomeningocele who is going to surgery later today for closure of the sac. Which of the following would be a priority nursing diagnosis before surgery?
    1. Alteration in parent-infant bonding.
    2. Altered growth and development.
    3. Risk of infection.
    4. Risk for weight loss.

23. Which of the following should the nurse include when teaching sexuality education to an adolescent with a spinal cord injury?
    1. "You can enjoy a healthy sex life and most likely conceive children."
    2. "You will never be able to conceive if you have no genital sensation."
    3. "Young men stop producing testosterone and sperm after their injury."
    4. "Young women lack estrogen and no longer ovulate after their injury."

24. The parent of a 6-year-old with a repaired myelomeningocele is in the clinic for her child's regular examination. The child has frequent constipation and has been crying at night because of pain in the legs. After an MRI, the diagnosis of a tethered cord is made. Which of the following should the nurse tell the parent?
    1. Tethered cord is a postsurgical complication.
    2. Tethered cord occurs during times of slow growth.
    3. Release of the tethered cord will be necessary only once.
    4. Offering laxatives and acetaminophen daily will help control these problems.

25. The nurse is caring for a newborn with a myelomeningocele who will have a surgical repair tomorrow. The nurse should do which of the following?
    1. Offer formula every 3 hours.
    2. Turn the infant back to front every 2 hours.
    3. Place a wet dressing on the sac.
    4. Provide pain medication every 4 hours.

26. Which of the following should the nurse do first when caring for an infant who just had a repair of a myelomeningocele?
    1. Weigh diapers for 24-hour urine output.
    2. Measure head circumference.
    3. Offer clear fluids.
    4. Assess for infection.

27. A newborn is diagnosed with a myelomeningocele at L2. Which of the following should be the priority nursing diagnosis for this infant at 12 hours of age?
    1. Altered bowel elimination related to neurological deficits.
    2. Potential for infection related to the physical defect.
    3. Altered nutrition related to neurological deficit.
    4. Disturbance in self-concept related to physical disability.

28. A 2-month-old has had a myelomeningocele repair and has been brought in by a parent for the well-child checkup and shots. Over the last week, the baby has had a high-pitched cry and has been irritable. Height, weight, and head circumference have been at the 50th percentile. Today height is at the 50th percentile, weight is at the 70th percentile, and head circumference is at the 90th percentile. The nurse should do which of the following?
    1. Tell the parent this is normal for an infant with a repaired myelomeningocele.
    2. Tell the parent this might mean the baby has increased intracranial pressure.
    3. Suspect the baby's intracranial pressure is low because of a leak.
    4. Refer the baby to the neurologist for follow-up care.

29. Which of the following should the nurse tell the parent of an infant with spina bifida?
    1. Bone growth will be more than that of babies who are not sick, because your baby will be less active.
    2. Physical and occupational therapy will be helpful to stimulate the senses and improve cognitive skills.
    3. Nutritional needs for your infant will be calculated based on activity level.
    4. Fine motor skills will be delayed because of the disability.

30. A 3-month-old with spina bifida is admitted to the nurse's unit. Which of the following gross motor skills should the nurse assess at this age?
    1. Head control.
    2. Pincer grasp.
    3. Sitting alone.
    4. Rolling over.

31. A 15-year-old with spina bifida is seen in the clinic for a well-child checkup. The teen uses leg braces and crutches to ambulate. Which of the following nursing diagnoses takes priority?
    1. Potential for infection.
    2. Alteration in mobility.
    3. Alteration in elimination.
    4. Potential body image disturbance.

32. A school-aged child is admitted to the unit preoperatively for bladder reconstruction. The child is latex-sensitive. Which of the following interventions should the nurse implement?
    1. Post a sign on the door and chart that the child is latex-allergic.
    2. Use powder-free latex gloves when giving care.
    3. Keep personal items such as stuffed animals in a plastic bag to avoid latex contamination.
    4. Use a disposable plastic-covered blood pressure cuff that will stay in the child's room.

33. Following surgical repair and closure of a myelomeningocele shortly after birth, which of the following is true of an infant?
    1. The infant will not need any long-term management and should be considered cured.
    2. The infant will no longer be at risk of urinary tract infections or movement problems.
    3. The infant will have continual drainage of cerebrospinal fluid, needing frequent dressing changes.
    4. The infant will need lifelong management of urinary, orthopedic, and neurological problems.

34. A newborn with a repaired myelomeningocele is assessed for hydrocephalus. What would the nurse expect if the infant has hydrocephalus?
1. Low-pitched cry and depressed fontanel.
2. Low-pitched cry and bulging fontanel.
3. Bulging fontanel and downwardly rotated eyes.
4. Depressed fontanel and upwardly rotated eyes.

35. The nurse is developing a plan of care for a child recently diagnosed with CP. Which of the following should be the nurse's priority goal?
1. Ensure the ingestion of sufficient calories for growth.
2. Decrease intracranial pressure.
3. Teach appropriate parenting strategies for a special-needs child.
4. Ensure that the child reaches full potential.

36. The nurse knows that teaching of parents of a child newly diagnosed with CP is successful when the parents state that CP is which of the following?
1. Inability to speak and drooling.
2. Poor dentition due to poor hygiene.
3. Involuntary movements of upper extremities only.
4. An increase in muscle tone and deep tendon reflexes.

37. The parent of a toddler newly diagnosed with CP asks the nurse what caused it. The nurse should answer which of the following?
1. Most cases are caused by unknown prenatal factors.
2. It is commonly caused by perinatal factors.
3. The exact cause is not known.
4. The exact cause is known in every instance.

38. Which of the following developmental milestones should the nurse be concerned about if a 10-month-old could not do it?
1. Crawl.
2. Cruise.
3. Walk.
4. Have a pincer grasp.

39. The parent of an infant asks the nurse what to watch for to determine if the infant has CP. The nurse should reply which of the following?
1. If the infant cannot sit up without support before 8 months.
2. If the infant demonstrates tongue thrust before 4 months.
3. If the infant has poor head control after 2 months.
4. If the infant has clenched fists after 3 months.

40. The parent of a young child with CP brings the child to the clinic for a checkup. Which of the parent's following statements indicates an understanding of the child's long-term needs?
1. "My child will need all my attention for the next 10 years."
2. "Once in school, my child will catch up and be like the other children."
3. "My child will grow up and need to learn to do things independently."
4. "I'm the one who knows the most about my child and can do the most for my child."

41. A child with spastic CP had an intrathecal dose of baclofen in the early afternoon. What is the expected result 3½ hours post dose that suggests the child would benefit from a baclofen pump?
1. The ability to self-feed.
2. The ability to walk with little assistance.
3. If the spasticity were decreased.
4. If the spasticity were increased.

42. The nurse is doing a follow-up assessment of a 9-month-old. The infant rolls both ways, sits with some support, pushes food out of the mouth, and pushes away when held. The parent asks about the infant's development. The nurse responds by saying which of the following?
    1. "Your child is developing normally."
    2. "Your child needs to see the primary care provider."
    3. "You need to help your child learn to sit unassisted."
    4. "Push the food back when your child pushes food out."

43. A child is admitted to the pediatric unit with spastic CP. Which of the following would the nurse expect this child to demonstrate? Select all that apply.
    1. Increased deep tendon reflexes.
    2. Decreased muscle tone.
    3. Scoliosis.
    4. Contractures.
    5. Scissoring.
    6. Good control of posture.
    7. Good fine motor skills.

44. A 3-year-old child with CP is admitted for dehydration following an episode of diarrhea. The nurse's assessment follows: awake, pale, thin child lying in bed, multiple contractures, drooling, coughing spells noted when parent feeds. T 97.8°F (36.5°C), P 75, R 25, weight 7.2 kg, no diarrheal stool for 48 hours. Which of the following nursing diagnoses is most important?
    1. Potential for skin breakdown: lying in one position.
    2. Alteration in nutrition: less than body requirements.
    3. Potential for impaired social support: mother sole caretaker.
    4. Alteration in elimination: diarrhea.

45. The parent of an infant with CP asks the nurse if the infant will be mentally retarded. Which of the following is the nurse's best response?
    1. "Children with CP have some amount of mental retardation."
    2. "Approximately 20% of children with CP have normal intelligence."
    3. "Many children with CP have normal intelligence."
    4. "Mental retardation is expected if motor and sensory deficits are severe."

46. Parents bring their 2-month-old into the clinic with concerns that the baby seems "floppy." The parents say the baby seems to be working hard to breathe. The nurse can see some intercostal retractions, although the baby is otherwise in no distress. The parents say the baby eats very slowly and seems to fatigue rapidly. They add there was a cousin whose baby had similar symptoms. The nurse would be most concerned with what possible complications?
    1. Respiratory compromise.
    2. Dehydration.
    3. Need for emotional support for the family.
    4. Feeding intolerance.

47. The mother of a newborn brings her infant in for a 2-week checkup. The mother relates that this is her first child, that the baby seems to sleep very often, and that the baby does not cry much. What question would the nurse ask the mother?
    1. "How many ounces of formula does your baby take at each feeding?"
    2. "How many bowel movements does your baby have in a day?"
    3. "How much sleep do you get every night?"
    4. "How long does the baby stay awake at each feeding?"

48. The mother of an infant diagnosed with Werdnig-Hoffmann disease asks the nurse what she could have done during her pregnancy to prevent this. The nurse explains that the cause of Werdnig-Hoffmann is which of the following?
    1. Unknown.
    2. Restricted movement in utero.
    3. Inherited as an autosomal recessive trait.
    4. Inherited as an autosomal dominant trait.

49. The parents of a toddler diagnosed with Werdnig-Hoffmann disease ask the nurse what they can feed their child that would be quality food. Which of the following would be good choices for the nurse to recommend?
    1. A hot dog and chips.
    2. Chicken and broccoli.
    3. A banana and almonds.
    4. A milkshake and a hamburger.

50. The parent of a child diagnosed with Werdnig-Hoffmann disease notes times of not being able to hear the child breathing. The nurse should first do which of the following?
    1. Check pulse oximetry on the child.
    2. Count the child's respirations.
    3. Listen to the child's lung sounds.
    4. Ask the parent if the child coughs at night.

51. A child presents with a history of having had an upper respiratory tract infection 2 weeks ago; complains of symmetrical lower extremity weakness, back pain, and muscle tenderness; and has absent deep tendon reflexes in the lower extremities. Which of the following is true regarding this condition?
    1. The disease process is probably bacterial.
    2. The recent upper respiratory infection is not important information.
    3. This may be an acute inflammatory demyelinating neuropathy.
    4. CN involvement is rare.

52. A child with GBS is admitted to the pediatric unit. The child has had lots of oral fluids but has not urinated for 8 hours. The nurse's first action would be to do which of the following?
    1. Check the child's serum blood-urea-nitrogen level.
    2. Check the child's complete blood count.
    3. Catheterize the child in and out.
    4. Run water in the bathroom to stimulate urination.

53. The nurse is planning care for a child who was recently admitted with GBS. Which of the following is a priority nursing diagnosis?
    1. Risk for constipation related to immobility.
    2. Chronic sorrow related to presence of chronic disability.
    3. Impaired skin integrity related to infectious disease process.
    4. Activity intolerance related to ineffective cardiac muscle function.

54. Which of the following should the nurse expect as an intervention in a child in the recovery phase of GBS?
    1. Assess for respiratory compromise.
    2. Assess for swallowing difficulties.
    3. Evaluate neuropsychological functioning.
    4. Begin an active physical therapy program.

55. A child has a provisional diagnosis of myasthenia gravis. Which of the following should the nurse expect in this child? Select all that apply.
    1. Double vision.
    2. Ptosis.
    3. Fatigue.
    4. Ascending paralysis.
    5. Sensory disturbance.

56. The nurse judges teaching as successful when the parent of a child with myasthenia gravis states which of the following?
1. "My child should play on the school's basketball team."
2. "My child should meditate every day."
3. "My child should be allowed to do what other kids do."
4. "My child should be watched carefully for signs of illness."

57. The parent of a 6-month-old calls the clinic for advice on how to treat the infant's constipation. The best advice the nurse can offer is which of the following?
1. Offer extra water every day.
2. Add corn syrup to two bottles a day.
3. Give the infant a glycerine suppository today.
4. Let the infant go 3 days without a stool before intervening.

58. A 6-year-old living in a rural area sustains a puncture wound and goes to the clinic. The child is missing shots for school. The nurse should do which of the following?
1. Administer tetanus immunoglobulin.
2. Start the child on an antibiotic.
3. Cleanse the wound with hydrogen peroxide.
4. Send the child to the emergency department.

59. A parent brings the 2-week-old to the clinic for a checkup. The infant has a brachial plexus injury. Which of the following should the nurse expect? Select all that apply.
1. A history of a normal vaginal delivery.
2. A small infant.
3. An absent Moro reflex on one side.
4. No sensory loss.
5. An associated clavicle fracture.

60. After surviving a motor vehicle accident but enduring a spinal cord injury, a patient is unable to walk but can use the arms, has no bowel or bladder control, and has no sensation below the nipple line. On the following figure, mark the vertebral/spinal cord area most likely injured.

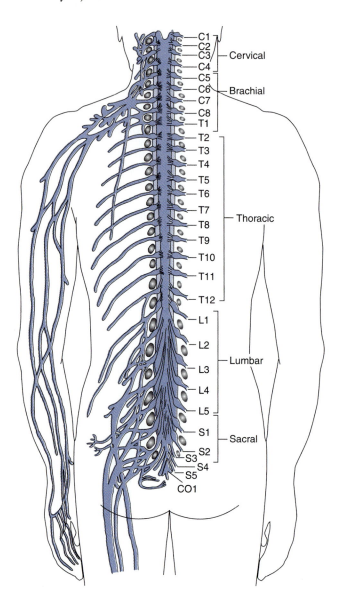

1. Sacral, S1–S5.
2. Cervical, C5–C7.
3. Thoracic, T1–T4.
4. Lumbar, L2–L5.
5. Cervical, C1–C5.
6. Thoracic, T5–T12.

61. Children with high-level spinal cord injuries may be afflicted with many complications, a serious one being autonomic dysreflexia due to unregulated sympathetic hyperactivity. Some of the causes of autonomic dysreflexia that the nurse should be aware of include which of the following? Select all that apply.
1. Decrease in blood pressure.
2. Abdominal distention.
3. Bladder distention.
4. Diarrhea.
5. Tight clothing.
6. Hypothermia.

1. 1. Paralysis of the facial nerve (CN VII) generally resolves within 2 to 4 weeks and has a good prognosis. Treatment is supportive.
   2. It would be very unusual for a healthy adolescent to have a stroke. One would also expect other symptoms.
   3. CN V (the trigeminal nerve) innervates the muscles of mastication.
   4. **This patient has Bell palsy, which is an idiopathic mononeuritis of CN VII (the facial nerve) that innervates the face and muscles of expression.**

   TEST-TAKING HINT: The test taker must know CNs and their actions.

2. 1. Neuropsychiatric symptoms include difficulty concentrating in school and emotional instability.
   2. **Fever, malaise, and weight loss are common presenting signs.**
   3. A rash is common, but with lupus it is usually a "butterfly" rash across the bridge of the nose. Maculopapular rashes are common but are usually on sun-exposed areas.
   4. Lupus nephritis requires urine output monitoring and is usually asymptomatic.

   TEST-TAKING HINT: The test taker must know the presenting signs and symptoms of systemic lupus erythematosus.

3. 1. **Muscular dystrophies are progressive degenerative disorders. The most common is Duchenne muscular dystrophy, which is an X-linked recessive disorder.**
   2. The weakness is progressive.
   3. The child will require assistance, and the need for it will increase with time and age.
   4. Daily therapy may be helpful in decreasing contractures, although it will not deter the disease progression.

   TEST-TAKING HINT: The test taker should know that muscular dystrophy is a progressive degenerative disorder.

4. 1. These symptoms are common with Down syndrome.
   2. Duchenne muscular dystrophy does not produce these symptoms.
   3. **The major complications of muscular dystrophy include contractures, disuse atrophy, infections, obesity, respiratory complications, and cardiopulmonary problems.**
   4. These symptoms are evidence of a possible head injury.

   TEST-TAKING HINT: The test taker should be able to identify signs and symptoms attributable to the loss of muscle function.

5. 1. This is the Romberg sign, which measures balance.
   2. This test measures balance and coordination.
   3. This test measures flexibility.
   4. **Children with muscular dystrophy display the Gower sign, which is great difficulty rising and standing from a squatting position due to the lack of muscle strength.**

   TEST-TAKING HINT: By eliminating cerebral activities, the test taker would know that the Gower sign assists in measuring leg strength.

6. 1. **Muscles become weaker, including those needed for respiration, and a decision will need to be made about whether respiratory support will be provided.**
   2. This is a progressive disease, which medications do not treat.
   3. Physical therapy will be part of the treatment plan, but respiratory support is a priority.
   4. The parents need to decide eventually if they will keep the child home or cared for in a nursing facility, but that is not an immediate concern.

   TEST-TAKING HINT: Pseudohypertrophic muscular dystrophy is a progressive neuromuscular disease with no cure.

7. 1. As the child with **muscular dystrophy** becomes less active, diet becomes more important. Attention should be paid to quality and quantity of food, so the child does not gain too much weight.
   2. Good-quality foods are important as the child continues to grow.
   3. Extra protein will not help the child recover from this disease.
   4. **As the child becomes less ambulatory, moving the child will become more of a problem. It is not good for the child to become overweight for several health reasons in addition to decreased ambulation.**

   TEST-TAKING HINT: Knowing that nutrition is important for every child as is awareness that as the child becomes less ambulatory, weight concerns arise.

8. 1. **Children who are active are usually able to postpone use of the wheelchair longer. It is important to keep using muscles for as long as possible, and aerobic activity is good for a child.**
   2. Use of a treadmill is not fun for children or adults, so keeping the child using the treadmill might be an issue.
   3. Any child with a chronic disease should be kept as active as possible for as long as possible.
   4. The goal is to keep the child as active as possible to prevent use of a wheelchair for as long as possible.

   TEST-TAKING HINT: Appropriate interventions for different kinds of chronically ill children can be similar, so think about what would be best for this child.

9. 1. **Genetic counseling is important in all inherited diseases. Duchenne muscular dystrophy is inherited as an X-linked recessive trait, meaning the defect is on the X chromosome. Women carry the disease, and males are affected. All female relatives should be tested.**
   2. **Women carry the disease, and males are affected. All female relatives should be tested.**
   3. Women carry the disease, and males are affected. All female relatives should be tested.
   4. **Women carry the disease, and males are affected. All female relatives should be tested.**
   5. Women carry the disease, and males are affected. All female relatives should be tested.

   TEST-TAKING HINT: Knowing that Duchenne muscular dystrophy is inherited as a X-linked trait excludes brother, uncle, and male cousins as carriers.

10. 1. Muscles become enlarged from fatty infiltration, so they are not stronger.
   2. **Difficulty climbing stairs, running, and riding a bicycle are frequently the first symptoms of Duchenne muscular dystrophy.**
   3. High fevers and tiredness are not early signs of muscular dystrophy but could be later signs as complications become more common.
   4. Respiratory infections and obesity are major complications as the disease progresses.

   TEST-TAKING HINT: Early symptoms have to do with decreased ability to perform normal developmental tasks involving muscle strength.

11. 1. This diagnosis would relate to the family and not to the child.
   2. This diagnosis would relate to the family and not to the child.
   3. The child does not have pain with the muscular dystrophy process.
   4. **The child would not be able to keep up with peers because of weakness, progressive loss of muscle fibers, and loss of muscle strength.**

   TEST-TAKING HINT: Knowing that the child has decreased strength helps to answer the question.

12. 1. The electromyelogram is part of the diagnostic work up, but muscle biopsy results classify muscle disorders.
   2. Nerve conduction velocity is part of the diagnostic workup, but muscle biopsy results classify muscle disorders.
   3. **Muscle biopsy confirms the type of myopathy that the patient has.**
   4. Creatine kinase is in muscle tissue and is found in large amounts in muscular diseases.

   TEST-TAKING HINT: Muscle biopsy is the definitive test for myopathies.

13. 1. **Spinal cord injury without radiographic abnormality results from the spinal cord sliding between the vertebrae and then sliding back into place without injury to the bony spine. It is thought to be the result of immature spines that allow for reduction after momentary subluxation.**
   2. On x-ray the spinal cord and body structure appear normal. The edema of the cord and resulting ischemia can cause neurological dysfunction below the level of the injury.
   3. Cervical injury is rare in children. The upper spine is more likely to be injured in small children than in adolescents.
   4. Young and preverbal children have difficulty expressing exactly what hurts and where, so physiological symptoms are also assessed.

   TEST-TAKING HINT: The test taker must understand the physiology of spinal cord injuries in children.

14. 1. Severe pain is unlikely, but the child may have pain at the injury site.
   2. An elevated temperature is not common in a spinal cord injury. In fact, most trauma patients are hypothermic in spite of high ambient temperatures.

3. **A spinal cord injury can occur at any level. The higher the level of the injury, the more likely the patient is to have respiratory insufficiency or failure. The nurse should be prepared to support the child's respiratory system.**
4. Spinal cord injury with an open or closed head injury does not cause an increase in intracranial pressure.

TEST-TAKING HINT: The test taker must know the signs of a spinal cord injury.

15. 1. Exposure to cold temperatures does not trigger an episode of autonomic dysreflexia.
2. **Autonomic dysreflexia results from an uncontrolled, paroxysmal, continuous lower motor neuron reflex arc due to stimulation of the sympathetic nervous system. It is a response that typically results from stimulation of sensory receptors such as a full bladder or bowel.**
3. Symptoms of autonomic dysreflexia are bradycardia, headache, and potentially life-threatening hypertension.
4. Symptoms of autonomic dysreflexia are bradycardia, headache, and potentially life-threatening hypertension.

TEST-TAKING HINT: The test taker must know what triggers autonomic dysreflexia and what the symptoms are.

16. 1. The infant is preverbal, so assessing clarity of speech is not age-appropriate or developmentally appropriate.
2. **Assessment for alteration in developmentally expected behaviors, such as stranger anxiety, is helpful. Interaction with staff is not to be expected due to stranger anxiety.**
3. Developmental delay is not the priority for assessment.
4. An 8-month-old infant is not expected to follow instructions.

TEST-TAKING HINT: The test taker must know about infant development.

17. 1. **Patients with complete spinal cord injury lose motor and sensory function below the level of the injury as a result of interruption of nerve pathways.**
2. Although spinal cord injury patients may suffer depression, it is not correct to state that all of them lose interest in normal activities.
3. Pain is absent below the level of the injury because of loss of sensory function.

4. Sparing of function below the level of the injury occurs only when there is partial spinal cord injury.

TEST-TAKING HINT: A spinal cord injury causes loss of motor and sensory function below the level of the injury.

18. 1. **Spinal cord injury patients experience many issues due to loss of innervation below the level of the injury. Skin integrity and incontinence are issues because of immobility and loss of pain receptors below the level of the injury.**
2. **Skin integrity and incontinence are issues because of immobility and loss of pain receptors below the level of the injury.**
3. Loss of motor activity is also a result of loss of innervation below the level of the injury.
4. Loss of voice is not a complication of T12 injury.
5. Flaccid paralysis occurs initially but changes to spasticity during the rehabilitation stage.

TEST-TAKING HINT: The test taker must know the long-term effects of spinal cord injury.

19. 1. The autonomic nervous system responds with arteriolar vasospasm, which results in an uncontrolled increase in blood pressure. The parasympathetic nervous system (vagus nerve) sends a stimulus to the heart resulting in bradycardia and vasodilation.
2. **The sympathetic nervous system responds to a full bladder or bowel resulting from an uncontrolled, paroxysmal, continuous lower motor neuron reflex arc. This response is usually from stimulation of sensory receptors (e.g., distended bladder or bowel). Because the efferent pulse cannot pass through the spinal cord, the vagus nerve is not "turned off," and profound symptomatic bradycardia may occur.**
3. Pain is not usually felt below the level of the injury, and pain elsewhere does not cause a severe headache.
4. In autonomic dysreflexia, the patient does not experience other symptoms.

TEST-TAKING HINT: Autonomic dysreflexia is usually caused by a full bladder or bowel.

20. 1. Sudden hypertension and bradycardia are symptoms of autonomic dysreflexia.
2. **Check to be certain that the bladder is not distended, which would trigger autonomic dysreflexia.**

3. The first intervention is to assess the bladder for fullness before administering any medication.
4. The first intervention is to assess the bladder for fullness before administering any medication.

TEST-TAKING HINT: The test taker must know which symptoms are suggestive of autonomic dysreflexia.

21. 1. **Before the surgical closure of the sac, the infant is at risk for infection. A sterile dressing is placed over the sac to keep it moist and help prevent it from tearing.**
    2. The infant's temperature will be taken, but prevention of infection is the priority.
    3. Prevention of infection is the priority. Once the temperature is taken, it can be determined if extra blankets are needed.
    4. Blood pressure is difficult to monitor in the newborn period. Prevention of infection is the priority.

TEST-TAKING HINT: Focus on the care and potential complications of an infant with spina bifida to answer the question correctly.

22. 1. This is certainly a possibility, but in the preoperative period risk of infection is the priority.
    2. Altered growth and development may occur, but in the preoperative period risk of infection is the priority.
    3. **A normal saline dressing is placed over the sac to prevent tearing, which would allow the cerebrospinal fluid to escape and microorganisms to enter and cause an infection.**
    4. It is normal in the first 2 weeks of life to lose up to 10% of birth weight. In fact, this infant may lose more weight because of surgery, but the priority is risk of infection.

TEST-TAKING HINT: The preoperative priority is risk of infection, especially when effort is necessary to keep a sterile saline dressing on the sac.

23. 1. **The reproductive system continues to function properly after a spinal cord injury. Much sexual activity and response occurs in the brain as well.**
    2. Conception does not depend on sensation in the genitals.
    3. Men continue to produce testosterone and sperm after a spinal cord injury.

4. Women continue to produce estrogen, and ovulation continues to occur.

TEST-TAKING HINT: Spinal cord injuries have little effect on reproduction.

24. 1. **Tethered cord is caused by scar tissue formation from the surgical repair of the myelomeningocele and may affect bowel, bladder, or lower extremity functioning.**
    2. Tethered cord occurs during growth spurts.
    3. Often the release of the tether will again become necessary.
    4. Laxatives and acetaminophen are temporary remedies, and they treat only the symptoms.

TEST-TAKING HINT: Tethering is caused by scar tissue from any surgical intervention and may recur as the child grows.

25. 1. A newborn may want formula every 2 to 4 hours but frequently is too sleepy to eat on a schedule.
    2. The infant should not be positioned on the back before surgery because of the potential to rupture the sac.
    3. **Priority care for an infant with a myelomeningocele is to protect the sac. A wet dressing keeps it moist with less chance of tearing.**
    4. Infants with myelomeningocele do not have pain because of lack of nerve innervations below the level of the defect.

TEST-TAKING HINT: Realizing the defect is on the back eliminates answer 2. Knowing newborns are sleepy and do not eat on a schedule eliminates answer 1.

26. 1. Weighing diapers for 24-hour urine output totals is important, but it is not the first thing to do following surgery.
    2. **Hydrocephalus occurs in about 90% of infants with myelomeningocele, so measuring the head circumference daily and watching for an increase are important. Accumulation of cerebrospinal fluid can occur after closure of the sac.**
    3. Clear fluids are offered after the infant is fully awake and there is no vomiting.
    4. Assessing for infection is important, but infection is not usually seen in the initial postoperative period.

TEST-TAKING HINT: The dynamics of the cerebrospinal fluid change after closure of the sac.

27. 1. Infants with myelomeningocele have altered bowel elimination as a result of their defect, but this is not the priority.
    2. **Because this infant has not had a repair, the sac is exposed. It could rupture, allowing organisms to enter the cerebrospinal fluid, so this is the priority.**
    3. These infants usually eat normally.
    4. The infant is too young to have a self-concept disturbance yet.

    TEST-TAKING HINT: Before surgery, the myelomeningocele is exposed, so risk of infection is much higher.

28. 1. The fact that the head circumference has changed so much might indicate increased intracranial pressure.
    2. **The increase in head size is one of the first signs of increased intracranial pressure; other signs include high-pitched cry and irritability.**
    3. The increase in head size is one of the first signs of increased intracranial pressure; other signs include high-pitched cry and irritability.
    4. This infant should be referred to the neurosurgeon, not the neurologist, and a computed tomography scan should be obtained to determine the cause of the increase.

    TEST-TAKING HINT: The test taker should know how fast an infant's head size changes.

29. 1. Bone growth is related to weight bearing as well as to secretion of the growth hormone. Decreased activity usually results in less bone growth.
    2. **Children with decreased activity due to illness or trauma are helped by physical and occupational therapy. The varied activities stimulate the senses.**
    3. This is partially true. Nutritional needs in children are also calculated based on growth needs.
    4. Many children with myelomeningocele have low-level defects, usually in the lumbar area, which do not affect upper body fine-motor skills.

    TEST-TAKING HINT: The test taker should know normal growth patterns.

30. 1. **A 3-month-old has good head control.**
    2. Pincer grasp occurs about 9 months.
    3. Sitting alone occurs about 6 months.
    4. Rolling over occurs about 4 months.

TEST-TAKING HINT: The test taker must know normal developmental milestones.

31. 1. This is certainly a possibility especially as the teen uses braces and can have some skin irritation.
    2. This is a nursing diagnosis to attend to now, because the teen uses braces and crutches.
    3. Because the teen is ambulatory, the teen probably has a lower-level defect, but even lower-level defects have some type of elimination issues.
    4. **As an adolescent on crutches and wearing braces, the teen would have the issue of body image disturbance, which must be addressed. This is a priority.**

    TEST-TAKING HINT: The test taker must know normal development.

32. 1. **Posting a sign on the door and charting that the child has a latex allergy is important so others will be aware of the allergy.**
    2. Do not use latex gloves with a person who has a latex allergy.
    3. Keeping personal items in a plastic bag does not keep latex away from the patient.
    4. A plastic cover for the blood pressure cuff is proper to use but is not related to the latex allergy.

    TEST-TAKING HINT: The test taker must know which supplies have latex and about contact allergies.

33. 1. Children with myelomeningocele have ongoing, lifelong, complex health-care needs.
    2. Children with myelomeningocele may have frequent urinary tract infections and mobility concerns.
    3. The surgical closure prevents the leakage of cerebrospinal fluid; dressing changes are necessary only during the postoperative period.
    4. **Although immediate surgical repair decreases infection, morbidity, and mortality rates, these children will require lifelong management of neurological, orthopedic, and elimination problems.**

    TEST-TAKING HINT: The test taker can eliminate answer 1 due to the complexity of myelomeningocele.

34. 1. An alteration in the circulation of the cerebrospinal fluid causes hydrocephalus. The anterior fontanel bulges because of an increase in cerebrospinal fluid, and an increase in intracranial pressure causes a

high-pitched cry in infants and downward deviation of the eyes, also called sunset eyes.
2. An alteration in the circulation of the cerebrospinal fluid causes hydrocephalus. The anterior fontanel bulges because of an increase in cerebrospinal fluid, and an increase in intracranial pressure causes a high-pitched cry in infants and downward deviation of the eyes, also called sunset eyes.
3. **An alteration in the circulation of the cerebrospinal fluid causes hydrocephalus. The anterior fontanel bulges because of an increase in cerebrospinal fluid, and an increase in intracranial pressure causes a high-pitched cry in infants and downward deviation of the eyes, also called sunset eyes. With sunset eyes the sclera can be seen above the iris.**
4. An alteration in the circulation of the cerebrospinal fluid causes hydrocephalus. The anterior fontanel bulges because of an increase in cerebrospinal fluid, and an increase in intracranial pressure causes a high-pitched cry in infants and downward deviation of the eyes, also called sunset eyes.

TEST-TAKING HINT: The test taker must know the difference in clinical signs of hydrocephalus in infants and older children. Infants' heads expand, whereas older children's skulls are fixed. The anterior fontanel closes between 12 and 18 months.

35. 1. Adequate calories are an appropriate goal, but the priority for a special-needs child is that the child develop to full potential.
2. Children with CP do not have increased intracranial pressure.
3. Teaching appropriate parenting strategies for a special-needs child is important and is done so the child can reach full potential.
4. **The priority for all children is to develop to their full potential.**

TEST-TAKING HINT: All of these are important goals, but determining the priority goal for a special-needs child is the key.

36. 1. Children may also have pseudobulbar involvement, which creates swallowing difficulties and recurrent aspiration.
2. Poor hygiene happens in clients with CP due to difficulty in oral hygiene because of increased muscle tone.
3. Abnormal involuntary movements usually involve the face, neck, trunk, and extremities.

4. **The primary disorder is of muscle tone, but there may be other neurological disorders such as seizures, vision disturbances, and impaired intelligence. Spastic CP is the most common type and is characterized by a generalized increase in muscle tone, increased deep tendon reflexes, and rigidity of the limbs on both flexion and extension.**

TEST-TAKING HINT: The test taker must know the definition of CP.

37. 1. **At least 80% of cases of CP result from unknown prenatal factors.**
2. It used to be thought that CP resulted from perinatal factors, but current knowledge is that CP results more commonly from existing prenatal brain abnormalities.
3. It used to be thought that CP resulted from perinatal factors, but current knowledge is that CP results more commonly from existing prenatal brain abnormalities.
4. Frequently, the exact cause is not known.

TEST-TAKING HINT: The test taker must know the latest information to answer this question correctly.

38. 1. **Most infants are able to crawl unassisted by 8 months.**
2. Infants learn to cruise (walk around holding onto furniture) at about 9 to 10 months.
3. Walking occurs on average at about 12 months.
4. Pincer grasp (thumb and forefinger) occurs at about 9 to 10 months.

TEST-TAKING HINT: The test taker must know developmental milestones.

39. 1. Children with CP frequently have developmental delays, including not being able to sit by themselves after 8 months. Sitting alone usually occurs by 6 months, so 8 months would be the outer limit of normal development and cause for concern.
2. Tongue thrust is common in infants younger than 6 months, but if it goes on after 6 months it is of concern.
3. Good head control is normally attained by 3 months.
4. **Clenched fists after 3 months of age may be a sign of CP.**

TEST-TAKING HINT: The test taker must know normal developmental milestones to identify those that are abnormal.

40. 1. The parent has an unrealistic picture of the child's future. The parent must help the

child achieve as much independence as possible in order to achieve full potential.
2. The child probably will never catch up to other children. That is part of the disorder, so the parent's role is to help the child achieve as much independence as possible.
3. This statement indicates that the parent understands the long-term needs of the child.
4. Parents do know the most about their children, but doing the most for the child is not the best way to manage the child's development. The child must become as independent as possible.

TEST-TAKING HINT: The test taker must understand the goals for children with chronic illnesses or disorders. One goal is to ensure that the child be diagnosed as early as possible so that interventions can be started. Another is to help the child realize as much potential as possible.

41. 1. The expected benefit from intrathecal baclofen is less spasticity, which allows the child to have more muscle control. This leads to more fine-motor control and ambulation. The onset of action is 30 minutes, and it peaks in 6 hours.
2. The expected benefit from intrathecal baclofen is less spasticity, which allows the child to have more muscle control. This leads to more fine motor control and ambulation. The onset of action is 30 minutes, and it peaks in 6 hours.
3. If baclofen were going to work for this patient, one could tell because spasticity would be decreased.
4. Baclofen should decrease, not increase, spasticity.

TEST-TAKING HINT: The test taker must know the purpose of baclofen.

42. 1. A 9-month-old should be able to sit alone, crawl, pull up, not push food out of the mouth (tongue thrust), and push away when held when wanting to get down. This child is not developing normally and must see the primary care provider.
2. A 9-month-old should be able to sit alone, crawl, pull up, not push food out of the mouth (tongue thrust), and push away when held when wanting to get down. This child is not developing normally and must see the primary care provider.
3. The mother will need help to teach the child how to sit alone.

4. Pushing food back into the mouth may be one strategy, but this is clearly abnormal in a 9-month-old.

TEST-TAKING HINT: The test taker must know normal developmental milestones. Rolling occurs about 4 months, sitting alone occurs at 6 months, and pushing food out of the mouth decreases by 4 months when the tongue thrust reflex wanes.

43. **1. Children with spastic CP have increased deep tendon reflexes.**
2. Children with spastic CP have increased muscle tone.
3. Children with spastic CP have scoliosis.
4. Children with spastic CP have contractures of the Achilles tendons, knees, and adductor muscles.
5. Children with spastic CP have scissoring when walking.
6. Children with spastic CP have poor control of posture.
7. Children with spastic CP have poor fine motor skills.

TEST-TAKING HINT: The test taker must know the typical signs of CP.

44. 1. This child is definitely at risk for skin breakdown, but alteration in nutrition is the priority. The child weights 15 pounds, which is normal for a 4-month-old. The child is severely underweight. The mother needs help to manage the coughing spells while the child is being fed.
2. This is the priority nursing diagnosis for this severely underweight child. Weight is average for a 4-month-old. The coughing episodes while feeding may indicate aspiration. The parent needs help to learn how to feed so less coughing occurs.
3. The parent needs support in caring for this child, but alteration in nutrition is the priority. The child weights 15 pounds, which is normal for a 4-month-old. The child is severely underweight. The parent needs help to manage the coughing spells while the child is being fed.
4. The child has not had a diarrheal stool for 48 hours, so the assumption is safe that the illness is over. The child weights 15 pounds, which is normal for a 4-month-old. The child is severely underweight. The parent needs help to manage the coughing spells while the child is being fed.

TEST-TAKING HINT: The test taker should convert the weight in kilograms to pounds

to have a better understanding of it. Knowing what a 3-year-old should weigh helps with answering this question.

45. 1. Children with CP have a range of intellectual abilities, from being profoundly retarded to having a high intelligence quotient. Many have normal intelligence. If a child has severe speech problems, some may assume that the child's intelligence is severely affected when that may not be true.
    2. Children with CP have a range of intellectual abilities, from being profoundly retarded to having a high intelligence quotient. Many have normal intelligence. If a child has severe speech problems, some may assume that the child's intelligence is severely affected when that may not be true.
    3. **Many children with CP have normal intelligence.**
    4. Children with CP have a range of intellectual abilities, from being profoundly retarded to having a high intelligence quotient. Many have normal intelligence. If a child has severe speech problems, some may assume that the child's intelligence is severely affected when that may not be true.

    TEST-TAKING HINT: Children with CP have a wide range of intellectual abilities.

46. 1. **This baby may have Werdnig-Hoffman disease, which is characterized by progressive generalized muscle weakness that eventually leads to respiratory failure. Respiratory compromise is the most important complication.**
    2. There is no history of being unable to ingest oral fluids; the baby is just a slow feeder.
    3. This is important, but respiratory compromise is a priority in this situation.
    4. There is no indication of feeding intolerance; the baby is just a slow feeder.

    TEST-TAKING HINT: Consider the ABCs in this situation: airway, breathing, and cardiac status. These are priorities when caring for clients.

47. 1. **Babies can lose up to 10% of birth weight but should regain it by 2 weeks of age. Knowing how much the baby eats can help the nurse determine if the infant is receiving adequate nutrition.**
    2. The number of bowel movements will also indicate whether the infant receives enough formula.

3. If the infant does not awaken during the night, then the mother may sleep all night. Most 2-week-olds feed every 2 to 4 hours day and night.
4. How long the infant stays awake is not the most important information. Most infants sleep about 20 hours per day.

TEST-TAKING HINT: The "red flags" in this question are that the baby sleeps a lot and does not cry much, both unusual behaviors. Follow-up questions need to be asked to determine if the infant is gaining weight as expected.

48. 1. Werdnig-Hoffmann disease is inherited as an autosomal-recessive trait.
    2. Werdnig-Hoffmann disease is inherited as an autosomal-recessive trait.
    3. **Werdnig-Hoffmann disease is inherited as an autosomal-recessive trait.**
    4. Werdnig-Hoffmann disease is inherited as an autosomal-recessive trait.

    TEST-TAKING HINT: The test taker needs to know how infants get this progressive disease.

49. 1. Hot dogs and chips are too high in sodium and fat.
    2. **Chicken is a good source of protein, and broccoli is a good choice for naturally occurring vitamins.**
    3. A banana is a food toddlers usually like. A child under 5 years should not eat nuts, however, because they are a choking hazard for a toddler who does not chew food well.
    4. A milkshake has a high amount of fat, as does a hamburger.

    TEST-TAKING HINT: The test taker must know good-quality foods that should be offered to children.

50. 1. The first intervention is to check the respiratory rate of the child to see if it is abnormal; then listen to the lung sounds, and then check pulse oximetry.
    2. **The first intervention is to check the respiratory rate of the child to see if it is abnormal; then listen to the lung sounds, and then check pulse oximetry.**
    3. The first intervention is to check the respiratory rate of the child to see if it is abnormal; then listen to the lung sounds, and then check pulse oximetry.
    4. The first intervention is to check the respiratory rate of the child to see if it is abnormal; then listen to the lung sounds, and then check pulse oximetry. Asking if

the child coughs at night would be helpful information as well.

TEST-TAKING HINT: The test taker would first count respirations to determine if the rate is normal for a child that age. Auscultation comes next, then pulse oximetry if needed.

51. 1. The disease etiology is frequently viral.
    2. Frequently a child has had recent viral infection prior to developing neurological symptoms.
    3. **This child probably has GBS, which is an acute inflammatory demyelinating neuropathy.**
    4. CNs are frequently involved.

TEST-TAKING HINT: Having a prior upper respiratory infection usually means this condition is not caused by bacteria, which eliminates answers 1 and 2. That leaves the choice between answers 3 and 4.

52. 1. Children with GBS frequently have urinary retention, so catheterization is necessary. Complications of GBS are usually respiratory and swallowing difficulties. Checking the serum blood urea nitrogen is a good thing to do, but not having voided in 10 hours is quite a lengthy time for a child.
    2. The complete blood count does not provide helpful information about urinary retention.
    3. **The child must be catheterized in and out to avoid the possibility of developing a urinary tract infection from urine in the bladder for too long.**
    4. Running water in the bathroom is a strategy used frequently to encourage patients to void. It takes time for it to work, however, and sometimes it does not have the intended results.

TEST-TAKING HINT: Urinary retention occurs with GBS and catheterization is necessary in a child who has had lots of fluids but not voided in 8 hours.

53. 1. The goal is to prevent complications related to immobility. Efforts include maintaining skin integrity, maintaining respiratory function, and preventing contractures. Constipation is a concern but not the primary one.
    2. Most children recover completely, so there is no chronic sorrow.
    3. **The goal is to prevent complications related to immobility. Efforts include maintaining skin integrity, maintaining**

respiratory function, and preventing contractures.
    4. GBS is a disease affecting the peripheral nervous system, not the cardiac muscle.

TEST-TAKING HINT: The test taker must have a basic understanding of GBS and know that it affects the peripheral nervous system.

54. 1. Assessing for respiratory compromise is critical in the acute phase of the disease process. Beginning active physical therapy is important for helping muscle recovery and preventing contractures.
    2. Assessing for swallowing difficulties is critical in the acute phase of the disease process. Beginning active physical therapy is important for helping muscle recovery and preventing contractures.
    3. GBS does not affect cognitive functioning.
    4. **Beginning active physical therapy is important for helping muscle recovery and preventing contractures.**

TEST-TAKING HINT: The test taker must know the normal progress of the disease. A hint is provided by the word "recovery" in the question.

55. 1. **Symptoms in a child with myasthenia gravis include fatigue, double vision, ptosis, and difficulty swallowing and chewing. This is an autoimmune disease triggered by a viral or bacterial infection. Antibodies attack acetylcholine receptors and block their functioning.**
    2. **Symptoms in a child with myasthenia gravis include fatigue, double vision, ptosis, and difficulty swallowing and chewing.**
    3. **Symptoms in a child with myasthenia gravis include fatigue, double vision, ptosis, and difficulty swallowing and chewing.**
    4. Symptoms in a child with myasthenia gravis include fatigue, double vision, ptosis, and difficulty swallowing and chewing.
    5. Symptoms in a child with myasthenia gravis include fatigue, double vision, ptosis, and difficulty swallowing and chewing.

TEST-TAKING HINT: The test taker must know the correct symptoms of myasthenia gravis.

56. 1. Children with myasthenia gravis should not play strenuous sports. They should learn strategies to decrease stress.
    2. **Meditation is a good strategy to learn to decrease stress.**

3. Children with myasthenia gravis can do many things other children do. They should be advised not to play strenuous sports, however, and they should learn how to control stress.

4. Children are watched for signs of illness because of the exacerbation of signs of myasthenia gravis.

TEST-TAKING HINT: The test taker must know the physiology of the illness.

57. 1. **Constipation means hard stools and infrequent passage. Adding extra water to the diet helps make the stool softer.**

2. It is not recommended to add corn syrup or honey to the bottle of a child younger than 12 months because of the danger of botulism.

3. It is not recommended to give an infant a glycerine suppository for hard infrequent stools; constipation should be managed with dietary changes.

4. Adding additional water daily is the easiest first step in handling constipation.

TEST-TAKING HINT: The test taker must know how to treat constipation in an infant, which is different from treating it in a child.

58. 1. **A child not fully immunized and who has a tetanus-prone wound should receive tetanus immunoglobulin to prevent tetanus. Tetanus-prone wounds include puncture wounds and those contaminated with dirt, feces, or soil.**

2. An antibiotic probably will be started, but administering tetanus immunoglobulin is the priority.

3. Wounds are routinely cleansed with soap and water. Hydrogen peroxide does not cleanse better.

4. This child can be cared for in the clinic.

TEST-TAKING HINT: The test taker must know about wound care and which wounds are considered contaminated.

59. 1. A brachial plexus injury in an infant (resulting from tearing or stretching of a nerve) usually occurs with large babies and breech delivery.

2. A brachial plexus injury in an infant (resulting from tearing or stretching of a nerve) usually occurs with large babies and breech delivery.

3. **The infant will have an absent Moro reflex on one side and no sensory loss.**

4. **The infant will have an absent Moro reflex on one side and no sensory loss.**

5. **The injury may be associated with a fractured clavicle.**

TEST-TAKING HINT: The test taker must know what a brachial plexus is and how an injury would affect it.

60. 1. S1–S5 is too low.
2. C5–C7 is too high, as the patient still has the use of the arms.
3. **Damage at T1–T4 manifests at or just below the nipple line. Every area below would be affected.**
4. L2–L5 is too low, as the patient has sensation only to the nipple line.
5. C1–C5 is too high, as the patient has the use of the arms and sensation to the nipple line.
6. Sensation ends at the nipple line, so T5–T12 is too low.

TEST-TAKING HINT: Deficits occur at and below the level of injury.

61. 1. A decrease in blood pressure does not contribute to autonomic dysreflexia. Increased blood pressure usually occurs with autonomic dysreflexia.
2. **Autonomic dysreflexia may be caused by abdominal pressure from a fecal impaction.**
3. **An overdistended bladder is usually the precipitating factor causing an increase in abdominal pressure.**
4. Fecal impaction and constipation, not diarrhea, can be causes of autonomic dysreflexia.
5. **Tight clothing can increase pressure to the central core of the body.**
6. Hyperthermia does not cause autonomic dysreflexia.

TEST-TAKING HINT: Autonomic dysreflexia most often occurs due to an irritating stimulus within the body below the level of spinal cord injury.

12

Orthopedic Disorders

Abduction
Adduction
Growth plate
Osteomyelitis

Pavlik harness
Pes cavus
Pes planus
Synovial fluid

ABBREVIATIONS

Developmental dysplasia of the hip (DDH)
Intravenous fluids (IVF)
Juvenile rheumatoid arthritis (JRA)
Nonsteroidal anti-inflammatory drugs
 (NSAIDs)

Osteogenesis imperfect (OI)
Patient-controlled analgesia (PCA)
Slipped capital femoral epiphysis (SCFE)
Systemic lupus erythematosus (SLE)

QUESTIONS

1. The nurse is assessing a 2-week-old for signs of DDH. The nurse should expect the infant to have which of the following?
   1. Excessive hip abduction.
   2. Femoral lengthening of an affected leg.
   3. Asymmetry of gluteal and thigh folds.
   4. Pain when lying prone.

2. An infant is in a Pavlik harness for treatment of DDH. While instructing the parents on preventing skin breakdown, the nurse should stress which of the following?
   1. Put socks on over the foot pieces of the harness to help stabilize the harness.
   2. Use lotions or powder on skin to prevent rubbing of straps.
   3. Remove harness during diaper changes for ease of cleaning diaper area.
   4. Check under the straps at least two to three times daily for red areas.

3. Which of the following conditions can occur in untreated DDH? Select all that apply.
   1. Duck gait.
   2. Pain.
   3. Osteoarthritis in adulthood.
   4. Osteoporosis in adulthood.
   5. Increased flexibility of the hip joint in adulthood.

4. The nurse is teaching about congenital clubfoot in infants. The nurse evaluates the teaching as successful when the parent states that clubfoot is best treated when?
   1. Immediately after diagnosis.
   2. At age 4 to 6 months.
   3. Prior to walking (age 9 to 12 months).
   4. After walking is established (age 15 to 18 months).

5. A parent asks the nurse to define talipes varus. The nurse tells the parent that it is which of the following?
   1. An inversion or bending inward of the foot.
   2. An eversion or bending outward of the foot.
   3. A high arch of the foot.
   4. A low arch (flatfoot) of the foot.

6. The nurse tells the parent that other conditions can be associated with congenital clubfoot? Select all that apply.
   1. Myelomeningocele.
   2. Cerebral palsy.
   3. Diastrophic dwarfism.
   4. Breech position in utero.
   5. Prematurity.
   6. Fetal alcohol syndrome.

7. When planning a rehabilitative approach for a child with osteogenesis imperfecta, the nurse should prevent which of the following? Select all that apply.
   1. Positional contractures and deformities.
   2. Bone infection.
   3. Muscle weakness.
   4. Osteoporosis.

8. A pregnant mother is told her fetus has OI. Which of the following classifications of OI is lethal in utero and in infancy?
   1. Type I.
   2. Type II.
   3. Type III.
   4. Type IV.

9. When counseling the parents of a child with OI, the nurse should do which of the following? Select all that apply.
   1. Discourage future children, because the condition is inherited.
   2. Provide education about the child's physical limitations.
   3. Give the parents a letter signed by the primary care provider explaining OI.
   4. Provide information on contacting the Osteogenesis Imperfecta Foundation.
   5. Encourage the parents to treat the child like their other children.
   6. Encourage use of calcium to decrease risk of fractures.

10. Which of the following factors are associated with SCFE? Select all that apply.
   1. Obesity.
   2. Female gender.
   3. African descent.
   4. Age of 5 to 10 years.
   5. Pubertal hormonal changes.
   6. Endocrine disorders.

11. Which of the following should be performed to make a diagnosis of SCFE?
   1. A history of hip trauma.
   2. A physical examination of hip, thigh, and knees.
   3. A complete blood count.
   4. A radiographic examination of the hip.

12. Which of the following should be included in teaching a family about postsurgical care for SCFE? Select all that apply.
    1. The patient will receive help with weight-bearing ambulation 24 to 48 hours after surgery.
    2. Monitoring of pain medication to prevent drug dependence.
    3. Instruction on pin site care.
    4. Offering low-calorie meals to encourage weight loss.
    5. Correct use of crutches by the patient.
    6. Outpatient physical therapy for 6 to 8 weeks.

13. Which of the following would the nurse assess in a child diagnosed with osteomyelitis? Select all that apply.
    1. Unwillingness to move affected extremity.
    2. Severe pain.
    3. Fever.
    4. Following a closed fracture of an extremity.
    5. Redness and swelling at the site.

14. The parent of a child diagnosed with osteomyelitis asks how the child acquired the illness. What is the nurse's best response?
    1. "Direct inoculation of the bone from stepping barefoot on a sharp stick."
    2. "An infection from a scratched mosquito bite carried the infection through the bloodstream to the bone."
    3. "The blood supply to the bone was disrupted because of the child's diabetes."
    4. "An infection of the upper respiratory tract."

15. A 10-year-old with osteomyelitis has been on intravenous antibiotics for 48 hours. The child is allergic to amoxicillin. Vital signs are: T 101.8°F (38.8°C), BP 100/60, P 96, R 24. Which of the following is the primary reason for surgical treatment?
    1. Young age.
    2. Drug allergies.
    3. Nonresponse to intravenous antibiotics.
    4. Physician preference.

16. The nurse expects the blood culture report of an 8-year-old with septic arthritis to grow which causative organism?
    1. *Streptococcus pneumoniae.*
    2. *Escherichia coli.*
    3. *Staphylococcus aureus.*
    4. *Neisseria gonorrhoeae.*

17. A 15-year-old is immobilized after SCFE surgery. Which of the following instructions should the nurse give the parents? Select all that apply.
    1. Continue upper body exercises to decrease loss of muscle strength.
    2. Do not turn the teen in bed when complaining of pain.
    3. Provide homework, computer games, and other activities to decrease boredom.
    4. Do most activities of daily living for the teen.
    5. Expect expressions of anger and hostility.
    6. Continue setting limits on behavior.

18. The parent of a 3-week-old states that the infant was recasted this morning for clubfoot and has been crying for the past hour. Which of the following interventions should the nurse suggest the parent do first?
    1. Give pain medication.
    2. Reposition the infant in the crib.
    3. Check the neurocirculatory status of the foot.
    4. Use a cool blow-dryer to blow into the cast to control itching.

19. A child has had surgery to correct bilateral clubfeet, and the cast has been removed. While instructing the parents about their child's future, the nurse should include which of the following statements? Select all that apply.
    1. "Your child will need to wear a brace on the feet 23 hours a day for at least 2 months."
    2. "Your child should see an orthopedic surgeon regularly until the age of 18 years."
    3. "Your child will not be able to participate in sports that require a lot of running."
    4. "Your child may have a recurrence of clubfoot in a year or more."
    5. "Most children treated for clubfeet develop feet that appear and function normally."
    6. "Most children treated for clubfeet require surgery at puberty."

20. Which parts of the body should the nurse assess on a child in a spica cast? See the following figure, and use the relevant label(s).

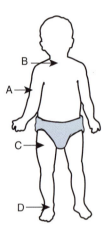

21. When a child is suspected of having osteomyelitis, the nurse can prepare the family to expect which of the following? Select all that apply.
    1. Pain medication is contraindicated so that symptoms are not masked.
    2. Blood cultures will be obtained.
    3. Pus will be aspirated from the subperiosteum.
    4. An intravenous line with antibiotics will be started.
    5. Surgery will be necessary.

22. Where should the top of the crutch bar be in relation to the axilla?

23. Select the numbers of inches lateral to the heel where a crutch should be placed.
    1. 1 to 3.
    2. 4 to 5.
    3. 6 to 8.
    4. 9 to 10.

24. Which of the following is most important when teaching a parent about preventing osteomyelitis?
    1. Parents can stop worrying about bone infection once their child reaches school age.
    2. Parents need to clean open wounds thoroughly with soap and water.
    3. Children will always get a fever if they have osteomyelitis.
    4. Children should wear long pants when playing outside because their legs might get scratched.

25. The nurse caring for a child with osteomyelitis assesses poor appetite. Which of the following interventions are most appropriate for this child? Select all that apply.
    1. Offer high-calorie liquids.
    2. Offer favorite foods.
    3. Do not worry about intake, as appetite loss is expected.
    4. Suggest intravenous removal to encourage oral intake.
    5. Decrease pain medication that might cause nausea.
    6. Offer frequent small meals.

26. The nurse on the pediatric floor is receiving a child with the possible diagnosis of septic arthritis of the elbow. Which of the following would the nurse expect on assessment? Select all that apply.
    1. Resistance to bending the elbow.
    2. Nausea and vomiting.
    3. Fever.
    4. Bruising of the elbow.
    5. Swelling of the elbow.
    6. A history of nursemaid's elbow as a toddler.

27. A 12-year-old diagnosed with scoliosis is to wear a brace for 23 hours a day. What is the most likely reason the child will not wear it for that duration?
    1. Pain from the brace.
    2. Difficulty in putting the brace on.
    3. Self-consciousness about appearance.
    4. Not understanding what the brace is for.

28. A spinal curve of less than _____ degrees that is nonprogressive does not require treatment for scoliosis.

29. A 13-year-old just returned from surgery for scoliosis. What nursing interventions are appropriate in the first 24 hours? Select all that apply.
    1. Assess for pain.
    2. Logroll to change positions.
    3. Get the teen to the bathroom 12 to 24 hours after surgery.
    4. Check neurological status.
    5. Monitor blood pressure.

30. A 9-year-old is in a spica cast and complains of pain 1 hour after receiving intravenous opioid analgesia. What should the nurse do first?
    1. Give more pain medication.
    2. Perform a neuromuscular assessment.
    3. Call the surgeon for orders.
    4. Tell the child to wait another hour for the medication to work.

31. A 14-year-old with osteogenesis imperfecta is confined to a wheelchair. Which nursing interventions will promote normal development? Select all that apply.
    1. Encourage participation in groups with teens who have disabilities or chronic illness.
    2. Encourage decorating the wheelchair with stickers.
    3. Encourage transfer of primary care to an adult provider at age 18 years.
    4. Allow the teen to view the radiographs.
    5. Help the teen set realistic goals for the future.
    6. Discourage discussion of sexuality, as the child is not likely to date.

32. After the birth of an infant with clubfoot, the nursery nurse should do which of the following when instructing the parents? Select all that apply.
    1. Speak in simple language about the defect.
    2. Avoid the parents unless providing direct care so they can grieve privately.
    3. Keep the infant's feet covered at all times.
    4. Present the infant as precious; emphasize the well-formed parts of the body.
    5. Tell the parent that defects could be much worse.
    6. Be prepared to answer questions multiple times.

33. The nurse should be suspicious of what condition in the following figure?_____

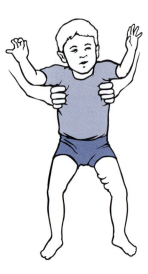

34. Name the harness in the following figure._____

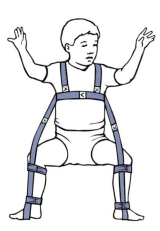

35. What condition is the harness used for in the following figure?_____

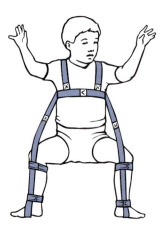

36. When instructing a family about care of an orthosis, the nurse should emphasize which of the following?
   1. Clean the brace with diluted bleach.
   2. Dry the brace over a heater or in the sun.
   3. Clean the brace weekly with mild soap and water.
   4. Return the brace to the orthopedic surgeon for cleaning.

37. When teaching parents about osteosarcoma, the nurse knows instruction has been successful when a parent says that this type of cancer is common in which age group?
   1. Infancy.
   2. Toddlers.
   3. School-age children.
   4. Adolescents.

38. A child with osteosarcoma is going to receive chemotherapy before surgery. Which of the following statements by the parents indicates they understand the side effect of neutropenia?
   1. "My child will be more at risk for diarrhea."
   2. "My child will be more at risk for infection."
   3. "My child's hair will fall out."
   4. "My child will need to drink more."

39. A 13-year-old with osteosarcoma is going to have an amputation of the affected limb. Which of the following is most important to discuss with a teenage patient?
   1. Pain.
   2. Spirituality.
   3. Body image.
   4. Lack of coping.

40. The best nursing intervention for a child with phantom pain after an amputation would be which of the following?
   1. Tell the child that the pain does not exist.
   2. Request a PCA pump from the physician for pain management.
   3. Encourage the child to rub the stump.
   4. Provide Elavil to help with pain.

41. Use the following labels to name the places on the bone in the following figure.

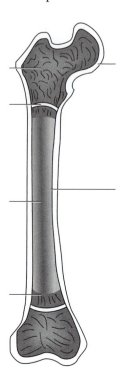

1. Epiphysis.
2. Diaphysis.
3. Epiphyseal plate.
4. Medullary cavity.
5. Calcaneus bone.
6. Compact bone.

42. The nurse is teaching an adolescent about Ewing sarcoma and indicates which of the following as a common site?
1. Shaft.
2. Growth plate.
3. Ball of the femur.
4. Bone marrow.

43. Which of the following nursing diagnoses is most important for a child with Ewing sarcoma who will be undergoing chemotherapy?
1. Risk for fluid volume deficit.
2. Potential for chronic pain.
3. Risk for skin impairment.
4. Ineffective airway clearance.

44. A child is going to receive radiation for Ewing sarcoma. Which of the following is the best nursing intervention to prevent skin breakdown during therapy?
1. Advise the child to wear loose-fitting clothes to minimize irritation.
2. Advise the child to use emollients to prevent dry skin.
3. Apply cold packs nightly to reduce the warmth caused by the treatments.
4. Apply hydrocortisone to soothe itching from dry skin.

45. A child with Ewing sarcoma is undergoing a limb salvage procedure. Which of the following statements indicates the parents understand the procedure?
1. "Our child will have a bone graft to save the limb."
2. "Our child will need follow-up lengthening procedures."
3. "Our child will need shorter shirt sleeves."
4. "Our child will not need chemotherapy."

46. A child with Ewing sarcoma is receiving chemotherapy and is experiencing severe nausea. The nurse has to administer Ativan at 0.04 mg/kg, and the child weighs 65 lb. What dose should the nurse administer? _____

47. The nurse is explaining about rhabdomyosarcoma cancer to an adolescent. From which of the following muscles does the cancer arise?
    1. Skeletal.
    2. Cardiac.
    3. Striated.
    4. Connective.

48. A child is diagnosed with stage IV rhabdomyosarcoma, and the parent asks what that means. The nurse provides which of the following explanations?
    1. The tumor is limited to the organ site.
    2. There is regional disease from the organ involved.
    3. There is distant metastatic disease.
    4. The disease is limited to the lymph nodes.

49. The nurse evaluates teaching as successful when the parent explains that an excisional biopsy is done to do which of the following?
    1. To find metastatic disease.
    2. To remove all metastatic disease.
    3. To confirm the type of metastatic disease.
    4. To treat metastatic disease.

50. It is recommended that a child with metastatic rhabdomyosarcoma undergo a bone marrow transplant. Education regarding life-threatening side effects should discuss:
    1. Diarrhea.
    2. Fever.
    3. Skin breakdown.
    4. Tumor shrinkage.

51. You are caring for a child with a retroperitoneal rhabdomyosarcoma. Select all the nursing diagnoses that apply.
    1. Acute pain.
    2. Risk for impaired urinary elimination.
    3. Impaired gas exchange.
    4. Self-care deficit.
    5. Risk for constipation.

52. The nurse is teaching the parent of a child newly diagnosed with JRA. The nurse would evaluate the teaching as successful when the parent is able to say that the disorder is caused by:
    1. The breakdown of osteoclasts in the joint space causing bone loss.
    2. The loss of cartilage in the joints.
    3. The buildup of calcium crystals in joint spaces.
    4. The immune-stimulated inflammatory response in the joint.

53. Which of the following would the nurse teach the adolescent is a complication of corticosteroids used in the treatment of JRA?
    1. Fat loss.
    2. Adrenal stimulation.
    3. Immune suppression.
    4. Hypoglycemia.

54. Which of the following would the nurse teach a patient when NSAIDs are prescribed for treating JRA?
    1. Take with food.
    2. Take on an empty stomach.
    3. Blood levels are required for drug dosages.
    4. Good oral hygiene is needed.

55. Chemotherapeutic agents such as methotrexate and cyclophosphamide are sometimes used to treat JRA. Why are these medications used?
    1. Effective against cancer, like JRA.
    2. Affect the immune system.
    3. Are similar to NSAIDs.
    4. Are absorbed into the synovial fluid.

56. One nursing diagnosis for JRA is impaired physical mobility. Select all nursing interventions that apply.
    1. Give pain medication prior to ambulation.
    2. Assist with range-of-motion activities.
    3. Encourage the child to eat a high-fat diet.
    4. Provide oxygen as necessary.
    5. Use nonpharmacological methods, such as heat.

57. The nurse is teaching the parent of a child diagnosed with SLE. The nurse evaluates the teaching as effective when the parent states:
    1. "The cause is unknown."
    2. "There is no genetic involvement."
    3. "Drugs are not a trigger for the illness."
    4. "Antibodies improve disease outcome."

58. A child is admitted to the pediatric unit with the diagnosis of SLE. On assessment, the nurse expects the child to have:
    1. Leukemia.
    2. Malar rash.
    3. Weight gain.
    4. Heart failure.

59. Which of the following is an important nursing intervention to teach about photosensitivity to the parents of a child with SLE?
    1. Regular clothing is appropriate for sun exposure.
    2. Sunscreen application is necessary for protection.
    3. Teenage patients cannot participate in outdoor sports.
    4. Water is important to reduce sensitivity.

60. Renal involvement is a side effect of latent SLE. Which of the following is an important nursing intervention to monitor in a child with renal involvement?
    1. Push fluids or start IVF.
    2. Check for uric salts in urine.
    3. Watch for hypotension.
    4. Check for protein in urine.

61. Because estrogen is a possible trigger for a SLE flare, advice for a teenager who may become sexually active includes which of the following. Select all that apply.
    1. Use Ortho Tri-Cyclen.
    2. Use Depo-Provera.
    3. Practice abstinence.
    4. Use condoms.
    5. Become pregnant.
    6. Use Ortho Evra.

62. A 6-year-old involved in a bicycle crash has a spleen injury and a right tibia/fibula fracture that has been casted. Which of the following are early signs of compartment syndrome in this child? Select all that apply.
    1. Edema.
    2. Numbness.
    3. Severe pain.
    4. Weak pulse.
    5. Anular rash

63. Nursing care of a child with a fractured extremity in whom there is suspected compartment syndrome includes which of the following? Select all that apply.
    1. Assess pain.
    2. Assess pulses.
    3. Elevate extremity above the level of the heart.
    4. Monitor capillary refill.
    5. Provide pain medication as needed.

64. The parent of a toddler asks the nurse to define greenstick fracture. Which of the following is the nurse's best explanation?
    1. It is a fracture located in the growth plate of the bone.
    2. Because children's bones are not fully developed, any fracture in a young child is called a greenstick fracture.
    3. It is a fracture in which a complete break occurs in the bone, and small pieces of bone are broken off.
    4. It is a fracture that does not go all the way through the bone.

65. A nurse is caring for a 5-year-old who has a fracture of the tibia involving the growth plate. When providing information to the parents, the nurse should indicate that:
    1. This is a serious injury that could cause long-term growth issues.
    2. The fracture usually heals within 6 weeks without further complications.
    3. The child will never be able to play contact sports.
    4. Fractures involving the growth plate require pain medication.

1. 1. In DDH, a newborn can have excessive hip adduction.
   2. In DDH, an appearance of femoral shortening is frequently present on the affected side.
   3. **In DDH, asymmetrical thigh and gluteal folds are frequently present.**
   4. Infants do not experience pain from this condition.

   TEST-TAKING HINT: If the test taker knows that DDH decreases smooth movement of the femoral head, then answers 1 and 2 can be eliminated because they indicate increased movement of the femur.

2. 1. Socks should be put on under the straps to prevent rubbing of the skin. The harness is stable if fitted correctly.
   2. Lotions and powders tend to cake and irritate under the straps. Their use is not recommended.
   3. The harness is not to be removed except in specific conditions and after instruction on removal and refitting. Diapering is easily done with the harness in place.
   4. **Checking under straps frequently is suggested to prevent skin breakdown.**

   TEST-TAKING HINT: The test taker can eliminate answer 1 because the question is about skin breakdown, not harness fit.

3. 1. **Due to abnormal hip joint function, the patient's gait is stiff and waddling.**
   2. **Due to abnormal femoral head placement, the patient may experience pain and decreased flexibility in adulthood.**
   3. **Due to abnormal femoral head placement, the patient may experience osteoarthritis in the hip joint in adulthood.**
   4. There is no increased risk for osteoporosis.
   5. There is no increased flexibility of the hip joint in adulthood.

   TEST-TAKING HINT: If the test taker knows that untreated DDH leads to decreased smooth movement of hip joint, answer 5 can be eliminated.

4. 1. **The best outcomes for clubfoot are seen if casting begins as soon as the diagnosis is made.**
   2. Although casting helps if started in the newborn period, the delay of even 4 to 6 months postpones the positive outcome.
   3. Infants of 9 months are already pulling up to stand and taking steps. Clubfoot puts weight on surfaces of feet that are not meant for weightbearing.

4. Clubfoot does not allow for normal gait, and the delay will decrease the likelihood of a successful outcome.

   TEST-TAKING HINT: The general principle of early treatment of orthopedic problems should lead to the correct answer.

5. 1. **Talipes varus is an inversion of the foot.**
   2. Talipes valgus is an eversion of the foot.
   3. Pes cavus is a high arch of the foot.
   4. Pes planus is flatfoot.

   TEST-TAKING HINT: The test taker must know the definition of terms.

6. 1. **There is an association between myelomeningocele and congenital clubfoot.**
   2. **There is an association between some forms of cerebral palsy and congenital clubfoot.**
   3. **There is an association between diastrophic dwarfism and congenital clubfoot.**
   4. Breech position is not associated with congenital clubfoot. It is associated with DDH.
   5. There is no association between prematurity and congenital clubfoot.
   6. Fetal alcohol syndrome is not associated with clubfoot.

   TEST-TAKING HINT: The test taker could look at other congenital deformities to gain a clue to an association to clubfoot.

7. 1. **A long-term goal in caring for a patient with OI is to prevent contractures and deformities.**
   2. There is no increased risk for bone infection in OI.
   3. **A long-term goal in caring for a patient with OI is to prevent muscle weakness.**
   4. **A long-term goal in caring for a patient with OI is to prevent osteoporosis.**

   TEST-TAKING HINT: The test taker should think about general nursing considerations for children with fractures and choose answers 1 and 3.

8. 1. Type I is the most common form. It is characterized by little deformity, variable fractures, blue sclera, hearing loss common in the 20s, and a normal life span.
   2. **Type II is lethal in utero and in infancy because of multiple fractures and deformities and underdeveloped lungs.**
   3. Type III is characterized by fractures, deformities, and short stature. Patients rarely live to age 30 years.

4. Type IV is similar to type I but not associated with blue sclera.

TEST-TAKING HINT: The test taker might be tempted to choose type IV, thinking that the higher number (IV) is the most severe form of OI.

9. 1. Genetic counseling should be provided as part of long-term care so that the parents can make an informed decision about future children.
   2. **The nurse should provide education about the child's physical limitations so that physical therapy and appropriate activity can be encouraged.**
   3. **OI is frequently confused with child abuse. Carrying a letter stating that the child has OI and what that condition looks like can ease the stressors of an emergency department visit.**
   4. **Osteogenesis Imperfecta Foundation is an organization that can provide information and support for a family with a child with the condition.**
   5. Children with OI must be treated with careful handling and cannot be allowed to participate in all activities that unaffected siblings are allowed.
   6. There is no support for the use of additional calcium to decrease fractures.

TEST-TAKING HINT: The test taker can eliminate answer 1 because it is based on the nurse's values, not necessarily those of the parents.

10. 1. **Obesity increases the risk of SCFE by stressing the physeal plate.**
    2. SCFE is more common in males.
    3. SCFE is more common in whites.
    4. SCFE is most common from the ages of 10 to 16 years.
    5. **SCFE is most common during pubertal hormone changes.**
    6. **SCFE is associated with endocrine disorders.**

TEST-TAKING HINT: If the test taker knows that SCFE is most common during rapid growth, answer 4 can be eliminated, and answer 5 can be chosen.

11. 1. In most cases of SCFE, there is no history of trauma to the hip.
    2. Physical examination may reveal some restriction of rotation of the hip, but it is not diagnostic.
    3. There is no change in blood laboratory values with SCFE. Radiographic examination is the only definitive tool for diagnosis of SCFE.

4. **Radiographic examination is the only definitive diagnostic tool for SCFE.**

TEST-TAKING HINT: The word "necessary" in the question should lead the test taker to the most definitive tool in assessing a hip, which is radiographic examination.

12. 1. Ambulation is to be non–weightbearing with crutches until range of motion is painless. This is usually 4 to 8 weeks.
    2. Pain medication is to be administered regularly during hospitalization to provide comfort to the patient and encourage cooperation with daily activities and ambulation. Drug dependence for the postoperative patient is not a significant concern.
    3. **The parents will be assessing pin sites for infection and stability upon discharge. Instructions on care should be demonstrated for and then by the parents.**
    4. Although obesity is often a factor in SCFE, the patient requires adequate caloric intake for healing and recovery postoperatively. Obesity issues can be addressed after surgical recovery.
    5. **Instruction on crutch usage will be given prior to discharge. Crutch walking will not be done during the early postoperative stage.**
    6. Outpatient physical therapy is not usually necessary.

TEST-TAKING HINT: The test taker should be able to rule out answer 2 by understanding the safe use of pain medication in the immediate postoperative period.

13. 1. **Pain in an extremity leads to resistance to movement.**
    2. **Pain is frequently severe in osteomyelitis.**
    3. **Fever is present in the acute phase of the illness.**
    4. Osteomyelitis can sometimes be seen after a direct inoculation of an open fracture. There is no increased risk after a closed fracture.
    5. **Redness and swelling occur because of the infection.**

TEST-TAKING HINT: The test taker can rule out answer 4 if it is understood that a closed fracture does not increase the risk of bone infection.

14. 1. **Although osteomyelitis can occur from direct inoculation, inoculation is not the most common cause.**

2. Infection through the bloodstream is the most likely cause of osteomyelitis in a child.
3. Although osteomyelitis can occur because of blood supply disruption, that is more likely to occur in older adults. Diabetes does increase the risk of osteomyelitis, but diabetes is more common in older adults.
4. A viral upper respiratory infection is not the most likely cause.

TEST-TAKING HINT: The age of the patient is important in choosing the most likely cause of the disease.

15. 1. All children with osteomyelitis are treated initially with intravenous antibiotics, regardless of age.
2. Although drug allergies are a concern, antibiotic choices can be made to accommodate patients with specific drug allergies.
3. **If a patient does not respond to an appropriate antibiotic within 48 hours, surgery may be indicated. This is the correct answer.**
4. Although there is some difference of opinion about the use of surgery in the treatment of osteomyelitis, the standard initial treatment is intravenous antibiotics.

TEST-TAKING HINT: Answer 4 should be eliminated because patient treatment should be based on evidence-based practice.

16. 1. *S. pneumoniae* is more common in children younger than age 5 years, but it is not the most common organism.
2. *E. coli* is more common in neonates, but it is also not the most common cause.
3. ***S. aureus* is a common organism found on the skin and is frequently the cause of septic arthritis.**
4. *N. gonorrhoeae* should be considered in sexually active patients, but it is not the most common organism.

TEST-TAKING HINT: The age of the patient is important in choosing the correct answer.

17. 1. **Immobilization can lead to a decrease in muscle strength. Upper body exercises should be continued soon after surgery.**
2. Although turning the patient in bed after surgery may be painful, it is essential that parents and the patient know that it is necessary to prevent skin ulcerations and promote healing.
3. **It is important for this patient to continue as many normal activities as**

possible. This should include schoolwork and leisure activities.
4. To promote independence that is essential for a teenager, this patient should be encouraged to continue activities of daily living.
5. **Some expressions of anger and hostility are normal, as this adolescent is losing some independence with this immobility.**
6. **Continuation of setting limits on behavior is important to keep as much normalcy as possible.**

TEST-TAKING HINT: The test taker needs to understand the developmental need for independence in this age group.

18. 1. The cause of the crying needs to be determined prior to administering pain medication.
2. Although this is a good choice, it is not the first intervention.
3. **Checking the neurocirculatory status of the foot is the highest priority.**
4. Although this is a good choice for cast discomfort, it is not the first choice.

TEST-TAKING HINT: The test taker should prioritize nursing interventions and know that safety needs are paramount.

19. 1. **After the final casting, bracing is required for 23 to 24 hours per day for 2 months. This decreases the likelihood of a recurrence.**
2. **Because clubfoot can recur, it is important to have regular follow-up with the orthopedic surgeon until age 18 years.**
3. After treatment, most children are able to participate in any sport.
4. **Even with proper bracing, there may be a recurrence.**
5. **Most children treated for clubfeet develop normally appearing and functioning feet.**
6. Most children do not require surgery at puberty.

TEST-TAKING HINT: If the test taker is aware that clubfoot can recur, providing instruction that includes long-term follow-up care will help in selecting answers.

20. **C, D. The nurse needs to assess areas under the cast for drainage through the cast and assess neurocirculatory status of the feet.**

TEST-TAKING HINT: The test taker should know to check for neurocirculatory status and wound drainage.

21. 1. Medication will be given regularly to help with the pain.
     2. **Blood cultures will be obtained.**
     3. **Pus will be aspirated from the subperiosteum.**
     4. **Antibiotics will be given via an intravenous line.**
     5. Surgery is indicated only when medication fails.

     TEST-TAKING HINT: If the test taker is unsure of specific care for osteomyelitis, standard nursing care for infection can lead to correct choices.

22. The crutch bar should not put pressure on nerves in the axilla.

     TEST-TAKING HINT: The axillae do not rest on the crutch bar.

23. 1. This position does not provide the best protection for balance and stability.
     2. This position does not provide the best protection for balance and stability.
     3. **This position provides the best protection for balance and stability.**
     4. This position does not provide the best protection for balance and stability.

     TEST-TAKING HINT: Consider the stance that is best for balance when standing.

24. 1. Osteomyelitis can occur in children older than school age.
     2. **Because bacteria from an open wound can lead to osteomyelitis, thorough cleaning with soap and water is the best prevention.**
     3. Children with osteomyelitis do not always have a fever.
     4. It is not necessary to require children to wear long pants whenever playing outside.

     TEST-TAKING HINT: The test taker can eliminate answers 1 and 3 because they do not address prevention.

25. 1. **High-calorie liquids are sometimes received better when the child has a poor appetite.**
     2. **Offering favorite foods can sometimes tempt the child to eat, even with a poor appetite.**
     3. Although decreased appetite is expected, it is something that needs nursing intervention in order to promote healing.
     4. An intravenous line is necessary for antibiotics, so it cannot be removed to encourage oral intake.
     5. Although some pain medications cause nausea, their use is important. If patients are in pain, they are not likely to want to eat.
     6. **Small, frequent meals might increase daily caloric intake.**

     TEST-TAKING HINT: Using routine nursing interventions for decreased appetite can lead to the correct answers.

26. 1. **Infection of the elbow joint can cause pain that leads to protecting the joint and resisting movement.**
     2. Infection of the elbow may cause generalized nausea and vomiting.
     3. Infection of the elbow frequently causes fever.
     4. There is no bruising with septic arthritis.
     5. **Septic arthritis can cause swelling of the joint.**
     6. There is no increased risk with a history of nursemaid elbow.

     TEST-TAKING HINT: The test taker can rule out answer 6, as risk of infection is not related to past injury.

27. 1. Putting on the brace is not painful.
     2. Putting on the brace is not difficult.
     3. **Children this age are very conscious of their appearance and of fitting in with their peers, so they might be very resistant to wearing a brace.**
     4. Although a child this age might not fully understand how the brace helps the condition, that would not be the most likely cause of noncompliance.

     TEST-TAKING HINT: The test taker must understand the development of children.

28. **20. A 20-degree spinal curve that is nonprogressive will not disfigure or interfere with normal functioning, so it is not treated with bracing or surgery.**

     TEST-TAKING HINT: The test taker must know about treatment for scoliosis.

29. 1. **General postoperative nursing interventions include assessing for pain.**
     2. **Specific to scoliosis surgery, logrolling is the means of changing positions.**
     3. Patients may not be upright less than 24 hours postoperatively.
     4. **It is essential to check neurological status in a patient who just had scoliosis surgery.**
     5. **General postoperative nursing interventions include assessing vital signs.**

     TEST-TAKING HINT: The test taker can use general postoperative care principles to lead to several correct answers.

30. 1. The nurse needs to assess the child prior to giving more pain medication.
2. **The nurse looks for the source of the pain by performing a neuromuscular assessment.**
3. If the neuromuscular assessment is normal, the nurse might need to call the surgeon for further orders.
4. The child should have relief from pain after 1 hour of receiving the intravenous medication, so waiting is not correct.

TEST-TAKING HINT: The surgeon should be called only after an assessment of the patient is done. The test taker can rule out answer 3.

31. 1. **This patient is trying to become more independent and trying to fit in with the peer group. Encouraging socializing with peers who face similar challenges alleviates feelings of isolation.**
2. **Decorating the wheelchair encourages the patient to assume independence in self-care.**
3. It is not necessarily appropriate to transfer health care at age 18 years. If the teen is with a provider who has known the patient and family most of the teen's life, it might be best to remain with that provider for several more years.
4. **Allowing the patient to view radiographs encourages the patient to assume self-care.**
5. **Helping the patient set realistic goals for the future encourages independence.**
6. It is appropriate for the nurse to discuss sexuality with this patient. Being confined to a wheelchair does not preclude dating or becoming intimate.

TEST-TAKING HINT: The test taker can use normal growth and development to help choose correct answers.

32. 1. **The parents will likely be shocked immediately after the birth of the child. To facilitate their understanding, the nurse should speak in simple terms.**
2. Avoiding the parents is not therapeutic.
3. The baby should be shown to the parents like all newborns, without hiding the clubfoot.
4. **The baby should be shown to the parents like all newborns, emphasizing the well-formed parts of the body.**
5. Negating the parents' grieving is not therapeutic.
6. **Information may need to be repeated as the family begins to absorb the information.**

TEST-TAKING HINT: The test taker can draw on therapeutic communication skills to choose correct answers.

33. **DDH. The asymmetry of the thigh folds suggests DDH.**

TEST-TAKING HINT: The age of the patient should be a clue to the answer.

34. **Pavlik harness. The Pavlik harness is used to treat DDH diagnosed in the newborn period.**

TEST-TAKING HINT: The harness places the hip joints in abduction.

35. **It is used for DDH. The Pavlik harness is used to treat DDH in neonates.**

TEST-TAKING HINT: Being able to answer previous questions correctly can sometimes help with later questions.

36. 1. The use of bleach can damage the brace.
2. Drying in direct sunlight or on a heater can warp the brace.
3. **An orthosis should be cleaned weekly with mild soap and water.**
4. The brace can be safely cleaned at home.

TEST-TAKING HINT: The test taker can rule out answer 4, because equipment care would not be confined to a physician's office.

37. 1. Osteosarcoma is a common cancer of adolescents.
2. Osteosarcoma is a common cancer of adolescents.
3. Osteosarcoma is a common cancer of adolescents.
4. **Osteosarcoma is a common cancer of adolescents.**

TEST-TAKING HINT: The test taker must remember that pediatric cancers usually develop during times of peak growth. Adolescence is the greatest time of peak bone growth.

38. 1. Diarrhea is a side effect of chemotherapy, not neutropenia.
2. **Neutropenia makes a patient more at risk for infection, because the immune system is compromised due to the chemotherapy.**
3. Alopecia is a side effect of chemotherapy.
4. Dehydration is a potential side effect of chemotherapy.

TEST-TAKING HINT: "Neutropenia" consists of *neutro-* (meaning neutrophils, a subset of the white blood cells) and *-penia* (meaning low or decreased).

39. 1. Pain is a common concern but adolescents are more concerned about their body image.
    2. In general, adolescents are more concerned with their body image and not spirituality.
    3. Body image is a developmental issue for adolescents and influences their acceptance of themselves and by peers.
    4. Body image is more of a concern for adolescents and should be addressed first by the nurse. Lack of coping is not a priority at this time.

    TEST-TAKING HINT: The question asks for specific versus general anticipatory guidance issues.

40. 1. This is not a helpful intervention.
    2. PCA is not necessary for phantom pain.
    3. Rubbing the stump is not helpful and possibly harmful to healing.
    4. Elavil is a medication for nerve pain that is helpful with relieving phantom pain.

    TEST-TAKING HINT: Knowing that phantom pain is due to nerve pain from the lost limb enables elimination of answer 2.

41.

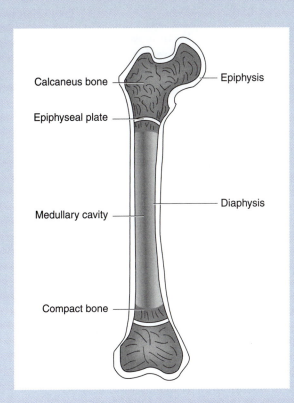

Calcaneus bone

Epiphyseal plate

Medullary cavity

Compact bone

Epiphysis

Diaphysis

TEST-TAKING HINT: The test taker should look at each word and think about the parts of the bone. Separate the parts of the words, and think about what their stems mean to help with locations.

42. **1. Ewing sarcoma is a bone tumor that affects the shafts of long bones.**
    2. Pediatric bone sarcomas do not affect the growth plate.
    3. This is a specific location of a specific bone. Ewing sarcoma can affect multiple bones.
    4. The bone marrow is a site for hematological cancers.

    TEST-TAKING HINT: It is important to be familiar with the physiology of bones to understand how bone sarcomas affect them. Ewing sarcoma is a rare cancer that affects a different part of the bone relative to osteosarcoma.

43. **1. Chemotherapy can cause nausea, vomiting, and possibly diarrhea, which contribute to fluid volume deficit.**
    2. Chemotherapy itself does not cause chronic pain.
    3. Radiation therapy has the potential for skin impairment.
    4. This is not an acute problem with chemotherapy.

    TEST-TAKING HINT: This is a general question asking for basic side effects of chemotherapy.

44. **1. Loose clothing helps reduce irritation on the sensitive irradiated skin.**
    2. Emollients are contraindicated during radiation because they can reflect the rays.
    3. Irradiated skin is very sensitive to extreme temperatures; a cold pack could cause pain.
    4. Hydrocortisone is not helpful for the radiation-induced itching; it is for atopic itching.

    TEST-TAKING HINT: The test taker must know what is most helpful for relieving irritation as a result of what radiation does to the skin. The question asks for what to do during therapy.

45. 1. Bone grafts are not part of limb salvage.
    2. Limb salvage requires the lengthening procedures to encourage the bone to continue to grow so the child will not have a short limb.
    3. This does not indicate understanding by the parents.
    4. Having a limb salvage does not mean the child will never require chemotherapy as part of the treatment.

TEST-TAKING HINT: A limb salvage means the limb is saved, but that is not the end of treatment for the child.

46. 1.1 mg. Change pounds to kilograms (2.2 lb = 1 kg: 65/2.2 = 29.5 kg). Then multiply kilograms by the dose of 0.04 mg/kg: 29.5 × 0.04 = 1.1 mg.

    TEST-TAKING HINT: Divide 65 lb by 2.2 to determine kilograms.

47. 1. Striated muscle is in many organs and sites of the body, thus leading to the multiple sites of the disease.
    2. Striated muscle is in many organs and sites of the body, thus leading to the multiple sites of the disease.
    3. **Striated muscle is in many organs and sites of the body, thus leading to the multiple sites of the disease.**
    4. There is no such muscle.

    TEST-TAKING HINT: The test taker must understand the basic locations for each muscle listed.

48. 1. This is stage I disease.
    2. This is stage II disease.
    3. **Stage IV disease means there is distant metastatic disease.**
    4. Lymph node involvement is not used as part of staging for rhabdomyosarcoma.

    TEST-TAKING HINT: The test taker must be familiar with the basic staging of cancers.

49. 1. Metastatic disease is confirmed by a combination of tests.
    2. A biopsy removes only a small piece of the tumor.
    3. **A biopsy confirms the histology of the tumor.**
    4. Chemotherapy, radiation, and surgery are required for treatment.

    TEST-TAKING HINT: A biopsy is used to get the basic information of any solid cancer. Additional tests and procedures are part of treatment and more extensive diagnosis.

50. 1. Diarrhea can be a side effect of chemotherapy, but it is not usually life-threatening.
    2. **Fever indicates infection that can be life-threatening after a bone marrow transplant.**
    3. Skin breakdown is usually not life-threatening.
    4. Skin shrinkage is expected with treatment, but it is not life-threatening.

TEST-TAKING HINT: The test taker must understand what a bone marrow transplant involves and how bone marrow suppression can have life-threatening effects.

51. 1. **Pain occurs due to pressure on the organs in the lower abdomen.**
    2. **A retroperitoneal tumor affects the organs of the lower abdomen, including the bowel and bladder.**
    3. A retroperitoneal tumor affects the organs of the lower abdomen, including the bowel and bladder. This tumor does not affect the lungs.
    4. There is no indication the child cannot administer self-help.
    5. **Because this tumor is in the lower abdomen, it puts pressure on the bowel causing constipation.**

    TEST-TAKING HINT: The test taker must understand the areas of the body. Having an idea of the organs involved will indicate possible problems that can arise when a tumor is in those locations.

52. 1. This is part of the normal breakdown and buildup of bone in the body.
    2. This is part of the process for osteoarthritis.
    3. This is the pathophysiology of calcium chondrosis.
    4. **JRA is caused by an immune response by the body on the joint spaces.**

    TEST-TAKING HINT: The test taker must understand JRA is an immune-modulated disorder and how the body attacks itself, causing destruction of the joint spaces.

53. 1. Long-term corticosteroid use causes fat deposits, especially in the back, face, and trunk.
    2. With the use of corticosteroids, there is adrenal suppression because the exogenous steroid causes the body to lower production of its own steroids.
    3. **Steroids cause immune suppression, which is the reason behind its use in JRA; it reduces the body's attack on itself.**
    4. Steroids cause hyperglycemia.

    TEST-TAKING HINT: The test taker must understand how immune system diseases work in order to know how treatments will be helpful. Consider how steroids work and their complications. Each answer listed, except the correct answer, is the opposite of the true side effects.

54. 1. NSAIDs can cause gastric bleeding with long-term use; food helps to reduce the exposure of the drug on the stomach lining.
2. NSAIDs can cause gastric bleeding with long-term use; food helps to reduce the exposure of the drug on the stomach lining.
3. NSAIDs do not require a blood level because they are available over the counter.
4. NSAIDs do not interfere with the oral cavity; however, other medications used for JRA cause oral ulcers.

TEST-TAKING HINT: The test taker must know what NSAIDs are and that they are available over the counter.

55. 1. JRA is not a type of cancer.
2. These drugs affect the immune system to reduce its ability to attack itself, as in the case of JRA.
3. These medications are not the same as NSAIDs.
4. They are not absorbed into the synovial fluid to treat JRA; they suppress the immune system.

TEST-TAKING HINT: There are some drugs that are used for other reasons outside of their usual use, like chemotherapeutic agents. Many drugs have multiple uses.

56. 1. Providing pain medication prior to ambulation helps decrease pain during ambulation.
2. Children with JRA need to do range-of-motion exercises to prevent joint stiffness.
3. A high-fat diet is not helpful for mobility.
4. Oxygen is usually not necessary with the diagnosis of JRA.
5. Using nonpharmacological methods such as heat helps with flexibility and pain.

TEST-TAKING HINT: By understanding the disease process of JRA, the test taker will know what interventions are needed to help alleviate pain and disability.

57. 1. SLE is a complex disease; there are many triggers, but how the disease develops is not known.
2. There is some correlation with family history.
3. There are multiple triggers for SLE, including prescription drugs.
4. Antibodies have nothing to do with SLE outcome.

TEST-TAKING HINT: Not all diseases have a known cause.

58. 1. This is not a clinical manifestation.
2. The "butterfly," or malar, rash is the most common manifestation of SLE.
3. Weight loss, not weight gain, is a symptom of SLE.
4. Heart failure is not a common manifestation, but it can occur after long-term disease that affects the heart muscle.

TEST-TAKING HINT: By understanding the pathophysiology of SLE, the test taker will be able to find the correct answer.

59. 1. Sun-protective clothing is important, including hats.
2. Sunscreen helps reduce accelerated burning due to sensitivity.
3. Participating in sports is important for normalcy and should be encouraged.
4. Water is important, but it does not affect photosensitivity.

TEST-TAKING HINT: In general, sunscreen is important for every question regarding sun exposure and photosensitivity.

60. 1. For renal impairment due to SLE, pushing fluids is not recommended.
2. Uric salts are a normal concentrate of urine.
3. Hypertension is a problem with renal involvement, not hypotension.
4. Protein in urine is a sign of renal impairment, even in nephrotic syndrome, in which the kidneys are losing protein.

TEST-TAKING HINT: The test taker must understand what can happen to the body when organs, such as the kidneys, fail.

61. 1. Ortho Tri-Cyclen contains estrogen; therefore, it is contraindicated.
2. Depo-Provera is progesterone, the only contraceptive that is approved for use.
3. Abstinence is always recommended to prevent pregnancy.
4. Condoms are always recommended.
5. Becoming pregnant is not recommended due to the need for estrogen to preserve the pregnancy.
6. Ortho Evra ("the patch") contains estrogen and is therefore not recommended.

TEST-TAKING HINT: The test taker must be familiar with the types of contraceptives and which contain combination hormones versus progesterone only.

62. 1. Edema, numbness or tingling, and pain are early signs of compartment syndrome.
    2. Edema, numbness or tingling, and pain are early signs of compartment syndrome.
    3. Edema, numbness or tingling, and pain are early signs of compartment syndrome.
    4. A weak pulse is a late sign of compartment syndrome.
    5. There is no rash with early compartment syndrome.

    TEST-TAKING HINT: The test taker can eliminate answers 3 and 5 because severe pain and rash are not signs of early compartment syndrome.

63. 1. In a recent fracture, the nurse should assess pain and provide treatment.
    2. Pain, pallor, and weak or absent pulses are all signs of compartment syndrome.
    3. Elevating the extremity is important to decrease edema prior to the onset of compartment syndrome. However, once compartment syndrome is suspected, the extremity should be kept at the level of the heart to facilitate arterial and venous flow.
    4. Weak or absent pulse is a sign of compartment syndrome, so monitoring capillary refill is important in assessment.
    5. Pain, pallor, and weak or absent pulses are signs of compartment syndrome. Pain should be treated.

    TEST-TAKING HINT: The test taker can eliminate answer 3 because it is important to keep the affected extremity at heart level to help arterial and venous blood flow.

64. 1. It is a fracture that does not go all the way through the bone.
    2. It is a fracture that does not go all the way through the bone.
    3. It is a fracture that does not go all the way through the bone.
    4. It is a fracture that does not go all the way through the bone.

    TEST-TAKING HINT: The test taker must know the definition of a greenstick fracture.

65. 1. Fractures of the growth plate are serious, as they can disrupt the growth process.
    2. Long-term follow-up is usually needed to evaluate limb discrepancies and potential joint abnormalities.
    3. The ability to participate in contact sports depends on many potential complications.
    4. The amount of pain medication needed in all fractures is determined by the patient.

    TEST-TAKING HINT: The test taker must know what determines how much pain medication is needed.

Leadership and Management

13

KEYWORDS

Advocacy
Assent
Confidentiality
Delegation
Ethical principles
Followership
Informed consent
Leadership

Malpractice
Management
Mentor
Nurse practice act
Priority
Risk management
Scope of practice

ABBREVIATIONS

Activities of daily living (ADLs)
Against medical advice (AMA)
Cardiopulmonary resuscitation (CPR)
Gastrointestinal (GI)
Glycosylated hemoglobin (HgA$_{1C}$)
Health Insurance Portability and Accountability Act (HIPAA)
Health maintenance organization (HMO)
Identification (ID)

Licensed practical nurse (LPN)
Peripherally inserted central catheter (PICC)
Prothrombin time (PT)
Registered nurse (RN)
Respiratory rate (RR)
United States (U.S.)

QUESTIONS

1. A 16-year-old is hospitalized for treatment of gunshot wounds acquired in gang conflict. The teen often shouts at the nurses and uses vulgar language. Which activity is the best example of patient advocacy?
   1. Accepting the rude behavior without comment.
   2. Avoiding entering the room except for scheduled treatments.
   3. Meeting all demands in order to achieve peace.
   4. Asking the teen to describe any fears about current treatment.

2. A 17-year-old is seen in the emergency department and diagnosed with a bowel obstruction. Despite the nurse's best attempt to explain the reason for a nasogastric tube, the adolescent refuses to let the nurse insert the tube. The parent's approach is also ineffective. Which of the following approaches would be most appropriate for the nurse to do first?
   1. Obtain an order for sedation, physically restrain the patient, and insert the tube.
   2. Page the physician, and document the patient's refusal to accept the nasogastric tube.
   3. Explain the AMA form to the adolescent and parent.
   4. Notify the hospital's patient advocate to meet with the adolescent and parent.

3. An infant returned from GI surgery 4 hours ago. The parent refuses pain medication for the baby and states, "The baby is crying because of hunger. Can I offer a bottle?" How should the nurse best advocate for the infant?
   1. Review the results of the observational pain scale with the parent, and explain why the infant must have nothing by mouth.
   2. Use nonpharmacological measures first to see if the pain rating of 8 (out of 10) decreases.
   3. Ask the parent to use the observational pain tool to measure the infant's pain.
   4. Call the physician to obtain an order to feed the infant.

4. At lunch, several nurses are discussing how difficult it is to care for a 16-year-old who constantly complains of pain, unrelieved by morphine via a patient-controlled analgesia pump. One nurse comments, "The teen is addicted to drugs; what do you expect!" Which of the following is the best response to this statement?
   1. "The teen should be moved to an adult unit, where the teen will be told what do."
   2. "We should make sure that the teen has a nursing student to give the staff some relief."
   3. "Perhaps we should call a team conference to review the pain complaints and treatment."
   4. "I think we should speak with the physician about changing to non-narcotic pain medications."

5. A case manager works in an outpatient clinic that administers palivizumab (Synagis) to premature infants at high risk for respiratory syncytial virus. Which outcome is most significant as an indication of effective treatment?
   1. Prevention of hospitalization.
   2. Optimum weight gain.
   3. Promotion of parent-infant bonding.
   4. Early detection and treatment of congenital defects.

6. A case manager is called to arrange for medical equipment and medications at discharge for a child with multiple social problems. Which problem is likely to have the greatest impact on discharge planning?
   1. The child and family are homeless.
   2. The child is not covered by insurance.
   3. The family cannot pay for medications.
   4. The child does not have a primary care provider.

7. A case manager coordinates outpatient care and referrals for patients in an HMO. Which outcome would indicate effective case management for a child with moderate to severe asthma?
   1. The child attends school regularly with few absences for the year.
   2. The child is able to tolerate a regular diet without constipation or diarrhea.
   3. The family does not fill prescriptions for prophylactic inhaled steroids.
   4. The child does not utilize the peak flowmeter when cared for at home.

8. Which of the following is a component of family-centered care?
   1. Reinforce all parenting practices.
   2. Accept all cultural practices and rituals.
   3. Guarantee that financial needs are met.
   4. Recognize family strengths.

9. Nurses are aware that current trends affecting health-care consumers include which of the following?
   1. Generally less informed about health-care issues than previous generations.
   2. Comfortable with health insurance benefits, services, and conditions.
   3. More trusting and less demanding of health-care organizations and staff.
   4. Expect to be more involved in decisions about health-care options.

10. A child and family are addressed by the nurse during admission to the pediatric unit. Which statement is the best example of a proactive service orientation?
   1. "Do you have any special questions or concerns that I can answer?"
   2. "It is important that you keep the crib side rails up at all times you are not at the bedside."
   3. "We ask that you restrict visitors to two persons at the bedside due to space limitations."
   4. "Because your child is on contact precautions, your child will have to remain in the room."

11. A seriously ill child is treated in the intensive care unit. Which aspect of care is the easiest for family members to evaluate and most important for consumer satisfaction?
   1. The compliance with standards.
   2. The efficiency of the medical equipment used in care.
   3. The relationship with the nurse and other staff.
   4. The accuracy of completion of medical orders.

12. An interdisciplinary team is assembled to review protocols for management of central intravenous lines. Which staff should be represented on the team?
   1. Experienced RNs and pharmacists.
   2. RNs, physicians, and pharmacists.
   3. RNs, LPNs, and physicians.
   4. Charge nurses and staff physicians.

13. The staff nurse is discharging an infant with a tracheostomy and gastrostomy to be cared for by parents at home. The case manager has arranged for home health supplies and services. Whose discussion would be of most direct benefit to ensure individualized care in the home?
   1. Case manager and community pediatrician.
   2. Case manager and home health company supervisor.
   3. Staff RN and medical supply company.
   4. Hospital staff nurse and home health nurse.

14. An experienced nurse notes that a patient is developing a rash shortly after the first dose of an intravenous antibiotic. Which team member should be called first?
   1. Physician.
   2. Pharmacist.
   3. Charge nurse.
   4. Unit manager.

15. It is a busy day on the pediatric unit, and the nurses are short-staffed. A school-age child is scheduled to undergo an invasive radiological procedure. Which staff member would be most appropriate to meet the child's support needs by accompanying the child?
   1. The staff nurse with the least busy assignment.
   2. The staff nurse assigned to this child.
   3. A volunteer grandparent who is on the unit.
   4. The child life–worker for the unit.

16. Which of the following activities would be most effective in helping a new nurse manager develop transformational leadership abilities in a rapidly changing practice setting?
    1. Select a mentor and a professional support group.
    2. Focus on activities that avoid change and involve minimal risk.
    3. Reward or correct followers to maintain current levels of practice.
    4. Use own judgment when making decisions, with little input from staff.

17. Which of the following activities best falls within the scope of management rather than leadership?
    1. Planning the staffing schedule for a 2-month period.
    2. Empowering the staff to meet patient care goals for the year.
    3. Encouraging staff to utilize reflective practice and self-awareness.
    4. Inspiring staff to develop a shared vision of quality patient care.

18. Tasks of followership that would be expected of a new nursing graduate include which of the following?
    1. Collaborates with others, honors standards, demonstrates individual accountability.
    2. Envisions organizational goals, affirms values, represents the group.
    3. Motivates others, develops standards, eliminates barriers to care.
    4. Evaluates system processes, recommends ways to improve the system.

19. The pediatric unit is re-evaluating the procedure used by staff to suction tracheostomies. Which activity demonstrates followership activities, appropriate to a recent nursing graduate?
    1. Rewrite the hospital policy and procedure for tracheostomy suctioning.
    2. Work with information technology to plan new computer screens for charting.
    3. Provide input on the feasibility and effectiveness of the new procedure.
    4. Hold in-services to educate staff on the techniques and rationale for the new procedure.

20. The nurse receives a telephone call from a staff member who works on another unit. The member is inquiring about the test results of a friend's child, who is hospitalized on the nurse's unit. Which response is appropriate?
    1. Summarize the test results as they are within the normal range.
    2. Move to a private phone to prevent being overheard before sharing the information.
    3. Decline to give out information.
    4. Direct the staff member to the test results in the hospital electronic medical record.

21. A pediatric hospital nurse receives a telephone call from an individual who is the parent of a child assigned to the nurse's care. Which action by the nurse is most correct?
    1. Verify the privacy code assigned to the child before giving any information.
    2. Decline to give out information over the telephone because no ID can be shown.
    3. Update the parent on the child's condition, as no family members are in the room.
    4. Take the parent's name and telephone number and give it to the other parent when visiting.

22. A nursing student records notes about a pediatric patient's condition in preparation for a clinical experience. Which of the following information is considered individually identifiable health-care information and cannot be attached to the notes?
    1. Date of birth.
    2. Medical diagnosis.
    3. Nursing diagnosis.
    4. Diagnostic test results.

23. If an employee has medical testing at a facility where that employee works, what is the appropriate way to access the test results?
1. Complete the authorization form and receive a copy of the results.
2. Get a fellow employee who works in that department to access the results.
3. Call a friend who has access to the records and ask for a copy of the test results.
4. Check the computer system for the test results.

24. For a school-age child who has Kawasaki disease and is taking aspirin, which laboratory value should be reported to the physician?
1. Blood, urea, nitrogen 18 mg/dL.
2. Hematocrit 42%.
3. Potassium 3.8 mEq/L.
4. PT 14.6 sec.

25. During a home visit to an 8-month-old infant in congestive heart failure on digoxin (Lanoxin), the nurse obtains assessment information. Which assessment indicates that the nurse needs to consult the physician?
1. The infant's apical pulse is 70 at rest.
2. After crying, the infant's heart rate is 170.
3. Respirations are 40 per minute at rest.
4. Capillary refill is <3 sec.

26. A premature infant with chronic lung disease is going home with complex care, including oxygen, tracheostomy suction, and gastrostomy feedings. Which of the following discharge planning activities will be most effective in promoting continuity of care?
1. Send the parents to meet staff at the nursing agency that will be providing care in the home.
2. Plan a team conference at the hospital before discharge to include parents and hospital and home health staff.
3. Ask the parents to meet with the hospital respiratory therapy staff to discuss adapting the home environment to meet equipment needs.
4. Teach parents how to care for the child by utilizing hospital equipment and protocols.

27. Which pediatric patient can benefit most by a primary nursing approach in which one nurse cares for the child whenever on duty and coordinates other staff care?
1. A patient admitted for a diagnostic workup of mononucleosis.
2. A patient who had surgery 1 day ago for appendicitis.
3. An infant treated with phototherapy for hyperbilirubinemia.
4. A toddler with leukemia, admitted for chemotherapy.

28. When caring for an infant admitted for pyloric stenosis surgery, which tasks would be appropriate for the RN to delegate to a nursing assistant? Select all that apply.
1. Physical assessment on admission.
2. Vital signs every 4 hours.
3. Discharge teaching for parents.
4. Bed, bath, and change of linens.
5. Daily weights.

29. The nurse is managing care of a school-age child with new-onset type I diabetes. Which tasks must be performed only by the RN and cannot be delegated to an LPN or nursing assistant? Select all that apply.
1. Teaching parents how to give subcutaneous injections of insulin.
2. Performing blood glucose monitoring before meals and bedtime.
3. Evaluating the child's response to insulin doses.
4. Determining the educational goals for the day.
5. Teaching the child signs for hypoglycemia and hyperglycemia.

30. Assigning the right task to the right person is a principle of nursing delegation and assignment. Which of the following scenarios best meets this principle?
    1. A 4-month-old with Down syndrome is assigned to a nurse whose own child died of heart disease due to Down syndrome 6 months ago.
    2. A child with a central intravenous line that occluded on the previous shift is assigned to a new LPN.
    3. A child newly diagnosed with acute leukemia is assigned to an experienced pediatric oncology nurse who floated to the general pediatric unit.
    4. A child with new-onset type I diabetes is assigned to an RN who has four other complex-care patients.

31. An experienced pediatric nurse relocates to a new city and state. In the new position, the nurse questions which skills and tasks can be performed by unlicensed nursing personnel. To obtain answers to this question, which resource is considered primary?
    1. Hospital policies and procedures manual.
    2. State nurses' association.
    3. Educational program for nursing assistants.
    4. State nurse practice act.

32. When caring for a patient in pain, which activity is appropriate to delegate to unlicensed nursing personnel?
    1. Coaching the patient during painful procedures.
    2. Assessment using a self-report pain scale.
    3. Evaluating pain after giving medication.
    4. Bathing the patient and hygiene measures.

33. After receiving the change-of-shift report, the nurse prioritizes care for the day. Which patient should the nurse assess first?
    1. 1-month-old admitted 1 day ago with fever and possible sepsis.
    2. 14-month-old with a tracheostomy admitted for respiratory syncytial virus bronchiolitis.
    3. 18-month-old with acute viral meningitis.
    4. 7-year-old 1 day after an appendectomy.

34. After a school bus accident, four elementary school children are delivered by ambulance to the emergency department. Only one emergency physician is on duty. Which child should be directed to the physician first by the triage nurse?
    1. The child who is crying uncontrollably and tries to move off the stretcher.
    2. The child with severe abdominal pain, anxious and responsive, blood pressure 100/60; heart rate 120; RR 28.
    3. The child with severe pain and distorted alignment of the right lower leg, indicating a possible fracture.
    4. The child who is unresponsive, with fixed and dilated pupils, blood pressure 58/44; heart rate 60; RR 10.

35. The nurse is providing care for an adolescent with complex needs after surgical correction of a severe bowel obstruction. On entering the room, the nurse prioritizes care and decides to complete which task first?
    1. Change the central intravenous line dressing, which is loose and gaping.
    2. Empty the ileostomy bag, which is moderately full of liquid stool.
    3. Change the gauze dressing around the Jackson-Pratt drain.
    4. Check for correct positioning of the nasogastric tube in the stomach.

36. An adolescent is received in the pediatric intensive care unit after scoliosis surgery. Using Maslow's hierarchy of needs as a guide, which problem takes priority?
    1. Hypotension related to analgesia.
    2. Fear of being left alone by parents.
    3. Frustration with postoperative immobility.
    4. Concern with the extensive skin incision.

37. A child is receiving continuous morphine by patient-controlled analgesia pump (basal and bolus) to control pain. Which side effect is the nurse's greatest concern?
    1. Sedation.
    2. Respiratory depression.
    3. Nausea and vomiting.
    4. Constipation.

38. Which of the following questions represents an ethical issue in nursing practice that cannot be resolved through research?
    1. How does the incidence of medication errors on the pediatric unit compare with the incidence of errors on the neonatal unit?
    2. Does the use of local anesthesia during circumcision make a difference in infants' pain scores, as measured on the face, legs, activity, cry, consolability (FLACC) scale?
    3. Is the emergency room nurse obligated to report suspicion of child abuse if signs of abuse are noted in the assessment?
    4. Which method of irrigating central venous lines results in less line obstruction and infection?

39. Shortly before a child's elective surgery, the parent tells the nurse, "I am having second thoughts about my child undergoing this surgery." The nurse respects the parent's concern and calls the surgeon. What ethical/moral principle is represented by this situation?
    1. Autonomy.
    2. Equality.
    3. Fidelity.
    4. Justice.

40. During a clinic visit, a child's mother tells the nurse, "I'm afraid of what my husband will do." Following an ethical decision-making process, the nurse's first step is to:
    1. Direct the mother to a center for abused women.
    2. Provide the phone number of the domestic violence hotline.
    3. Clarify what the mother means by her statement.
    4. Ask the mother, "Why does your husband feel this way?"

41. Which situation would be appropriate to refer to the hospital ethics committee?
    1. The physician recommends that a young child in the end stages of terminal cancer be taken off the ventilator. The parents, who are divorced and have joint custody of the child, have different views about whether to discontinue the ventilator.
    2. A child in end-stage renal failure is placed on the renal transplant list. The parents are asked to sign permission for surgery after a cadaver kidney is located. One parent is out of town and gives telephone consent.
    3. After initial therapies have failed, a child with leukemia is evaluated for a new cancer protocol. The child, age 8 years, gives assent for the new treatment, and his parents give consent as well.
    4. Parents are shocked when their child is diagnosed with a malignant bone tumor. The orthopedic surgeon discusses the options of limb amputation and a limb-salvage procedure. The parents are asked to consider each option.

42. Organizational policies on the security of computer data mandate that system users keep which of the following pieces of user information confidential?
    1. Name.
    2. ID.
    3. Password.
    4. Credentials.

43. The nurse is charting on the computer at the nursing station when a parent exits a nearby room and asks for help because the child has vomited. Which immediate action is best?
    1. Immediately assist the parent.
    2. Put the computer in "suspend mode" so that the screen is blank and then assist the parent.
    3. Finish recording information and exit out of the computer before assisting the parent.
    4. Continue charting and call another team member to assist the parent.

44. If a staff member has the right to access the computer system, the member has a right to view which of the following health records?
    1. Personal health records.
    2. Health records of immediate family members.
    3. Health records of patients assigned to their care.
    4. Health records of patients' family members.

45. Individually identifiable health information may not be:
    1. Faxed.
    2. Mailed.
    3. Copied.
    4. Sold.

46. Which patient is able to give informed consent for a surgical procedure in many U.S. states?
    1. 13-year-old abused male.
    2. 15-year-old pregnant female.
    3. 16-year-old cancer patient.
    4. 17-year-old college freshman.

47. Which of the following situations would be considered failure to obtain informed consent?
    1. Parents who speak Spanish receive information about their child's surgery from the surgeon using a telephone language-line Spanish translator.
    2. Bilingual parents sign the consent form for a lumbar puncture. Later, they tell a Spanish-speaking nurse, "We do not understand why they are doing this test."
    3. The physician addresses the benefits of a procedure with a child's parents but gets called away. Later, the physician returns to finish the discussion before parents sign the consent.
    4. Only one parent of a child is present in the hospital to sign the surgical consent. The other parent is out of town on business.

48. Staff members working with school-age children believe it is important for each child to understand and agree to medical treatment, especially when treatment is part of research protocols. The term for this process is:
    1. Assent.
    2. Informed consent.
    3. Confidentiality.
    4. Emancipation.

49. When explaining the procedure to the parent of a child undergoing surgery, the provider must give the following information as part of informed consent. Select all that apply.
    1. Date and time the specific procedure will be performed.
    2. Alternative therapies.
    3. Benefits that are likely to result from the procedure.
    4. Names and titles of all staff members who will be in the operating room.
    5. The patient and family may withdraw consent at any time.

50. When making assignments for the oncoming shift on the pediatric unit, the charge nurse assigns a float RN from another unit to care for an infant with complex needs. What is the legal responsibility of the charge nurse in this situation?
    1. Assurance of scope of practice.
    2. Duty to orient, educate, and evaluate.
    3. Patient's rights and responsibilities.
    4. Determination of nurse/patient ratios.

51. After the parent leaves the side rail down, a hospitalized toddler falls from the crib and suffers a skull fracture. Earlier that day, the nurse had discussed the importance of side rails with that parent and recorded the discussion in the nursing notes. Which element of malpractice is missing in this case?
    1. Relationship with the patient.
    2. Breach of duty of care.
    3. Injury.
    4. Damage.

52. The legal basis for nursing activities may be at the local, state, or national level. The nurse should check the agency's policy and procedure manual as the primary legal authority for which of the following?
    1. Whether an RN can initiate a blood transfusion.
    2. Sharing of patient-sensitive information.
    3. Legal protection when providing CPR to a non-patient.
    4. Procedure for flushing a central venous line.

53. Assault and battery is considered an intentional tort that may leave the nurse liable for malpractice. Which situation might be considered assault and battery of a child?
    1. The nurse sticks a hysterical infant five times in an attempt to start a PICC line, although the parent verbally refuses to allow the procedure to continue after the third try.
    2. A 2-year-old screams while being restrained for a dressing change of a complex burn wound.
    3. A nurse attempts to administer an oral antibiotic to a young child who then spits the entire dose of medication out on the sheet.
    4. A postoperative school-age child refuses when told to get out of bed and walk in the hall four times a day.

54. The nurse makes an error by giving the wrong medication to a patient. An incident report is completed per hospital policy. What information should the nurse chart in the medical record?
    1. Description of the specific occurrence and treatment given.
    2. Completion of the incident report.
    3. Date, time, and name of person completing the incident report.
    4. Nothing.

55. Which of the following events should be reported to a risk management committee by documentation?
    1. A nurse administered a double therapeutic dose of medication based on an incorrect physician order.
    2. A patient's heparin lock became clotted between intermittent medication doses.
    3. A toddler dislodged the intravenous catheter, resulting in an occluded intravenous line.
    4. An uncooperative child spit out an undeterminable amount of oral medication despite the nurse's best effort.

56. Which of the following events represents a departure from safe practice as defined by risk management?
    1. A nurse double-checks an insulin dose with a nursing assistant before administration to the patient.
    2. The physician writes an illegible order, then draws a line through it, initials it, and prints the same information above the line.
    3. The nurse repeats a verbal order back to the physician and asks for verification of accuracy.
    4. A nurse asks another RN to double-check a dose of morphine before administering the drug via intravenous push.

57. The diabetes clinic conducts a disease management program for children with type I diabetes. Which test is the most valid indicator of compliance with the diabetes regimen?
    1. Fasting blood glucose level.
    2. Fingerstick glucose for 24 hours.
    3. Urine ketone strip.
    4. HgA$_{1C}$ assay.

58. A charge nurse overhears a staff nurse make an erroneous statement to a parent in the hallway. Which initial approach by the charge nurse should follow the observation?
    1. Discuss the correct information with the parent.
    2. Discuss the observation with the manager of the unit.
    3. Write a description of the incident and share it with the staff nurse.
    4. Ask the staff nurse to describe the situation in private.

59. Which situation should be referred by the pediatric nursing staff to the nurse manager?
    1. Several staff members plan to get together to celebrate the end of a successful year working on the unit.
    2. Staff members complain about the cafeteria food and want a broader menu.
    3. Patients with occluded saline locks are repeatedly being transferred from the emergency department to the pediatric unit.
    4. Nursing staff members who have joined the union are in disagreement with union policies.

60. A 9-year-old patient on the pediatric unit is immobilized in a spica cast. When the parents are absent, the child presses the call light constantly. Which action would be most appropriate to meet the child's needs?
    1. Consult with the charge nurse to obtain a 24-hour sitter for the child.
    2. Speak with the parents and ask them not to leave the bedside.
    3. Refer to the child life–worker for bedside play activities.
    4. Obtain a social service referral to meet emotional needs.

61. A young child hospitalized with asthma is ready for discharge. A home nebulizer is ordered by the physician. In order to obtain the nebulizer, a referral should be made to which staff member?
    1. Case manager.
    2. Nurse manager.
    3. Materials management staff.
    4. Child life staff.

1. 1. Acceptance of the teen's humanity does not mean acceptance of inappropriate or rude behavior. The nurse also has rights and should communicate to the teen how the behavior is being interpreted.
2. Avoidance of the teen is likely to further alienate and isolate the teen, increasing fears and concerns.
3. Meeting all demands may not be appropriate in this situation. Nursing staff members need to negotiate, clarify, and explain which behaviors are acceptable, without reinforcing negative behavior.
4. **All patients have the right to be informed and participate in care decisions. Assessment of needs is the first step in providing culturally congruent care and education.**

TEST-TAKING HINT: Patient advocacy is based on protecting the basic rights of patients in the health-care system. Understanding the disease process and its treatment is one of these rights. As in all aspects of care, assessment of the patient's questions and fears is the beginning of patient education.

2. 1. This approach involves little advocacy for the patient, because it bypasses rather than supports self-determination.
2. This approach would be used only after other methods to communicate with the patient have been attempted.
3. This is the least effective approach, because if the adolescent leaves against medical advice, no care will be received.
4. **Because of the patient's age, the teen should be treated as an adult. The nurse best promotes self-determination by making additional attempts to elicit any fears and concerns that are preventing effective care. The patient advocate may be able to gain this information.**

TEST-TAKING HINT: Patient advocacy includes promoting the rights of the patient, in this case the right to self-determination and informed consent. Utilizing the patient advocate in this situation is an effective way to further determine why the patient is refusing care.

3. 1. **As the advocate for the infant and parent, the nurse has the responsibility to educate the parent about the infant's condition after surgery, the rationale for having nothing by mouth, and the assessment and treatment of pain. By being informed, the parent can make educated assessments and decisions, collaborating with the nurse to meet the infant's needs.**
2. A pain rating of 8 indicates severe pain and the need for pharmacological and non-pharmacological pain control measures.
3. Although the parent should be educated about the pain tool, the parent should not be accountable to use the tool to measure the infant's pain.
4. If the infant had major GI surgery, it would be contraindicated to feed the infant immediately postoperatively.

TEST-TAKING HINT: Advocacy helps to ensure that pain and other postoperative needs are met by nursing staff. Because parents have the legal authority to consent for their child's treatment, it is critical that they be fully informed and understand the child's postoperative status and rationale for treatment.

4. 1. Passing responsibility for care to another unit where staff do not know the teen is unlikely to resolve problems with care.
2. Recruiting a student who is less experienced in the care of complex pain patients is unlikely to resolve problems with care.
3. **As a patient advocate, the nurse is responsible for recognizing when current approaches are ineffective and working with other staff members to develop effective care. Planning a team conference is one way to brainstorm new approaches.**
4. If morphine does not relieve the pain, this answer is unlikely to be effective.

TEST-TAKING HINT: As a patient advocate, the nurse promotes the rights of this patient to optimum treatment and pain relief. Because pain is a complex phenomenon, a multidisciplinary approach is often helpful to come up with new and more effective approaches.

5. 1. **Palivizumab is an antibody administered monthly to premature and other high-risk infants during respiratory syncytial virus season. The goal is prevention of serious respiratory syncytial virus bronchiolitis requiring hospitalization.**
2. Although weight gain is an important health outcome for rapidly growing premature infants, it is not the focus of a clinic for respiratory syncytial virus prophylaxis.

3. Promotion of parent infant bonding is a goal for nurses working with infants; however, this is not the focus of a clinic for respiratory syncytial virus prevention.

4. Early detection and treatment of congenital problems is important for the health of premature infants, but it is not the focus of a clinic for respiratory syncytial virus prevention.

TEST-TAKING HINT: Because of the expense and special authorization needed from third-party payers, palivizumab (Synagis) is often administered in specialty clinics. Case managers work with clinic patients to coordinate care, promote cost savings, use resources efficiently, and improve patient outcomes.

6. 1. **Homelessness is likely to have the greatest impact on discharge planning because all other aspects of care revolve around this issue.**

2. The social worker can assist the family in applying for medical aid due to low income.

3. Discharge medications can often be secured through the assistance of the social worker and hospital pharmacy.

4. The child can be referred to a clinic that works with indigent patients for follow-up and continued care.

TEST-TAKING HINT: Homelessness affects all other issues and requires social services in both the community and hospital.

7. 1. **Regular school attendance is a positive outcome of case management because asthma can result in frequent absences from school.**

2. Diet is rarely a problem in asthma and would not be an indication of compliance with care.

3. This situation is considered a negative outcome, because children with moderate or severe asthma need inhaled steroids to decrease lung inflammation.

4. This situation is a negative outcome. Peak flowmeters should be used to monitor lung function and guide treatment decisions.

TEST-TAKING HINT: The goal of case management in asthma is improved health outcomes, including prevention of exacerbations of illness. School attendance, prevention of hospital admissions, regular checkups, early diagnosis of illness, and compliance with medications are indicators of effective case management.

8. 1. Parenting practices are respected as long as children's needs are met; however, this may not be true of all parenting practices. Parent education and negotiation may be required.

2. There may be times that cultural practices directly conflict with medical treatments; therefore acceptance is based on compatibility.

3. Although financial support for families is included in family-centered care guidelines, there is no guarantee that all financial needs will be met.

4. **Recognizing and building on family strengths is an important component of family-centered care.**

TEST-TAKING HINT: All pediatric healthcare organizations include family-centered care as part of their patient rights documents. Family-centered care includes recognizing the family as the constant in the child's life, creating parent/professional collaboration, encouraging parent-to-parent support, and building on family strengths.

9. 1. Today's health-care consumer is better educated, often from searching the Internet, and expects to receive more information from providers.

2. In contrast, many patients are dissatisfied or confused about benefits under their health insurance plans.

3. To the contrary, data show that patients are more demanding and aggressive in situations involving health care.

4. **Data show that current health-care consumers expect to participate more in decisions about medical treatment.**

TEST-TAKING HINT: Consider the effect of societal trends, such as Internet access, advertising and marketing, increased rights of women and minorities, changes in insurance and HMOs, and increasing diversity.

10. 1. **This is a proactive statement with a "ready to help" image.**

2. This statement provides information about crib safety.

3. This statement provides information about visiting policies.

4. This statement provides information about isolation policies.

TEST-TAKING HINT: A service orientation focuses on customer satisfaction. Proactive statements with a "ready to help" image include such phrases as "How may I help you?", "I'd be happy to...", and "It's my pleasure...".

11. 1. Consumers are frequently unable to judge this aspect of care.
    2. This is not a known aspect of care for most family members.
    3. **Consumers always have the ability to evaluate the quality of the relationship with the person delivering the service.**
    4. Family members as consumers seldom have the information to judge this aspect of care.

TEST-TAKING HINT: Although consumers are frequently unable to judge or evaluate the quality of interventions, they always have the ability to evaluate the quality of the relationship with the person delivering the service. Most consumer complaints resolve around problems with staff, such as feeling ignored, disrespected, or being treated poorly.

12. 1. The team should be composed of these staff members; however, this answer omits physicians, who write the orders for the central intravenous line.
    2. **Because all three of these disciplines are involved in care of central intravenous lines, this answer is the most complete.**
    3. In many locations, LPNs are not authorized to care for central intravenous lines and would not be involved in this care. Furthermore, this answer omits pharmacists, who are concerned with medication administration through these lines.
    4. Involving only persons at the leadership level may lead to omission of valuable input from staff RNs, resident physicians, and other disciplines such as pharmacy.

TEST-TAKING HINT: Involving all team members who have responsibilities related to this activity helps to ensure that all important factors are considered. When members of all involved disciplines participate in decision making, they are more likely to agree to any changes made.

13. 1. These team members have oversight for assessing, planning, and evaluating care of the child but do not provide direct nursing care in the hospital or home.
    2. Both of these team members are in managerial roles, which are essential for providing resources, but may not guarantee an individualized approach to care.

3. Planning for home-care supplies is an important function but not as broad as that provided by other team members.
    4. **If the goal is individualized care, the best team members to discuss this child's care are the two staff members with the most direct care-taking responsibilities—the hospital staff nurse and the home health nurse.**

TEST-TAKING HINT: The key to deciding among staff members is the phrase "individualized care." Which two team members will be in most direct contact with the child and family? These staff members are most likely to know the individual characteristics of the child and family members.

14. 1. **Development of an allergic reaction, which is most likely happening in this situation, requires prompt treatment to prevent complications such as anaphylaxis. The physician should be called first so that prompt treatment can be ordered.**
    2. The pharmacist cannot change the drug without a physician's order.
    3. Although the charge nurse should be informed in a timely manner, the nurse has the responsibility to communicate directly with the physician when an allergic reaction is suspected.
    4. This incident may or may not require communication to the unit manager.

TEST-TAKING HINT: Problem solving requires knowledge of clearly delegated roles and duties. Only the physician has the authority to prescribe an antihistamine. Furthermore, the nurse has the legal responsibility to notify the physician of any complication, such as a rash.

15. 1. The child does not know that nurses have other patient assignments and may not feel supported. Additionally, this arrangement takes the staff nurse away from assigned patients.
    2. In a short-staffed situation, it may be impossible to take a nurse off the floor for even a short radiological procedure. Care of other assigned patients may be compromised.
    3. A volunteer may not be able to support the child adequately in an unfamiliar situation and may have difficulty coping with the stress of an intrusive procedure.
    4. **Helping children cope with intrusive or frightening procedures is part of the**

job description of the child life–worker. This answer has the added advantage of maintaining staff nurse numbers on the unit.

TEST-TAKING HINT: The best answer considers the staffing needs of the unit as well as the individual support needs of the child. In answers 1 and 2, staffing may be compromised by sending a nurse off the unit. In answer 3, the volunteer may not be able to support the child adequately. Because support during intrusive procedures is a common function of the child life–worker, answer 4 is most likely to provide the child with maximum support without reducing nursing staffing.

16. 1. **A mentor can model new behavior and coach the new nurse manager while providing support during new experiences.**
    2. The novice nurse leader/manager must be willing to change, grow, and take risks.
    3. Transformational leadership involves inspiring new visions rather than maintaining the status quo.
    4. A good leader gathers input from all levels of staff when making decisions.

    TEST-TAKING HINT: Transformational leadership is best in changing environments. This leadership style involves creativity, change, risk, shared vision, and attention to the importance of people. The challenges of developing these leadership abilities are best met by the novice leader/manager who has the support of a mentor who can serve as a coach, teacher, and resource person.

17. 1. **Managers coordinate and utilize resources. Planning for staffing is an example of both coordination and utilization of staff.**
    2. Empowerment of staff best fits within the scope of leadership.
    3. Encouraging self-reflection is a motivational activity included in leadership theories.
    4. Leaders help to transform organizations through motivation and inspiration of employees.

    TEST-TAKING HINT: Management is defined as a process of coordinating activities and utilizing resources to achieve goals. Actions tend to be more specific, such as preparing the staffing schedule. Leadership is a broader concept, involving staff

empowerment, system redesign, ethics, and increased motivation.

18. 1. **These followership activities are appropriate for a new graduate nurse.**
    2. These activities are leadership and management tasks, appropriate for the experienced practitioner.
    3. These tasks fall within the scope of leadership and management.
    4. These tasks require experience in an organization and are appropriate for leaders and managers.

    TEST-TAKING HINT: Bleich's tasks of leadership, management, and followership are included in the examples above. The new nursing graduate would be expected to demonstrate good followership before taking on leadership and management tasks.

19. 1. Writing policies and procedures is an advanced activity, performed by nurse managers.
    2. Designing systems for charting is an advanced task, requiring experienced staff.
    3. **Testing a new procedure falls within the scope of a new practitioner and is an appropriate followership activity.**
    4. Staff educators are experienced staff members whose responsibility is to plan in-service education.

    TEST-TAKING HINT: Because the new graduate focuses on followership tasks, the key to answering this question is to determine whether actions fall within the scope of leadership, management, or followership. Testing out a new procedure is most clearly a followership task.

20. 1. Providing information to a staff member who is not involved in the patient's care is a violation of privacy and must be avoided.
    2. It is a violation of privacy to share information with others without the patient/family permission.
    3. **The pediatric nurse cannot legally share this information, but the parent can choose to do so. This response does not violate the patient/family right to privacy.**
    4. It is a clear violation of privacy to access electronic medical records without a need to know this information to provide care. Because the staff member is not involved in the child's care, that person cannot legally access the child's medical information.

    TEST-TAKING HINT: Sharing clinical information is guided by the "need to know" in order to care for a patient. In this case, the staff member works on another unit and is not caring for the friend's child. "Need to know" does not exist here.

21. 1. **The nurse is correct to verify the privacy code, which is given only to the child's legal guardians, before relating medical information over the telephone.**
    2. The nurse is incorrect to deny information to individuals who have a right to know such information.
    3. Failure to verify the caller's right to receive information is a violation of the patient's right to privacy and confidentiality.
    4. The nurse is incorrect to deny information if the caller can provide proper ID.

    TEST-TAKING HINT: Institutions can reduce violation of a patient's privacy and confidentiality by allowing access to patient data only by individuals who are legally allowed to receive it. Most hospitals maintain privacy of data by assigning a privacy code, which is given to immediate family members, or maintaining a list of persons who are allowed information. Verification of a caller's right to receive information should be made by the nurse before giving out information over the telephone.

22. 1. **Date of birth is information that can be used to identify an individual and should not be attached to students' notes.**
    2. The medical diagnosis is not considered individually identifiable information.
    3. A nursing diagnosis is not considered individually identifiable information.
    4. Diagnostic test results are not considered individually identifiable information.

    TEST-TAKING HINT: Information that can be used to identify an individual includes name, birth date, social security number, and medical record number. Attaching this information to health-care data violates patient confidentiality and privacy.

23. 1. **Employees who seek access to their own medical records must follow the same procedures as any patient treated by the health-care facility.**
    2. This action violates federal laws regarding protected health information, because the employee does not have a "need to know" to provide care.
    3. This action constitutes a privacy violation, because the friend does not have a "need to know" to provide care.

4. Clinical information systems should be accessed only as necessary to provide patient care. This does not include access to personal records.

    TEST-TAKING HINT: Federal guidelines require that all patients access their personal medical records following the same procedures. The standard for accessing patient information is a "need to know" for the performance of the job.

24. 1. This value is in normal range. Normal blood, urea, nitrogen is 10–20 mg/dL. For a patient on aspirin, an elevated blood, urea, nitrogen value might be a result of chronic GI bleeding.
    2. This value is in normal range. Normal hematocrit values are 37–47 (females) and 42–52 (males). Hematocrit values decrease if bleeding occurs.
    3. This value is in normal range. Normal potassium values are 3.5–5.0 mEq/L. The nurse monitors for a decrease in potassium.
    4. **This value indicates an increase in PT and should be reported to the physician. Normal range is 11–12.5 seconds. Prolonged bleeding time can be a side effect of aspirin.**

    TEST-TAKING HINT: Two variables must be considered when answering this question: which laboratory values are abnormal and what changes are likely to be seen with aspirin, due to the side effect of bleeding.

25. 1. **Bradycardia (heart rate below 90–110 beats/min in infants) is a common sign of digoxin toxicity. The provider should be notified.**
    2. Increased heart rate after crying is a normal finding in an infant.
    3. This is a normal RR in an infant. Tachypnea, a complication in congestive heart failure, is usually defined as an RR greater than 60–80 breaths per minute.
    4. This is a normal capillary refill (<2–3 sec). Delayed capillary refill is a sign of complications in congestive heart failure.

    TEST-TAKING HINT: Digoxin is a potentially dangerous drug because of the narrow margin of safety between therapeutic and toxic doses. Accidental overdose is possible because such small doses are given to infants (usually less than 1 mL).

26. 1. This activity is appropriate but does less than other answers to promote continuity of care because it omits hospital staff.

2. By including parents, hospital staff, and home-care staff, a joint team conference is the best option to promote continuity of care.
3. Adaptation of the home environment is important in the discharge process, but it is not focused on the goal of continuity of care.
4. Teaching parents how to care for the child in the hospital is an important first step to home care, but it does less than other options to meet the goal of continuity of care.

TEST-TAKING HINT: The question focuses on effective promotion of continuity of care. Although other answers are important in planning for home care, only answer 2 involves all family and staff members, promoting continuity between hospital and home.

27. 1. Primary nursing is less important in this situation. This child is likely to have a short hospital stay, without readmission.
2. Appendicitis, without complications, usually results in early discharge or a short hospital stay. Continuity of staff is less important.
3. The hospital treatment of hyperbilirubinemia is likely to be very short, because this condition can also be treated in the home. Primary nursing is less important.
4. **This child is likely to be admitted for repeated hospitalizations and over a longer period of time than other patients. Having a close relationship with one or a few nurses can lead to increased satisfaction for all.**

TEST-TAKING HINT: The advantage of primary nursing is continuity in the relationship between the child/family and the nurse. A more individualized approach can be provided, leading to more holistic care. This approach is most valuable for patients with repeat hospitalizations and longer stay.

28. 2, 4, 5.
1. RNs should perform all admission assessments. By law, this function cannot be delegated.
2. **Determination of vital signs is within the scope of practice of the nursing assistant and is an appropriate task for the RN to delegate.**
3. RNs perform all patient teaching. Therefore, it is not appropriate to delegate this task to a nursing assistant.
4. **ADLs are appropriate for the RN to delegate to a nursing assistant.**
5. **Daily weights are appropriate for the RN to delegate to a nursing assistant.**

TEST-TAKING HINT: The test taker must know which tasks can be assigned to nursing assistive personnel. Baseline assessments and patient teaching are never delegated and must be completed by the RN. Vital signs and ADLs are within the scope of practice of a nursing assistant and may be delegated.

29. 1, 3, 4, 5.
1. **All education must be completed by the RN and cannot be delegated. This includes insulin administration.**
2. Blood glucose monitoring is within the scope of practice of an LPN and nursing assistant and can be delegated by the RN.
3. **Evaluation of a patient's responses to treatments and medications must be completed by the RN and cannot be delegated.**
4. **Determining the plan of care, including educational goals, must be completed by the RN. This task is not within the scope of practice of the LPN or nursing assistant.**
5. **Teaching the child about hypoglycemia and hyperglycemia is the responsibility of the RN and cannot be delegated.**

TEST-TAKING HINT: Determining the plan of care and patient teaching are functions that are only within the scope of practice of the RN and cannot be delegated to an LPN or nursing assistant.

30. 1. This might not be the best match between patient and nurse, if the emotions of the nurse who recently lost a child are still overwhelming.
2. A new-graduate LPN might not be intravenous certified and would probably have little experience with central intravenous line malfunctions. Some states exclude LPNs from working with central intravenous lines.
3. **Even though the pediatric oncology nurse has floated to the pediatric unit, this patient's care involves routine skills and knowledge used in the nurse's oncology practice. This makes this assignment the best example of "right task to right person."**
4. Extensive teaching is involved for a child with new-onset diabetes. The nurse with a

very busy assignment is not likely to have the time required for teaching.

TEST-TAKING HINT: The "right task" is one that can be safely and effectively assigned to the nursing staff person who has the knowledge and skills required. In answers 1 and 4, the nurse may be distracted by interpersonal or environmental factors. In answer 2, the new-graduate LPN may not have the skills. Answer 3 is the best answer because the oncology nurse is likely to have the needed knowledge and skills.

31. 1. The hospital's policies and procedures must be based on the state's nurse practice act and is a secondary resource.
    2. The nurses' association in each state focuses on the welfare of nurses, not the legal scope of practice.
    3. Educational programs for nursing assistants must take scope of practice into consideration, but they are not the legally defining bodies.
    4. **Each state establishes legal guidelines for health-care professionals in various roles. These guidelines are in the state's nurse practice act, which is the ultimate legal document.**

TEST-TAKING HINT: The word "primary" is the key to answering this question. Each state has its own definition of scope of practice for different nursing roles. These are legal definitions, passed by the state legislature and are therefore the primary sources of information.

32. 1. Rules of management dictate that the RN does not delegate the function of patient teaching.
    2. Rules of management dictate that the RN does not delegate the function of assessment.
    3. Rules of management dictate that the RN does not delegate the function of evaluation.
    4. **The nursing assistant may help the patient in hygiene matters, including bathing.**

TEST-TAKING HINT: When answering delegation questions, follow the rules of nursing management. The RN does not delegate assessment, teaching, or evaluation to unlicensed personnel such as nursing assistants.

33. 1. Fever is likely to be the most acute problem of this infant, but it is not life-threatening.

2. **Following the ABCs (airway-breathing-circulation), this baby has the greatest potential for a life-threatening complication if the tracheostomy becomes obstructed by mucus.**
3. Although fever and discomfort may need prompt attention, neither one is life-threatening.
4. Pain is the critical assessment area for this child, but it is not life-threatening

TEST-TAKING HINT: The question is asking the nurse to prioritize care based on physiological parameters. The infant in answer 2 presents the greatest possibility for an acute life-threatening complication— respiratory obstruction. Although other patients are acutely ill, their conditions are more stable and unlikely to be life-threatening.

34. 1. This child is experiencing a psychological crisis. The child is alert and mobile, behavior that indicates there are no severe physical injuries.
    2. **Presentation indicates possible abdominal injury and internal bleeding in early shock. With immediate attention, the injuries may be treatable; therefore, this child should be seen first.**
    3. Relief of pain is this child's immediate priority, which is not life-threatening.
    4. Although this child is the sickest, presentation indicates irreversible brain injury; therefore, this child would not be the first priority for treatment.

TEST-TAKING HINT: Physiological injuries always take priority over psychological issues, eliminating answer 1. If a patient cannot be saved, the patient does not need to be seen first, eliminating answer 4. Of the two remaining answers, the child in answer 2 is the most unstable and should be treated first.

35. 1. **The best method for preventing contamination of the central intravenous line site is to complete this procedure first. This lessens the likelihood of spreading microorganisms from the GI track to the central line. The possible complication of sepsis is most life-threatening.**
    2. Accurate measurement of output and maintaining patency of the ileostomy bag are lower priority than preventing sepsis of the central intravenous line.

3. Maintaining patency of the Jackson-Pratt drain and dressing is lower priority than maintaining asepsis of the central intravenous line.
4. Correct positioning of the nasogastric tube is lower priority than prevention of sepsis.

TEST-TAKING HINT: Determine which principle of care supersedes the others. In this case, maintaining sterility of the central intravenous line takes precedence over accuracy of output, patency of an abdominal dressing, or nasogastric tube position.

36. 1. **Physiological needs take priority over other needs; therefore, hypotension is the priority need.**
2. Fear of being alone falls within the "security" category, which is lower than physiological needs.
3. Frustration with immobility falls within the "self-esteem" category, which is lower than physiological needs.
4. Body image concerns fall within the category of "self-esteem," which is lower than physiological needs

TEST-TAKING HINT: Maslow's hierarchy begins with physiological needs and proceeds to safety and security, love and belonging, self-esteem, and self-actualization. Hypotension is the only clear physiological need listed.

37. 1. Sedation is to be expected and is not the greatest concern.
2. **Airway and breathing complications are the most serious side effects.**
3. As long as the nurse is careful to prevent aspiration, nausea and vomiting are less serious side effects.
4. Constipation is a more long-term and less serious side effect.

TEST-TAKING HINT: Prioritizing following the ABCs (airway-breathing-circulation) indicates that respiratory depression is the most dangerous side effect of treatment.

38. 1. This question can be answered by collecting data on medication errors on each unit and comparing the data.
2. This research question can be answered by comparing pain scores for infants with and without local anesthesia.
3. **This is a legal/ethical issue that is guided by state mandates and the nurse's values of altruism and justice.**
4. This question involves a nursing treatment (irrigation) and patient outcomes

(line obstruction and infection) that can be determined through action and data collection.

TEST-TAKING HINT: This question involves ethical principles such as altruism (doing good for another), human dignity (each individual has intrinsic worth), and justice (treat persons equally).

39. 1. **Autonomy is the right to make one's own decisions; in this case, the right of the parent to make decisions about the child's surgery. As legal guardian, the parent has the right to choose or not choose for the child to undergo an elective procedure.**
2. Equality is the value for uniformity or evenness between cases or patient. This is not directly related to the situation.
3. Fidelity means keeping promises or agreements. While important in any nurse-parent interaction, it is not the focus of this situation.
4. Justice is the moral principle of fairness. Although this is a universal principle of care, it is not the main issue in this situation.

TEST-TAKING HINT: By knowing the meaning of each principle or value, the test taker can select the correct one.

40. 1. This answer is based on the assumption that the couple's relationship involves abuse; however, this has yet to be established.
2. Only after the nurse clarifies that the mother is experiencing violence will this answer be appropriate.
3. **Clearly identifying the problem, as suggested in this answer, is the first step in the ethical decision-making process.**
4. This statement is an example of the consideration of causative factors; however, the problem has not been clearly identified yet.

TEST-TAKING HINT: Ethical decision making follows steps that closely resemble the nursing process: identify the problem, consider causative factors, explore answers for action, develop a plan, implement the action, and evaluate the results.

41. 1. **This situation involves differences of opinion among persons who have a legal responsibility to make decisions for the child. Consultation by the multidisciplinary members of the ethics committee may help caregivers reach an agreement.**

2. Routine care and consent are involved in this situation. No ethical dilemma is apparent.
3. Chemotherapy protocols require parental consent and, when appropriate, child assent before implementing. In this situation, all are in agreement about care; therefore, no ethical dilemma is involved.
4. Parents in this situation are given information and asked to make decisions about two possible courses of treatment. Although each course has advantages and disadvantages, both are acceptable for treating the diagnosis. Unless parents disagree on what course to pursue, there is no ethical dilemma.

TEST-TAKING HINT: Ethics committees provide a forum for discussing different views, especially when caregivers, patients, or providers differ in their preferences for treatment. A situation most likely to be reviewed by a committee is one involving differences of opinion about what should be done for a child.

42. 1. The user name can often be linked to the system user's real name and is not considered confidential.
    2. The user ID can often be linked to the system user's real name and is not considered confidential.
    3. **A password uniquely identifies a user and provides access to data appropriate to the user. System users must maintain confidentiality of their password.**
    4. The credentials of the system user are not considered confidential.

    TEST-TAKING HINT: System users must never share their passwords. When the nurse signs onto a system, data and information that are entered can be traced to that nurse's password. The nurse is accountable for all actions linked to that password.

43. 1. Although this action gives immediate attention to the patient, it violates confidentiality of patient information by leaving the computer screen open.
    2. **Changing the computer to suspend mode requires only a few seconds. This answer is the best choice, because confidentiality is maintained and the patient receives prompt attention.**
    3. The amount of information left to be recorded is unknown, and completing charting may delay the assistance needed by the parent.

4. How soon will another staff member be able to assist the patient? Because this information is unknown, meeting patient needs may be delayed.

TEST-TAKING HINT: Two issues are involved: meeting patient needs in a timely manner and maintaining confidentiality of patient information. This clinical situation does not appear to be a true emergency. Therefore, confidentiality takes priority and should be maintained by closing the computer screen before leaving the computer unattended.

44. 1. Although staff members may have access to their own records, HIPAA regulations disallow personal access that bypasses institutional policies and procedures.
    2. As in answer 1, this access is disallowed under HIPAA regulations.
    3. **The right to access information is based on the need to know this information to provide patient care. Staff must have access to records of assigned patients in order to provide care.**
    4. As in answers 1 and 2, this access is disallowed under HIPAA regulations.

    TEST-TAKING HINT: In order to maintain patients' rights and confidentiality of health-care information, HIPAA regulations spell out the standard for accessing patient information—a need to know for the performance of the job.

45. 1. Individually identifiable health information, such as patient name or ID number, may be shared via fax with other health-care personnel who have a need to know the information to provide care.
    2. As in answer 1, this information may be mailed to others who have a need to know to provide proper care.
    3. Following the "need to know" rule, individually identifiable information may be copied, as long as confidentiality is maintained.
    4. **Selling information, such as lists of names and addresses, is disallowed by law, because the purpose of sharing the information is not the provision of care.**

    TEST-TAKING HINT: The key to sharing or utilizing health information that can be traced to an individual patient is the "need to know" to provide individual health care. Confidentiality must be maintained, and providers may not benefit financially by selling such information.

46. 1. Abuse alone is not a basis for emancipation.
2. **Pregnant minors are considered emancipated minors in many U.S. states and are able to give informed consent.**
3. A diagnosis of cancer is not a basis for emancipation.
4. Attending college is not a basis for emancipation.

TEST-TAKING HINT: Emancipated minors are individuals younger than 18 years of age who are able to give valid informed consent. State statutes mandate who can be considered emancipated. Examples include pregnant females and adolescents treated for substance abuse or communicable disease.

47. 1. Use of a competent translator does not violate the method of obtaining informed consent.
2. **This situation violates the principle of informed consent. Despite signing the written consent form, the parents state a lack of understanding of the procedure.**
3. As long as full information is revealed to parents, the timing of information can vary. This situation does not violate the principle of informed consent.
4. It is acceptable for either parent to sign the consent, if both have custody of the child. This practice does not violate the principle of informed consent.

TEST-TAKING HINT: The primary care provider is responsible for informing the legal guardian of a pediatric patient about a procedure and its potential benefits and risks. Criteria that must be satisfied for informed consent are: the person giving consent must understand the procedure, expected outcomes, risks or side effects, and alternate treatments; and a person who is considered legally capable, such as a legal guardian or parent, must give consent.

48. 1. **Assent is the process by which children give their consent for medical treatment. Assent does not have the same legal implications as informed consent, which is given by parents or legal representatives.**
2. Children younger than 18 years cannot give legal informed consent unless they are emancipated minors. Parents serve as children's legal representatives and give informed consent.

3. Confidentiality is one component of the consent process, but it is not a term used to designate the consent process.
4. Emancipation is a different process than consent for treatment. Emancipated minors may include pregnant adolescents and minors seeking treatment for substance abuse or communicable diseases.

TEST-TAKING HINT: The test taker must understand the legal implications of informed consent. Informed consent is based on legal capacity, voluntary action, and comprehension. Unless a child is an emancipated minor, he or she does not have the legal capacity to give informed consent. However, a child younger than 18 years may be able to comprehend the implications of treatment and give voluntary assent.

49. 2, 3, 5.
1. Although this is helpful information for a patient, it is not required on the informed consent form.
2. **Alternative treatments are part of the informed consent process.**
3. **Benefits likely to result from the procedure are part of the process of informed consent.**
4. Only the names of the persons performing the procedure are required for informed consent.
5. **The statement that the patient may withdraw consent at any time is required for informed consent.**

TEST-TAKING HINT: Information required for informed consent includes: an explanation of the procedure, risks involved, benefits likely to result, options other than the procedure, name of the person(s) performing the procedure, and statement that the patient may withdraw consent at any time.

50. 1. Scope of practice refers to the legally permissible boundaries of practice and is applicable to all RNs. In this situation, it is the float nurse's lack of familiarity with care, rather than scope of practice, that influences the legal responsibility of the charge nurse.
2. **The charge nurse has a duty to orient the float nurse to the pediatric unit, educate the nurse on any unfamiliar procedures, and evaluate the float nurse's competency to provide care.**
3. The patient's right to competent care can be maintained as long as the assignment of the float nurse is implemented to meet care standards.

4. In this situation, the established nurse/patient ratio may be maintained and is not the primary issue raised by floating a nurse from another unit.

TEST-TAKING HINT: Floating nurses from one clinical unit to another to fill a staffing vacancy can be an effective strategy, if floating guidelines are met. The charge nurse is responsible for ensuring that the floating nurse has the required competencies for working on the unit and is supported in carrying out the assigned care. This legal responsibility includes the supervisory duty to orient, educate, and evaluate the floating staff.

51. 1. The nurse has a relationship with the patient because the nurse has been assigned to care for the child in the hospital. This element is present.
    2. **Breach of duty of care is missing in this case, because the nurse met the standard of care. The nurse educated the parent on the importance of side rail safety before the incident occurred.**
    3. The element of injury is present in this case, because the child suffered a skull fracture.
    4. The child sustained damage in this case, as evidenced by the skull fracture.

TEST-TAKING HINT: In order for malpractice to be proved, four elements must be present: the nurse has a relationship with the patient by being assigned to care for the patient; the nurse failed to observe a standard of care in the specific situation; the patient sustained harm, injury or damage; and the harm must have occurred as a direct result of the nurse's failure to act in accordance with the standard of care.

52. 1. Each state's nurse practice act defines the scope of nursing practice, such as what level of practitioner can initiate a blood transfusion.
    2. The national HIPAA is in place to ensure that providers protect the privacy and security of health information.
    3. Each state has a Good Samaritan act to protect health-care workers who give assistance in emergency situations.
    4. **The local agency's policy manual would describe acceptable procedures for performing specific skills, such as flushing a central venous line. These procedures serve as the legal standard of care.**

TEST-TAKING HINT: The nurse needs to know major laws that govern practice, at both state and national levels. Where these laws exist, they serve as the primary legal authority for care. Examples include nurse practice acts, Good Samaritan acts, HIPAA, Patient Self-Determination Act, and child and elder abuse reporting. The legal basis for most specific technical procedures can be found in agencies' policy and procedure manuals.

53. 1. **The parent's refusal to allow the nurse to continue constitutes a revocation of informed consent; therefore, the nurse is acting without permission. Additionally, the nurse should consult the agency policy and procedure manual regarding the number of attempts allowed in this procedure.**
    2. Normal toddler behavior is being exhibited here. This response might occur despite use of analgesics, parental presence, and other coping measures.
    3. Many young children have difficulty taking oral medication, and this situation falls within normal parameters.
    4. Initial refusal of a painful activity is typical behavior for a school-age child, but it can often be overcome by motivational and diversional measures.

TEST-TAKING HINT: Battery is intentional physical contact that is wrongful in some way, such as causing embarrassment or injury or done without permission. In pediatrics, the parent gives consent for the child and must give permission for a procedure of this type.

54. 1. **After an error occurs, the nurse should document what occurred and what was done to solve or treat the problem.**
    2. The fact that an incident report was completed should not be documented in the patient medical record.
    3. No information regarding the incident report should be documented in the patient medical record.
    4. The facts concerning the medication error should be recorded, because of the effect on the patient's health status.

TEST-TAKING HINT: An incident report helps an organization track patient care–related problems. The facts of what occurred, the effect on the patient, and the treatment given should be recorded.

55. 1. **Administration of a medication dose outside the therapeutic range is an execution error and should be reported as a critical incident. The nurse is held responsible for administering the wrong dose, just as the physician is responsible for ordering the wrong dose.**

2. This event is not considered to be a nursing error because it is not under the control of the nurse, if proper flushing protocol has been followed. Rather, it is a complication of intravenous therapy.

3. This event is a complication of intravenous therapy and is not a nursing error.

4. This event is an example of the challenges of giving oral medications to uncooperative children and is not considered a nursing error.

TEST-TAKING HINT: The goal of risk management is to promote quality patient care and minimize adverse outcomes. Medication errors are monitored through incident reporting. Events that represent a departure from safe practice, with or without resulting harm to the patient, should be reported.

56. 1. **This answer is an example of a violation of the policy for administering a high-risk drug such as insulin. Policy dictates that another RN (not a nursing assistant) double-check the dose before administering.**

2. This is an example of a potential error that was corrected appropriately before it was completed.

3. This is an example of appropriate verification of orders.

4. This is an example of appropriate double-checking of a high-risk drug.

TEST-TAKING HINT: The goal of risk management is to create an awareness of potential risk factors and set up various mechanisms to control and/or eliminate risk. The protocol for high-risk medications, including insulin, is to check the dose with another RN before administering.

57. 1. Fasting blood glucose level may be used as a diagnostic test.

2. Fingerstick blood glucose values reflect compliance over the previous 1–2 days, making this test less valid as a long-term indicator of compliance. This test allows for short-term adjustment of the therapeutic regimen.

3. Urine ketones are measured to detect diabetic ketoacidosis.

4. **HgA$_{1C}$ reflects the average blood glucose level over 3 months, making it the most valid indicator.**

TEST-TAKING HINT: Blood glucose levels are the best indicators of compliance with insulin, diet, and exercise regimens in diabetes. Long-term measurements, such as HgA$_{1C}$, are better indicators than short-term levels, such as fasting glucose or fingerstick glucose checks.

58. 1. The charge nurse needs to validate correct understanding of what was observed by speaking with the staff nurse before addressing the parent.

2. Until validation with the staff, the charge nurse does not know whether a problem has occurred.

3. Verbal assessment and validation of the situation should occur before a written reprimand.

4. **Validation of information that was actually communicated to the parent should be the next step. This should come from the staff nurse in a private discussion.**

TEST-TAKING HINT: Before disciplinary action is taken in regard to any personnel situation, the charge nurse should give the staff member the opportunity to discuss the situation from the personal viewpoint.

59. 1. Social interactions among staff are not necessarily within the jurisdiction of the nurse manager.

2. The cafeteria is not a responsibility of nursing administration, and staff would better facilitate change by giving input directly to this department.

3. **This is a patient care issue that will take some investigation and correction on a unit-to-unit level. Pediatric unit and emergency department managers should be involved. This situation is most appropriate to refer to nurse managers.**

4. Union policies are separate from hospital administration and nursing management.

TEST-TAKING HINT: Focus on the role of the nurse manager and the activities under that role. Only answer 3 focuses on events that are within the job description of the nurse manager.

60. 1. Employing a sitter is not a cost-effective solution because the child is not in danger when adults are out of the room.

2. Parents need break times to deal with the stress of having a hospitalized child. It is unreasonable to expect them to stay at the bedside 24 hours a day.

3. The role of the child life–worker is to help hospitalized children meet normal developmental needs. Referring to them is the most appropriate action.

4. The behavior shown is normal and does not indicate unusual social or emotional needs. Therefore, a social service consult is not indicated.

TEST-TAKING HINT: The child has difficulty only on the occasions that parents are absent, indicating a need for attention from staff or the diversion of play activities. A child life–worker is the best staff person to meet these needs.

61. **1. The role of case manager includes ordering medical equipment for discharge; therefore, this is an appropriate referral.**

2. Most nurse manager activities are broader in scope than discharge planning.

3. Materials management stocks hospital supplies but is usually not involved in discharge supplies.

4. Child life staff members focus on emotional needs during hospitalization and would not be involved in this aspect of discharge planning.

TEST-TAKING HINT: The test taker must know the role of each staff member listed. Obtaining equipment for discharge is an important role of the case manager.

Pharmacology

14

KEYWORDS

Acetaminophen (Tylenol)
Albuterol (Proventil)
Amoxicillin (Amoxil)
Amoxicillin/clavulanate potassium
 (Augmentin)
Amphotericin B
Anticholinergic
Baclofen
Benadryl (diphenhydramine)
Benzoyl peroxide
Carbamazepine (Tegretol)
Chlorhexidine (Hibiclens)
Ciprofloxacin (Cipro)
Collagenase (Santyl)
Cyclophosphamide (Cytoxan)
Dalteparin sodium (Fragmin)
Deferoxamine (Desferal)
Dexamethasone (Decadron)
Diclofenac (Voltaren)
Digoxin (Lanoxin)
Diltiazem (Cardizem)
Erythromycin
Filgrastim (Neupogen)
Gamma globulin
Gentamycin
Growth hormone
Ibuprofen

Ifosfamide
Indomethacin
Intradermal
Isotretinoin (Accutane)
Levothyroxine (Synthroid)
Lindane (Kwell, G-Well)
Mesna (Mesnex)
Metoclopramide (Reglan)
Morphine (morphine sulfate)
Nasal decongestant
NPH insulin
Oxybutynin (Ditropan)
Pancreatic enzymes
Penicillin
Phenytoin (Dilantin)
Prednisone
Prostaglandin E
Pyrantel pamoate (Antiminth)
Ribavirin (Virazole)
Rifampin (Rifadin)
Salicylic acid
Sulfamethoxazole (Septra)
Sympathomimetic
Terbinafine (Lamisal)
Vancomycin
Vastus lateralis

ABBREVIATIONS

grain (gr)
gram (g)

milligram (mg)
pound (lb)

CONVERSIONS

1 fl ounce = 30 mL (mL) (fluid volume)
1 g = 15 gr
1 g = 1000 mg
1 gr = 60 mg (or 65 mg for Tylenol or aspirin)
1 in = 2.54 cm

1 kg = 2.2 lb
1 L = 1000 mL
1 lb = 454 g
1 lb = 16 ounces
1 mg = 1000 mcg
1 ounce = 28 g (weight)

QUESTIONS

1. After sustaining a closed head injury, a child is admitted to the pediatric intensive care unit. The child is ordered to receive phenytoin (Dilantin) 100 mg intravenously for seizure prophylaxis. Which of the following interventions should be done when administrating this drug?
   1. Mix it in dextrose 5% in water and give over 1 hour.
   2. Administer as an intravenous bolus using a syringe pump no faster than 50 mg/min.
   3. An inline filter should not be used.
   4. Monitor temperature prior to and after administration.

2. The parent of a child who is being discharged from the clinic wants to know if there is a difference between Advil and ibuprofen, saying "I can buy ibuprofen over the counter at a cheaper price than the Advil that was ordered." What is the nurse's best response?
   1. "Advil and ibuprofen are two different drugs with similar effects."
   2. "There is no difference between the two medications, so you should use whichever one is cheaper."
   3. "Similarities exist between the drugs, but you need to consult the physician about the specific order."
   4. "Ibuprofen is usually cheaper, so you should use it."

3. A nurse is caring for an adolescent with diabetes. The nurse gives the adolescent NPH insulin at 0730. What time would the nurse most likely see signs and symptoms of hypoglycemia?
   1. 0930 to 1030.
   2. 1130 to 1430.
   3. 1130 to 1930.
   4. 1530 to 1930.

4. Morphine sulfate 2 mg IV q2h prn for pain is ordered for a 12-year-old who has had abdominal surgery. Which of the following is the most appropriate nursing action?
   1. Administer the morphine sulfate using a syringe pump over 1 hour.
   2. Encourage the child to do incentive spirometer every hour during the day and when awake at night.
   3. Ask the physician to change the medication to Demerol (meperidine).
   4. Administer the morphine sulfate with Benadryl (diphenhydramine) to prevent itching.

5. The parent of a child who is being treated for *Haemophilus influenzae* meningitis tells the nurse that the family is being treated prophylactically with rifampin (Rifadin). Which of the following should the nurse include in teaching about this medication?
   1. "The drug will change the color of the urine to orange-red, so you should protect your undergarments as it will cause staining."
   2. "Adverse effects of the drug may cause urinary retention."
   3. "The drug is given to treat meningitis."
   4. "You will need to continue taking the drug for 7 days."

6. A 2-year-old child has been prescribed amoxicillin (Amoxil) three times a day for treatment of pharyngitis. Which of the following statements by the parent indicates the parent knows how to give the medication?
   1. "If I miss giving my child a dose at lunch, I will double up on the dose at night."
   2. "I will give the medication at breakfast, lunch, and dinner."
   3. "I know that amoxicillin (Amoxil) is a chewable tablet, but sometimes my child likes to swallow it whole."
   4. "I will continue giving the amoxicillin (Amoxil) for 10 days even if my child's cough gets better."

7. A nurse is caring for a child who is receiving amphotericin B intravenously daily for a fungal infection. Prior to starting the therapy, the nurse should review which of the following?
   1. Aspartate aminotransferase and alanine aminotransferase levels.
   2. Serum amphotericin level.
   3. Serum protein and sodium levels.
   4. Blood, urea, and nitrogen and creatinine levels.

8. Which of the following are specific toxicities to gentamycin?
   1. Hepatatoxicity.
   2. Ototoxcity.
   3. Anaphylaxis.
   4. Neurological.

9. A nurse is administrating vancomycin intravenously to a child and sets the pump to infuse the medication over 90 minutes. Which of the following adverse reactions is the nurse trying to prevent?
   1. Vomiting.
   2. Headache.
   3. Flushing of the face, neck, and chest.
   4. Hypertension.

10. The parents of an 8-year-old come to the clinic and ask the nurse if their child should receive growth hormone to boost short stature. Which is the nurse's best response?
    1. "Growth hormone only works if the child has short bones."
    2. "Can your child remember to take the pills every day?"
    3. "Scientific evidence is required before growth hormone can be started in children."
    4. "How tall do you think your child should be?'

11. A child has been receiving prednisone for the past 3 weeks, and the parent wants to stop the medication. What is the nurse's best response?
    1. "There should be no problem in stopping the medication since the child's symptoms have gone away."
    2. "It is dangerous for steroids to be withdrawn immediately."
    3. "Your child may develop severe psychological symptoms when prednisone is stopped."
    4. Stopping the prednisone will require serum blood work."

12. A child who has been diagnosed with hypothyroidism is being started on levothyroxine (Synthroid). Which of the following should be included in the nurse's teaching plan about this medication?
   1. The child will have more energy the next day after starting the medication.
   2. Optimum effectiveness of the medication may not occur for several weeks.
   3. The medication should be taken once a day at any time.
   4. The medication should be taken with milk.

13. A child is going to start growth hormone therapy. Which of the following should the nurse include in the discharge teaching plan?
   1. The child is expected to grow 3 to 5 inches during the first year of treatment.
   2. The parents must measure the child's weight and height daily.
   3. The parents must remember that once the growth hormone therapy is started, they will need to continue the therapy until the child is 21 years old.
   4. There are no side effects from taking growth hormones.

14. The nurse is caring for a child with diabetes. There is an order for Humalog insulin for this child. The nurse knows that the onset of Humalog insulin is which of the following?
   1. 1 to 2 hours.
   2. 30 minutes to 1 hour.
   3. 10 to 15 minutes.
   4. 2 to 4 hours.

15. A child has been started on metoclopramide (Reglan) for gastric esophageal reflux disease. Which of the following should the nurse include in the teaching plan?
   1. This drug increases gastrointestinal motility.
   2. The drug decreases tone in the lower esophageal sphincter.
   3. The drug prevents diarrhea.
   4. The drug induces the release of acetylcholine.

16. High-dose prednisone is given to a 5-year-old with leukemia as part of the treatment protocol. The nurse will monitor the child for which of the following?
   1. Diabetes.
   2. Deep vein thrombosis.
   3. Nephrotoxicity.
   4. Hepatotoxicity.

17. A nurse is administering cyclophosphamide (Cytoxan) to a child with leukemia. Which of the following actions by the nurse would be appropriate?
   1. Monitoring serum potassium levels.
   2. Checking for hematuria.
   3. Obtaining daily weights.
   4. Getting neurological checks every 4 hours.

18. A nurse is giving ifosfamide as chemotherapy for a child who has leukemia. Mixed in with the ifosfamide is mesna (Mesnex). The nurse knows that mesna is given for which of the following reasons?
   1. Combination chemotherapy.
   2. An antiarrhythmic.
   3. Prevent hemorrhagic cystitis.
   4. Increase absorption of the chemotherapy.

19. Chelation therapy is used to prevent organ damage from the presence of too much iron in the body as a result of frequent transfusions. Which of the following should a nurse anticipate to be prescribed in chelation therapy?
   1. Dalteparin sodium (Fragmin).
   2. Deferoxamine (Desferal).
   3. Diclofenac (Voltaren).
   4. Diltiazem (Cardizem).

20. Filgrastim (Neupogen) is given to a child who has received chemotherapy. The nurse knows that this drug is given for which of the following reasons?
    1. Reduce fatigue level.
    2. Prevent infection.
    3. Reduce nausea and vomiting.
    4. Increase mobilization of stem cells.

21. A child comes to the clinic for diphtheria, pertussis, and tetanus and inactivated poliovirus vaccines. The child has a temperature of 101°F (38.3°C). The nurse should take which of the following actions?
    1. Withhold the vaccines, and reschedule when the child is afebrile.
    2. Administer Tylenol, and give the vaccine.
    3. Give the vaccine, and instruct the parent to give Tylenol every 4 hours for the next 2 days.
    4. Have the physician order an antibiotic and give the vaccine.

22. A child comes to clinic with a pediculosis infestation. The nurse instructs the parent to do which of the following to treat the problem?
    1. Apply lindane (Kwell) to the scalp, leave it in place for 4 minutes, and then add water.
    2. Apply chlorhexidine (Hibiclens) to the scalp with sterile gloves.
    3. Apply terbinafine (Lamisal) as a thin layer to the scalp twice a day.
    4. Apply collagenase (Santyl) to the scalp with cotton applicator.

23. Amoxicillin (Amoxil) 250 mg by mouth every 8 hours is prescribed for a child who weighs 42 lb. The nurse knows that the safe pediatric dosage is 25 to 90 mg/kg/day. The nurse determines that:
    1. The prescribed dose is too low.
    2. The prescribed dose is too high.
    3. The prescribed dose is within a safe range.
    4. There is not enough information to determine the safe dose.

24. A child with a heart defect is placed on a maintenance dose of digoxin (Lanoxin) elixir. The dose is 0.07 mg/kg/day, and the child's weight is 16 lb. The medication is to be given two times a day. The nurse prepares how much digoxin (Lanoxin) to be given to the child?
    1. 0.25 mg.
    2. 0.37 mg.
    3. 0.5 mg.
    4. 2.5 mg.

25. Ciprofloxacin (Cipro) 300 mg is ordered for a child with a urinary tract infection. The medication comes 250 mg/5 mL. The nurse has determined that the dosage prescribed is safe. How much of the medication will the nurse prepare to give to the child?
    1. 1.2 mL.
    2. 3 mL.
    3. 6 mL.
    4. 12 mL.

26. A nurse is caring for a child with congenital heart disease who is being treated with digoxin (Lanoxin). The nurse knows that which of the following needs to be included in the family's discharge teaching?
    1. Make sure the medication is taken with food.
    2. Repeat the dose of the medication if the child should vomit.
    3. Take the child's pulse prior to administrating the medication.
    4. Weigh the child daily.

27. The nurse informs a parent of a teenager that the most effective treatment of acne is with which of the following medications?
    1. Salicylic acid.
    2. Benzoyl peroxide.
    3. Chlorhexidine (Hibiclens).
    4. Collagenase (Santyl).

28. A nurse is caring for an adolescent female who is going to be treated with isotretinoin (Accutane) for acne. Which of the following does the nurse know is true about the medication?
    1. The adolescent needs to apply a thin layer to the skin affected with acne twice a day.
    2. The use of a tanning bed will be an added benefit to help dry up the acne.
    3. The adolescent needs to have a pregnancy test done prior to starting treatment.
    4. The adolescent needs to keep the lips moistened to prevent inflammation.

29. A nurse is caring for a child with spastic cerebral palsy. Which of the following medications should be used for the treatment of spasticity?
    1. Dexamethasone (Decadron).
    2. Baclofen.
    3. Diclofenac (Voltaren).
    4. Carbamazepine (Tegretol).

30. After administrating a narcotic, the nurse will monitor the child for pain relief. Which of the following assessments should be a priority in addition to pain relief?
    1. Respirations.
    2. Bowel sounds.
    3. Blood pressure.
    4. Oxygen saturation.

31. The nurse is to administer eardrops to a 5-year-old who has a draining ear. Which of the following is the correct method of instillation?
    1. Pull the pinna of the ear downward and back for instillation.
    2. Place cotton tightly in the ear after instillation.
    3. Have the child remain upright after instillation.
    4. Pull the pinna of the ear upward and back for instillation.

32. A physician has ordered amoxicillin (Amoxil) 500 mg intravenous piggyback every 8 hours for a child with tonsillitis. Which of the following actions by the nurse is appropriate?
    1. Call the physician, and question the order because the route is incorrect.
    2. Give the medication as ordered.
    3. Call the physician because the dosing frequency is incorrect.
    4. Call the physician, and question the dose of the drug.

33. A child who has been diagnosed with conjunctivitis is ordered to have eye ointment applied three times a day. Which of the following should the nurse do first?
    1. Remove any discharge from the affected eye.
    2. Ensure the ointment is at room temperature.
    3. Hold the tip of the eye ointment parallel to the eye.
    4. Wash hands.

34. Decongestant nasal drops are prescribed for a child with nasopharyngitis. The nurse should include which of the following instructions for the parents about the nasal drops?
    1. "Do not use the drops for any other family member."
    2. "Administer the drops as often as necessary until the nasal congestion subsides."
    3. "Insert the dropper tip as far back as possible to make sure you get the medication in the nasal passage."
    4. "You can save the drops for the next time your child has the same symptoms."

35. A child has been started on sulfamethoxazole (Septra) for treatment of a urinary tract infection. How should the medication be given?
    1. At breakfast and dinner.
    2. With a snack.
    3. With water.
    4. With a cola beverage.

36. A 22-lb child is to receive treatment for Kawasaki syndrome. The physician has ordered an intravenous infusion of gamma globulin 2 g/kg over 12 hours. Which of the following doses is correct?
    1. 11 g.
    2. 20 g.
    3. 22 g.
    4. 44 g.

37. A 7-year-old is diagnosed with head lice. The physician has ordered lindane (G-Well) shampoo to be used once to treat the lice. The nurse knows that the shampoo is used only once for which of the following reasons?
    1. Causes hypertension.
    2. Associated seizures.
    3. Associated with elevated liver functions.
    4. Can cause alopecia.

38. Each member of the family of a child diagnosed with pinworms is prescribed a single dose of pyrantel pamoate (Antiminth). Which of the following should the nurse teach the parents regarding administration of this drug?
    1. Fever and rash are common adverse effects.
    2. The medication kills the eggs in about 48 hours.
    3. The drug may stain the feces red.
    4. The dose may be repeated in 2 weeks.

39. A 6-month-old is prescribed 2.5% hydrocortisone for topical treatment of eczema. The nurse instructs the parent not to use the cream for more than a week. What is the primary reason for this instruction?
    1. Adverse effects, such as skin atrophy and fragility, can occur with long-term treatment.
    2. If, after a week there is no improvement, then a stronger dose is required.
    3. The drug loses its efficacy after prolonged use
    4. If no improvement is seen after a week, an antibiotic should be prescribed.

40. A 15-kg child is started on amoxicillin/clavulanate potassium (Augmentin) for treatment of cellulitis. The dose is 40 mg/kg/day, given three times a day. The nurse has a bottle of Augmentin that indicates there is 200 mg/5 mL. How many milliliters must the nurse draw up for each dose?
    1. 2.5 mL.
    2. 5 mL.
    3. 15 mL.
    4. 20 mL.

41. A child with hives is prescribed diphenhydramine (Benadryl) 5 mg/kg per day in divided doses over 6 hours. The child weighs 40 lb. How many milligrams should the nurse give with each dose?
    1. 4.5 mg.
    2. 11.45 mg.
    3. 22.75 mg.
    4. 50 mg.

42. A child is receiving furosemide (Lasix) 20 mg daily. The parent asks the nurse what is the best time of day for giving the medication. The nurse indicates which of the following times?
    1. 8:00 a.m.
    2. 12 noon.
    3. 6:00 p.m.
    4. Bedtime.

43. A school nurse administers albuterol (Proventil) to a 10-year-old who is having an acute asthma attack. Which of the following assessment findings should the nurse observe?
    1. Decrease in wheezing.
    2. Decrease in respiratory rate from 34 to 22.
    3. Decrease in dyspnea.
    4. Decrease in heart rate.

44. A child in the emergency room is being treated with albuterol (Proventil) aerosol mist treatments for an acute asthma attack. She requires treatment every 2 hours. Which of the following adverse effects of the medication should the nurse expect?
    1. Lethargy and bradycardia.
    2. Decreased blood pressure and dizziness.
    3. Nervousness and tachycardia.
    4. Increased blood pressure and fatigue.

45. A child with cystic fibrosis is placed on an oral antibiotic to be given four times a day for 14 days. Which of the following schedules is the most appropriate for the child?
    1. 8 a.m., 12 p.m., 4 p.m., 8 p.m.
    2. 7 a.m., 1 p.m., 7 p.m. 12 midnight.
    3. 9 a.m., 1 p.m., 5 p.m., 9 p.m.
    4. 10 a.m., 2 p.m., 6 p.m., 10 p.m.

46. An adolescent is about to have a tuberculin skin test. Which is the best area for this intradermal test?
    1. Upper thigh.
    2. Scapular area.
    3. Back.
    4. Ventral forearm.

47. A hospitalized child is to receive 75 mg of acetaminophen (Tylenol) for fever of 101°F (38.3°C). If the acetaminophen (Tylenol) is 80 mg per 0.8 mL, how much will the nurse administer?
    1. 0.75 mL.
    2. 1.5 mL.
    3. 2.5 mL.
    4. 3 mL.

48. Which of the following is a toxic reaction in a child taking digoxin (Lanoxin)?
    1. Weight gain.
    2. Tachycardia.
    3. Nausea and vomiting.
    4. Seizures.

49. A 10-month-old with heart failure weighs 10 kg. Digoxin (Lanoxin) is prescribed as 10 mcg/kg/day to be given every 12 hours. How much is given as each dose?
    1. 10 mcg.
    2. 50 mcg.
    3. 100mcg.
    4. 500 mcg.

50. A preterm neonate is admitted to the hospital. The physician orders indomethacin. The nurse informs the parents that the medication is given for which of the following reasons?
 1. To encourage ductal closure.
 2. To prevent hypertension.
 3. To promote release of surfactant.
 4. To protect the immature liver.

51. Administration of which of the following drugs is most important in treating an infant with transposition of the great vessels?
 1. Digoxin (Lanoxin).
 2. Antibiotics.
 3. Prostaglandin E.
 4. Diuretics.

52. Penicillin is given to a 2-year-old prior to dental work. The child weighs 22 lb. The order is for 25 mg/kg to be given 2 hours before the procedure. The penicillin comes in 250 mg/5 mL. How much of the medication will the nurse administer?
 1. 2.5 mL.
 2. 5 mL.
 3. 10 mL.
 4. 15 mL.

53. Which of the following is the most common adverse reaction from erythromycin?
 1. Weight gain.
 2. Constipation.
 3. Mouth sores.
 4. Nausea and vomiting.

54. A child who weighs 20 kg is to receive 8 g of gamma globulin for the treatment of idiopathic thrombocytopenia purpura. The order is to give the gamma globulin over 12 hours. The concentration is 8 g in 300 mL of normal saline. How many milliliters per hour will the child receive?
 1. 12 mL/hr.
 2. 25 mL/hr.
 3. 50 mL/hr.
 4. 40 mL/hr.

55. The treatment for a child with sinus bradycardia is atropine 0.02 mg/kg/dose. How much should the nurse give a child who weighs 20 kg?
 1. 0.02 mg.
 2. 0.04 mg.
 3. 0.2 mg.
 4. 0.4 mg.

56. A nurse is giving atropine for sinus bradycardia. The nurse knows that atropine is which of the following?
 1. Anticholinergic.
 2. Beta-adrenergic agonist.
 3. Bronchodilator.
 4. Sympathomimetic.

57. A nurse is caring for an 11-month-old who has received atropine to treat sinus bradycardia. The nurse knows that a common adverse reaction to atropine is which of the following?
 1. Diarrhea.
 2. Increased urine output.
 3. No tears when crying.
 4. Lethargy.

58. A nurse is caring for a child with cystic fibrosis. Which of the following should the nurse include in teaching the parents about administrating pancreatic enzymes?
    1. The enzymes may be chewed or swallowed.
    2. The capsules may be opened and sprinkled over acidic food.
    3. Give the same amount of the medicine with meals and snacks.
    4. Store the enzymes in the refrigerator.

59. A child who has been diagnosed with enuresis has been started on oxybutynin (Ditropan). The nurse knows that common side effects of oxybutynin (Ditropan) are which of the following?
    1. Increase in heart rate and blood pressure.
    2. Sodium retention and edema.
    3. Constipation and dry mouth.
    4. Insomnia and hyperactivity.

60. Ribavirin (Virazole) is prescribed for a hospitalized child with respiratory syncytial virus. The nurse prepares to administer the medication by which of the following routes?
    1. Oral.
    2. Subcutaneous.
    3. Intramuscular.
    4. Oxygen tent.

61. A 5-year-old is admitted to the pediatric unit. The child has an infusion of dextrose 5% via a line with a volume control chamber on a pump. The nurse knows that this system is used for administration of intravenous solutions for which of the following reasons?
    1. Prevents accidental fluid overload.
    2. Reduces the potential for bacterial infection.
    3. Makes administering of intravenous fluids easier.
    4. Is less costly.

1. 1. Mix intravenous doses in normal saline as mixtures precipitate with dextrose 5% in water.
   2. **Phenytoin (Dilantin) should be given slowly (1–2 mg/kg/min) via pump. Rapid infusion may cause hypotension, arrhythmias, and circulatory collapse.**
   3. An inline filter is recommended.
   4. Continuous monitoring of electrocardiogram, blood pressure, and respiratory status is essential because of potential side effects.

   TEST-TAKING HINT: The test taker must know both the side effects of the drug and how to administer it safely.

2. 1. This does not answer the parent's question.
   2. This is not a true statement as Advil is enteric-coated, and not all ibuprofens are enteric-coated.
   3. **This response answers the question and tells the parent the physician is the only one who can change a name brand to a generic drug.**
   4. The nurse should not make that judgment. The physician should be consulted.

   TEST-TAKING HINT: The nurse needs to answer the parent's question and be aware that a physician chooses name brand or generic.

3. 1. Peak time for regular insulin is 2 to 3 hours.
   2. Peak time for Semilente insulin is 4 to 7 hours.
   3. **Peak time for NPH insulin is 4 to 12 hours.**
   4. Peak time for Lente is 8 to 12 hours.

   TEST-TAKING HINT: NPH insulin works in an intermediate range; select an appropriate period.

4. 1. Giving morphine sulfate over 1 hour takes too long to relieve the pain. It can be given by slow intravenous push.
   2. **Because morphine sulfate can depress respirations and the child has just had abdominal surgery, deep breathing should be encouraged.**
   3. Demerol (meperidine) is not used in children because of the risk of induced seizures.
   4. One of the side effects of morphine sulfate is itching, and Benadryl (diphenhydramine) is a good medication to give as needed in case of itching. It should not be given together with the morphine sulfate.

   TEST-TAKING HINT: The test taker must be aware of the major side effects of

morphine and type of patient who is receiving the morphine.

5. 1. **Rifampin (Rifadin) causes an orange-red discoloration of body fluids, including urine. Knowledge of this can decrease anxiety when it occurs.**
   2. Urinary retention is not a side effect. Rifampin (Rifadin) is metabolized in the liver and should be used with caution in patients with elevated liver enzymes.
   3. The drug is ordered prophylactically to guard against developing meningitis.
   4. The drug is given for 2 days as prophylactic treatment.

   TEST-TAKING HINT: Associate the "R" in rifampin (Rifadin) with the red in orange-red body fluids.

6. 1. Missed doses should be given as soon as possible and not doubled with the next dose.
   2. Doses of antibiotics should be taken at regular intervals over 24 hours without interrupting sleep to maintain maximum blood levels.
   3. Attempting to have the child take it whole could cause the child to aspirate.
   4. **A full course of the antibiotic must be taken to decrease the risk of resistance to the antibiotic or recurrence of the infection.**

   TEST-TAKING HINT: The test taker must know specific information about antibiotic therapy.

7. 1. Liver damage is not associated with amphotericin therapy.
   2. Levels of the drug are not done.
   3. By giving the drug, there should not be a change in sodium or protein levels.
   4. **The drug tends to be nephrotoxic. Elevation of blood, urea, and nitrogen and creatinine levels indicates renal damage. If elevated, the physician must be notified to determine if the drug must be withheld for the day.**

   TEST-TAKING HINT: This drug is nephrotoxic. Some nurses refer to the drug as "amphoterrible."

8. 1. Hepatic and neurological toxicities are more common in fluoroquinolones.
   2. **Nephrotoxicity and ototoxicity are the most significant adverse effects.**
   3. Allergic reactions are more commonly associated with sulfonamides.

4. Hepatic and neurological toxicities are more common in fluoroquinolones.

TEST-TAKING HINT: Aminoglycosides cause kidney damage and loss of hearing. Levels are checked before and after dosing so that toxicity can be prevented.

9. 1. Vomiting is a side effect and is not related to the rate of infusion.
   2. Headache is not related to the rate of infusion.
   3. **"Red man syndrome" or "red neck syndrome" is flushing of the face, neck, and upper chest associated with too rapid an infusion of vancomycin. This can be prevented with infusing the vancomycin over 90 to 120 minutes and pretreating the patient with Benadryl (diphenhydramine) prior to the infusion.**
   4. Hypotension with shock can result from a histamine release from rapid infusion.

TEST-TAKING HINT: "Red man syndrome" is a side effect of too rapid an infusion of vancomycin.

10. 1. Only long bones are affected.
    2. Growth hormone is available as a parenteral medication and is given intramuscularly or subcutaneously.
    3. **Growth hormone is approved for use only in children to treat a documented lack of growth hormone.**
    4. The nurse must first answer the parents' question about growth hormone.

TEST-TAKING HINT: Recall the reason for giving growth hormone.

11. 1. Abrupt withdrawal can cause severe side effects.
    2. **Abrupt cessation of long-term steroid therapy can cause acute adrenal insufficiency that could lead to death. Long-term steroid use can cause shrinkage of the adrenal gland, which decreases the production of the hormone.**
    3. Central nervous system symptoms such as confusion and psychosis are adverse effects of steroids.
    4. Gradual tapering of the dosages will prevent severe side effects, and no blood work is required.

TEST-TAKING HINT: The test taker must know about abrupt withdrawal of steroids and the effects on the adrenal gland.

12. 1. The energy level takes much longer than 1 day to increase.
    2. After starting therapy, peak levels of the drug may not be expected for many weeks to months. Patients need to know this to prevent them from stopping the medication because they think it is not working.
    3. **The drug works best when taken on an empty stomach; the patient should select a time each day when the stomach is empty. In children, just prior to bed may be the best time, as most children do not eat prior to bedtime.**
    4. The drug works best when taken on an empty stomach. Taking it with milk should be contraindicated.

TEST-TAKING HINT: Answers 1 and 2 are opposites, and the answer will be one or the other answers.

13. 1. **The expected growth rate with growth hormone therapy is 3 to 5 inches in the first year.**
    2. Height and weight are measured monthly.
    3. Growth hormone is discontinued when optimum adult height is attained and fusion of the epiphyseal plates has occurred.
    4. Side effects include glucose intolerance, hypothyroidism, adrenocorticotropic hormone deficiency, hypercalciuria, renal calculi, gastrointestinal upsets, and intracranial tumor growth.

TEST-TAKING HINT: Answer 2 is not correct as "must" is too strong. Answer 4 states "no side effects," and this is unrealistic. To choose the correct answer, the test taker must rely on knowledge of growth hormones.

14. 1. Humalog insulin has an onset of 1 to 2 hours and is intermediate-acting.
    2. Regular insulin has an onset of 30 minutes to 1 hour.
    3. **Humalog insulin is rapid-acting and has an onset of 10 to 15 minutes.**
    4. No insulin has an onset of 2 to 4 hours. Ultralente insulin has an onset of 2 to 6 hours and is a long-acting insulin.

TEST-TAKING HINT: Review the onset, peak, and duration of all types of insulin.

15. 1. **Metoclopramide (Reglan) is a gastrointestinal stimulant that increases motility of the gastrointestinal tract, shortens gastric emptying time, and reduces the risk of the esophagus being exposed to gastric content.**

2. A decreased esophageal sphincter increases the risk of gastric contents being regurgitated upward in the esophagus.
3. There can be an increase in diarrhea because of the increase in gastrointestinal motility.
4. Methylscopalamine blocks effects of acetylcholine and relaxes sooth muscles.

TEST-TAKING HINT: Gastroesophageal reflux disease results in backward flow of gastric contents, so it is logical that a drug prescribed should promote forward movement of gastric content.

16. 1. **One of the side effects of high-dose steroids can be diabetes mellitus. The child needs to be evaluated so prompt treatment can be initiated. The diabetes is self-limiting and after the steroids are discontinued should no longer be present. Other side effects include mood changes, hirsutism, trunk obesity, thin extremities, gastric bleeding, poor wound healing, hypertension, immunosuppression, insomnia, and increased appetite.**
2. This is not a side effect of steroids. Deep vein thrombosis is related to clotting abnormalities.
3. This is not a side effect of steroids.
4. This is not a side effect of steroids.

TEST-TAKING HINT: Review side effects of high-dose steroid use.

17. 1. There should not be a change in potassium level, as the drug does not cause potassium loss.
2. **Hemorrhagic cystitis is a major side effect of cyclophosphamide (Cytoxan); by checking the urine for blood, appropriate interventions can be made.**
3. Weights are obtained daily with clients receiving chemotherapy because of nausea and vomiting.
4. There are no central nervous system side effects with cyclophosphamide (Cytoxan).

TEST-TAKING HINT: Review major side effects of cyclophosphamide.

18. 1. Mesna (Mesnex) is not a chemotherapeutic agent.
2. Mesna (Mesnex) does not prevent arrhythmias.
3. **Mesna (Mesnex) is a detoxifying agent used as a protectant against hemorrhagic cystitis induced by ifosfamide and cyclophosphamide (Cytoxin).**

4. There is no medication that increases absorption of chemotherapy.

TEST-TAKING HINT: Review the action of mesna (Mesnex).

19. 1. Dalteparin sodium (Fragmin) is an anticoagulant used as prophylaxis for postoperative deep vein thrombosis.
2. **Deferoxamine (Desferal) is an antidote for acute iron toxicity.**
3. Diclofenac (Voltaren) is an anti-inflammatory drug.
4. Diltiazem (Cardizem) is an antianginal agent for chronic stable angina.

TEST-TAKING HINT: Deferoxamine (Desferal) is used to prevent iron overload.

20. 1. Chemotherapy may cause anemia which can compound the feeling of fatigue rather than reduce fatigue.
2. The drug does not prevent infection, but it does increase the number of neutrophils.
3. The drug may cause nausea and vomiting rather than reduce it.
4. **The drug mobilizes stem cells to produce neutrophils.**

TEST-TAKING HINT: Recall the function of the neutrophils and how to stimulate them.

21. 1. **Because fever is a side effect of the vaccine, the immunization should be withheld as it would be difficult to determine if the fever was due to the vaccine or another febrile illness. Immunizations can be given when the child has a low-grade fever.**
2. Diagnose the problem before giving the vaccine. Just giving the Tylenol would not allow a diagnosis to be made, as it may mask symptoms.
3. Giving the Tylenol would decrease the temperature, but the nurse would not be able to determine if there was another illness present.
4. The nurse would not want to give an antibiotic until a bacterial infection was diagnosed.

TEST-TAKING HINT: Immunizations should not be given when a child has a higher fever than 100.5°F (38°C).

22. 1. **Lindane (Kwell) is the drug of choice because it is well absorbed by the central nervous system of the parasite (lice) and results in death.**
2. Chlorhexidine (Hibiclens) is a skin cleanser. Clean gloves, not sterile gloves, should be used in treating lice.

3. Terbinafine (Lamisal) is an oral or nasal antifungal agent for the treatment of tinea infections.
4. Collagenase (Santyl) is an enzyme used in skin débriding.

TEST-TAKING HINT: Associate the nature of the parasite with the drug and application method.

23. 1. The dose prescribed is within a safe dosing range.
    2. The dose prescribed is within a safe dosing range.
    3. **750 mg/day is between 477.25 mg/day and 954.5 mg/day. The nurse first must determine what the safe dosage range is.**
       Convert pounds to kilograms by dividing by 2.2 kg (2.2 kg = 1 lb)
       42 lb ÷ 2.2 = 19.09 lb
       Dosing parameters:
       25 mg/kg/day × 19.09 = 477.25 mg/day
       50 mg/kg/day × 19.09 = 954.5 mg/day
       Dosing frequency:
       250 mg × 3 doses (every 8 hours) = 750 mg/day
    4. There is enough information to determine the safe dose.

TEST-TAKING HINT: First change pounds to kilograms. Calculate safe-dose parameters by using the safe-dose range identified in the question.

24. 1. **0.25 mg.**
       Convert pounds to kilograms by dividing by 2.2 kg (2.2 kg = 1 lb)
       16 kg ÷ 2.2 = 7.27 kg
       Calculate the dosage by weight:
       0.07 mg/day × 7.27 = 0.5 mg/day
       Divide the dose by 2 because it is to be given 2 times a day:
       0.5 mg/day ÷ 2 doses = 0.25 mg for each dose
    2. Change the pounds to kilograms; the correct answer is 0.25 mg.
    3. Change the pounds to kilograms; the correct answer is 0.25 mg.
    4. Change the pounds to kilograms; the correct answer is 0.25 mg.

TEST-TAKING HINT: Change the pounds to kilograms. The total amount is to be given twice a day, so calculate each dose.

25. 1. The formula to determine the correct answer is:
       Desired over Available × Volume = amount to be given

2. The formula to determine the correct answer is:
   Desired over Available × Volume = amount to be given
3. **Desired over Available × Volume = amount to be given**
   $$\frac{300mg}{250mg} \times 5 \text{ mL} = 6 \text{ mL}$$
4. The formula to determine the correct answer is:
   Desired over Available × Volume = amount to be given

TEST-TAKING HINT: Use the formula to determine the correct answer.

26. 1. Digoxin (Lanoxin) should not be taken with food. Administer the medication 1 hour before or 2 hours after a meal.
    2. The dose should not be repeated if the child vomits.
    3. **The child's pulse should be monitored before each dose. The dose should be withheld according to the physician's parameters.**
    4. Checking weight is not related to the medication.

TEST-TAKING HINT: Know the principles of giving digoxin (Lanoxin). Knowing that the drug is given to decrease the heart rate and increase cardiac output should be a key to the answer involving checking pulse.

27. 1. Salicylic acid is used in the treatment of corns.
    2. **Benzoyl peroxide inhibits growth of *Propionibacterium acnes* (a gram-positive microorganism). It is effective against inflammatory and anti-inflammatory acne.**
    3. Chlorhexidine (Hibiclense) is a cleaning agent.
    4. Collagenase (Santyl) is a débriding agent.

TEST-TAKING HINT: The test taker needs to know the specific treatment for acne.

28. 1. The drug is not topical.
    2. The patient should avoid ultraviolet light to prevent the risk of developing cancer.
    3. **It is mandatory to have a pregnancy test done before starting treatment as spontaneous abortions and/or fetal abnormalities have been associated in pregnancy with the use of isotretinoin (Accutane).**
    4. Inflammation of the lips is a side effect of isotretinoin (Accutane), but moisture will not prevent the inflammation.

TEST-TAKING HINT: Consider birth defects associated with isotretinoin (Accutane).

29. 1. Dexamethasone (Decadron) is a corticosteroid used to decrease inflammation. Spinal cord–related spasms are not caused by inflammation.
    2. Baclofen is used to treat the spasticity in cerebral palsy. It is a centrally acting muscle relaxant.
    3. Diclofenac (Voltaren) is a nonsteroidal anti-inflammatory drug.
    4. Carbamazepine (Tegretol) is an antiepileptic used to treat seizures.

TEST-TAKING HINT: Spasticity affects the muscles.

30. **1. The primary purpose of administrating an opioid analgesic is to relieve pain. Side effects placing the child at greatest risk are respiratory depression and decreased level of consciousness.**
    2. Bowel sounds should be assessed because some opioids, such as morphine, can decrease gastric motility, but this is not as high a priority as decrease in respirations.
    3. Blood pressure could decrease and would be assessed, but it is not as high a priority. Decrease in blood pressure occurs after decrease in respiratory effort.
    4. Oxygen saturation will be decreased after decrease in respiratory effort.

TEST-TAKING HINT: The critical word in this question is "priority." Associate side effects from a drug that have highest priority and will require nursing actions.

31. 1. Pull the pinna down and back for a child younger than age 3 years.
    2. Placing the cotton in the ear tightly should be painful. The cotton could act as a wick and not allow the medication to absorb. It will not help in the administration of the eardrops.
    3. Having the child stay in an upright position after instillation does not affect administration of the eardrops.
    4. The correct way to administer eardrops in a child older than 3 years of age is to pull the pinna up and back, the same as for an adult.

TEST-TAKING HINT: In infants, the ear canal is curved upward; therefore, the pinna should be pulled down and back. With children older than 3 years of age, the canal curves downward and forward; therefore, the pinna should be pulled up and back.

32. **1. Amoxicillin is given only orally, so the order should be questioned.**
    2. The dose cannot be given because the route is incorrect.
    3. The dosing frequency is correct.
    4. There is not enough information to determine if the dose is correct.

TEST-TAKING HINT: Focus on the route, dose, and frequency when administrating a medication.

33. 1. This is correct, but it is not done first.
    2. This is correct, but it is not done first.
    3. This is correct, but it is not done first.
    4. The procedure for instilling eye ointment begins with washing hands followed by donning clean gloves.

TEST-TAKING HINT: The keyword in the question is "first." Washing hands has the highest priority.

34. **1. The medication should not be shared because of the risk of spreading the infection to another family member.**
    2. The medication should be given only as prescribed. More frequent use could cause adverse reactions.
    3. Inserting the dropper as far back as possible into the nasal canal could cause injury to the child.
    4. Medications should not be saved for future illness, as the drug may not be appropriate.

TEST-TAKING HINT: The test taker must have specific knowledge of instillation of nasal drops.

35. 1. Sulfamethoxazole (Septra) should be given on an empty stomach.
    2. Sulfamethoxazole (Septra) should be given on an empty stomach.
    3. Sulfamethoxazole (Septra) should be administered with a full glass of water on an empty stomach. If nausea and vomiting occur, giving the drug with food may decrease gastric distress.
    4. Carbonated beverages should be avoided because they may irritate the bladder.

TEST-TAKING HINT: The test taker must know how to administer sulfamethoxazole (Septra).

36. 1. First convert pounds to kilograms. The correct answer is 20 g.
    2. Convert pounds to kilograms: 2.2 kg = 1 lb
    Divide 22 pounds by 2.2 kg
    22 lb. ÷ 2.2 kg = 10 kg

Calculate the dose:
2 g/kg = 2 g × 10 kg = 20 g
3. First convert pounds to kilograms. The correct answer is 20 g.
4. First convert pounds to kilograms. The correct answer is 20 g.

TEST-TAKING HINT: Convert pounds to kilograms before starting any calculations.

37. 1. Hypertension is not associated with lindane (Kwell).
   2. Lindane (Kwell) with topical use is associated with seizures after absorption.
   3. Lindane (Kwell) is not associated with elevated liver functions.
   4. Lindane (Kwell) does not cause alopecia.

TEST-TAKING HINT: Lindane (Kwell) is used as a second-line treatment for lice. Be aware of the reasons it should not be used a second time.

38. 1. Common adverse effects are headaches and abdominal complaints.
   2. Pyrantel pamoate (Antiminth) is effective against adult worms, and additional treatment is needed to kill the emerging parasites.
   3. Pyrvinium pamoate (Antiminth) stains feces.
   4. As the first treatment kills the adult worms, a second treatment is done in 2 weeks to treat emerging parasites.

TEST-TAKING HINT: Review medications used to treat pinworms and how they are administrated.

39. **1. Hydrocortisone cream should be used for brief periods because it can thin the skin and cause skin breakdown.**
   2. Higher concentrations of hydrocortisone are contraindicated.
   3. The drug does not lose its efficacy.
   4. An antibiotic is inappropriate for the treatment of eczema.

TEST-TAKING HINT: Focus on the concentration of the hydrocortisone and the effects on the skin.

40. 1. Incorrect calculation.
   2. The dose is calculated by multiplying the weight by the milligrams. That result is divided by the three doses. The milligrams are then used to determine the milliliters based on the concentration of the drug.
   40 mg × 15 kg = 600 mg/3 doses =
   200 mg/dose
   The concentration of the drug is 200 mg/5 mL, so the answer is 5 mL

3. Incorrect calculation.
4. Incorrect calculation.

TEST-TAKING HINT: Identify the key components of the question.

41. 1. First convert pounds to kilograms; multiplying by 5 mg by weight gives the amount of milligrams per hour.
   2. First convert pounds to kilograms; multiplying by 5 mg by weight gives the amount of milligrams per hour.
   3. First convert 40 pounds to kilograms by dividing the pounds by 2.2 kg (2.2 kg = 1 lb)
   40 ÷ 2.2 = 18.18 kg
   Multiply 5 mg by the weight (18.18) gives the amount of milligrams for 24 hours
   18.18 kg × 5 mg = 90.9 mg/day
   Divide the total milligrams (90.9 mg) by 4, as that is the number of doses
   90.9 mg ÷ 4 = 22.75 mg
   4. First convert pounds to kilograms; multiply by 5 mg by weight gives the amount of milligrams per hour.

TEST-TAKING HINT: Convert pounds to kilograms, and then identify the key components needed to determine the answer.

42. **1. The onset of Lasix is 20 to 60 minutes. It peaks at 60 to 70 minutes, with a duration of 2 hours. By 24 hours, 50% is eliminated. Because the child may not respond as expected, the mother should be instructed to give the Lasix at 8:00 a.m. to avoid interruption of sleep with frequent urination.**
   2. Noon is more appropriate than 6:00 p.m. and bedtime.
   3. Because 50% remains in the body, a cumulative effect could disrupt the child's sleep-rest pattern.
   4. An onset of 20 to 60 minutes results in a direct interruption of the sleep-rest pattern.

TEST-TAKING HINT: Knowledge of pharmacokinetics is necessary to determine the best time to administer Lasix. Knowing the drug is a diuretic assists in determining a time that avoids disrupting the sleep-rest pattern.

43. **1. The symptoms of an acute asthma attack are related to constriction of the airway, which leads to dyspnea and an increased respiratory rate. The albuterol (Proventil) is a beta-adrenergic agent that relaxes the smooth muscles of the bronchial tree, which will decrease the wheezing.**

2. The respiratory rate should return to normal. A rate of 22 is considered high.
3. Albuterol (Proventil) will decrease dyspnea when the wheezing is relieved.
4. Tachycardia is a side effect of albuterol (Proventil).

TEST-TAKING HINT: The test taker must know the primary outcome of the drug action.

44. 1. The side effect of albuterol (Proventil) is tachycardia, not bradycardia.
2. Decreased blood pressure is not expected. Dizziness may occur from the tachycardia.
3. **Potential side effects of this medication are stimulation of the central nervous system and cardiovascular system. Tachycardia is the most frequent side effect of albuterol (Proventil).**
4. Increased blood pressure can occur, but the child will not experience lethargy until exhausted, which is a later effect.

TEST-TAKING HINT: Albuterol (Proventil) has a major side effect of tachycardia, which worsens with increased doses.

45. 1. The antibiotic should be given every 6 hours to maintain blood levels of the antibiotic. This schedule means that the antibiotic should be given every 4 hours, with 12 hours between the last night dose and the first morning dose.
2. **Antibiotics should be scheduled to maintain therapeutic blood levels and not interfere with the child's sleep. This schedule allows for dosing every 6 hours during the day and allows the child to get 7 hours of uninterrupted sleep.**
3. This is basically the same interval of dosing as answer 1.
4. This is the same interval of dosing as answers 1 and 2.

TEST-TAKING HINT: Determine the best timing to maintain the best therapeutic drug levels.

46. 1. The upper thigh is used for subcutaneous and intramuscular injections.
2. The scapular area and back are used for allergy skin testing.
3. The scapular area and back are used for allergy skin testing.
4. **The ventral forearm is the preferred site for the tuberculin skin test.**

TEST-TAKING HINT: The test taker must know sites of administration of medications in children.

47. 1. **Desired over Available × Volume = Desired dose**
$$\frac{75 \text{ mg} \times 0.8 \text{ mL}}{80 \text{ mg}} = 0.75 \text{ mL}$$
2. Desired over Available × Volume = Desired dose.
3. Desired over Available × Volume = Desired dose.
4. Desired over Available × Volume = Desired dose.

TEST-TAKING HINT: The test taker must know the correct formula and then use the information in the question to determine the answer.

48. 1. Weight gain is not a toxic reaction.
2. Bradycardia is a side effect. Tachycardia is not a reaction.
3. **Digoxin (Lanoxin) toxicity in infants and children may present with nausea, vomiting, anorexia, or a slow, irregular, apical heart rate.**
4. Seizures are not a toxic reaction that occur with digoxin (Lanoxin).

TEST-TAKING HINT: The test taker must know common toxic effects of digoxin (Lanoxin), which is used frequently in children with heart defects.

49. 1. Use the desired amount divided by what you have times the amount available.
2. **10 kg × 10 mcg/kg/day = 100 mcg ÷ 2 doses a day = 50 mcg/dose.**
3. Use the desired amount divided by what you have times the amount available.
4. Use the desired amount divided by what you have times the amount available.

TEST-TAKING HINT: The test taker must know the correct formula to use.

50. 1. **Preterm neonates with good renal function may receive indomethacin, a prostaglandin inhibitor, to encourage ductal closure.**
2. Hypertension is a side effect of indomethacin.
3. A prostaglandin inhibitor does not affect surfactant in the lungs.
4. The drug may cause nephrotoxicity.

TEST-TAKING HINT: Apply pathophysiology of the preterm neonate to the drug.

51. 1. Digoxin (Lanoxin) is given to treat congestive heart failure.
2. Antibiotics are used if there is an infection and prophylactically with invasive procedures.

3. Prostaglandin E is necessary to maintain patency of the patent ductus arteriosus and improve systemic arterial flow in children with inadequate intracardiac mixing.

4. Diuretics are given to treat congestive heart failure.

TEST-TAKING HINT: The test taker must know the pathophysiology of the defect, and determine the most important treatment to improve cardiac function.

52. 1. Determine the child's weight in kilograms; then multiply the child's weight by 25 mg.
2. Determine the child's weight in kilograms; then multiply the child's weight by 25 mg.
3. **Determine the child's weight in kilograms by dividing 44 lb by 2.2 (2.2 kg = 1 lb). Then determine how many milligrams need to be given by multiplying the child's weight in kilograms by 25 mg.**
   44 lb ÷ 2.2 kg = 22 kg
   22 kg × 25 mg = 500 mg
   Use the formula: Desired over Available × Volume = Desired dose
   $$\frac{500 \text{ mg}}{250 \text{ mg}} \times 5 \text{ mL} = 10 \text{ mL}$$
4. Determine the child's weight in kilograms; then multiply the child's weight by 25 mg.

TEST-TAKING HINT: The test taker must know the correct formula to use.

53. 1. Weight gain is not a side effect of erythromycin.
2. Diarrhea, not constipation, is an adverse reaction to erythromycin.
3. Mouth sores are not an adverse reaction.
4. **Common adverse reactions to erythromycin include nausea, vomiting, diarrhea, abdominal pain, and anorexia. Erythromycin should be given with a full glass of water and after meals. Because these gastrointestinal adverse reactions occur commonly, it may be necessary to give erythromycin with food.**

TEST-TAKING HINT: The test taker must know the major side effects of this drug are gastrointestinal.

54. 1. Take the total volume and divide it by the number of hours.
2. **Take the total volume (300 mL) and divide it by the number of hours (12 hours)**
   300 mL ÷ 12 hours = 25 mL/hr
3. Take the total volume and divide it by the number of hours.

4. Take the total volume and divide it by the number of hours.

TEST-TAKING HINT: The test taker must know the correct formula to use.

55. 1. Take the dose of atropine times the child's weight.
2. Take the dose of atropine times the child's weight.
3. Take the dose of atropine times the child's weight.
4. **Take the dose of atropine (0.02 mg/kg) times the child's weight (20 kg)**
   0.02 mg/kg × 20 kg = 0.4 mg

TEST-TAKING HINT: Atropine is a medication given during a code situation, so the test taker must know how to calculate the dosing.

56. 1. **Atropine is an anticholinergic drug. It blocks vagal impulses to the myocardium and stimulates the cardioinhibitory center in the medulla. It increases heart rate and cardiac output.**
2. This is not the classification of atropine.
3. This is not the classification of atropine.
4. This is not the classification of atropine.

TEST-TAKING HINT: The test taker must know the classification of major drugs.

57. 1. There should be constipation, rather than diarrhea, because of decrease in smooth muscle contraction of the gastrointestinal tract.
2. There should be urinary retention due to decrease in smooth muscle contractions of the gastrourinary tract.
3. **Atropine dries up secretions and also lessens the response of ciliary and iris sphincter muscles in the eye, causing mydriasis.**
4. Atropine usually causes paradoxical excitement in children, so lethargy should not occur.

TEST-TAKING HINT: The test taker must know the side effects based on the action of the drug.

58. 1. The enzymes must be swallowed whole. Retention in the mouth may cause mucosal irritation and stomatitis.
2. **When administrating enzymes to infants, the capsule may be opened and sprinkled over an acidic food, such as applesauce or mashed fruit.**
3. The child should take the same amount of enzymes with each meal and half the dose with each snack.

4. There is no need to refrigerate the medication.

TEST-TAKING HINT: By knowing that enzymes are capsules, the test taker should eliminate answer 1 as capsules are not chewed.

59. 1. There may be tachycardia but no hypertension.
2. There is no sodium retention, so there will be no edema.
3. **Common side effects are constipation and dry mouth as the oxybutynin (Ditropan) has an atropine-like effect.**
4. Adverse effects from overdose may have some central nervous system effects like nervousness that cause insomnia and hyperactivity.

TEST-TAKING HINT: Oxybutynin (Ditropan) has an atropine-like effect that causes vasoconstriction symptoms.

60. 1. Ribavirin (Virazole) is not given orally.
2. Ribavirin (Virazole) is not given subcutaneously.
3. Ribavirin (Virazole) is not given intramuscularly.
4. **Ribavirin (Virazole) is an antiviral respiratory medication used in the hospital for children with severe respiratory syncytial virus. Administration is via hood, face mask, or oxygen tent.**

TEST-TAKING HINT: The test taker must know that this medication is aerosolized.

61. 1. **The volume control chamber functions as a safety device. No more than 2 hours of solution is placed in the chamber at a time. If the pump should be programmed incorrectly, the child would get only 2 hours of fluids; then the pump would alarm. The nurse is thereby alerted that the pump was programmed incorrectly.**
2. This is not a measure to prevent infection.
3. The rationale for using a particular protocol for administration of intravenous fluids should not be based on conveniences of the nurse, but rather on safety.
4. This is more costly because it requires additional or different tubing.

TEST-TAKING HINT: The test taker must know safety issues for administration of intravenous fluids with children.

QUESTIONS

1. Which outcome is expected in a breast-fed newborn?
   1. Voids spontaneously within 12 hours of life.
   2. Loses 10% of body weight in the first 5 days.
   3. Regains birth weight by the 10th day of life.
   4. Awakens spontaneously for all feedings.

2. The average newborn weighs 3400 g. The nurse will tell the parents that the baby weighs_____ lb.

3. The posture of a healthy term newborn is described by which word?
   1. Hypotonic.
   2. Asymmetric.
   3. Opisthotonic.
   4. Flexion.

4. The nurse is working in the newborn nursery and accidentally bumps the crib of one of the babies. This baby demonstrates an asymmetric tonic neck reflex. The nurse sees this baby in which posture?
   1. Extends trunk upward and lifts head.
   2. Oscillating movements of the ankles and knees.
   3. A "fencing" posture.
   4. Extension and abduction of extremities and fanning of fingers.

5. The parent of a newborn wants to know what the newborn screening test does. What is the nurse's best response?
   1. "Not all states do newborn screening."
   2. "All states test for phenylketonuria and hypothyroidism."
   3. "Babies are screened at 48 hours of age."
   4. "The baby who is taken home within 24 hours is not screened."

6. A family is adopting a 3-year-old child from Russia. What suggestions can be given to the parents for incorporating the child? Select all that apply.
   1. Learn as much about the child as possible before adoption.
   2. Expect conflict and determine how to work through it with the child.
   3. Do not discuss the biological parents with the child.
   4. Discuss your expectations with the child.
   5. Try to maintain a part of the child's original family name.

7. When the parents of a 5-year-old tell the child they are divorcing, the parents need to be aware of behaviors that the child may demonstrate. Select all that apply.
   1. Increased self-esteem, bragging.
   2. Changes in sleep and appetite.
   3. Feelings of abandonment.
   4. Develops dictatorial attitude.
   5. Verbalizes feelings about divorce-related changes.

8. The mother of a 6-month-old is going back to work. The nurse should make which of the following suggestions for ways to evaluate day care. Select all that apply.
   1. Larger day-care centers with more services.
   2. High health and safety requirements.
   3. Caretakers who are loving and kind.
   4. Challenging activities for all the children.
   5. Child care ratios that maximize staff use.
   6. Small class size.

9. Match each genetic term with its definition and function.
   1. Congenital   A. Morphogenic defect of an organ
   2. FISH analysis   B. Recognized pattern of malformation
   3. Genome   C. Present at birth
   4. Malformation   D. Clinically exhibited characteristic
   5. Phenotype   E. Fluorescent in situ hybridization
   6. Syndrome   F. Complete genetic information of organism

10. Parents are concerned that their provider suspects Turner syndrome in their newborn. What physical characteristics can the nurse point out that lead to this suspicion?
    1. Cleft lip and palate.
    2. Weak, high-pitched cry.
    3. Webbed neck and lymphedema.
    4. Long arms and small genitalia.

11. A pregnant teen is to have prenatal genetic testing. She is afraid of needles and wants to know the least invasive way she can get the genetic testing done. The nurse should suggest which testing procedure?
    1. Triple marker screen.
    2. Ultrasound examination.
    3. Amniocentesis.
    4. Chorionic villus sampling.

12. Parents are told by the genetic counselor that they have a 1:4 probability of having a second child with cystic fibrosis (CF). They already have one child who is affected. The parents state their risk is lower now than when they had the previous child. What should the nurse tell the parents about the 1:4 probability?
    1. Each pregnancy is an independent event.
    2. The probability of having another child with CF is twice as likely as it was when they had the first child.
    3. The probability of having a healthy child is twice as likely with this pregnancy.
    4. The probability of miscarrying is greater now than with the previous pregnancy.

13. A nurse is working in the obstetrics/gynecology clinic, and a young woman tells the nurse she is pregnant. She states she is concerned that her boyfriend may be "slow" mentally. The nurse should do which activity first?
    1. Develop a pedigree.
    2. Take a family history.
    3. Inform the provider about the concern.
    4. Refer the client for genetic counseling.

14. The nurse is caring for a school-aged child with leukemia. The child's complete blood count is very low. The parents are Jehovah's Witness. The nurse should recognize that the family faces which dilemma?
    1. Numerous dietary kosher laws exist.
    2. A belief that only Allah cures illness.
    3. The parents may want the child to have anointing of the sick.
    4. Opposed to transfusions and vaccines.

15. The nurse is working in a large clinic for low-income children in Florida. In the clinic are many families of different cultures. The families are first-generation and have many beliefs about health that were learned in their native countries. Match the culture with the health-care belief.

1. Haitians	A. Religion and medicine strongly interwoven
2. Cubans	B. Nutrition is important in good health
3. Latinos, Chicanos	C. Illness has a supernatural origin (voodoo)
4. Puerto Ricans	D. Believe hot-cold theory of illness
5. Native Americans	E. Seek help from *curandero* (healer)

16. The nurse is working in a clinic, and the next patient is an infant with deaf parents. In addition to providing an interpreter for the deaf, the nurse should incorporate what additional aid in her communication with the family?
    1. Talk as done with hearing families.
    2. Maintain good eye contact to let them read the nurse's lips.
    3. Explain procedures thoroughly.
    4. Recommend a trained hearing dog.

17. A teenager is legally blind. The teen is wearing thick glasses and is carrying some school books. What question should the nurse ask the teen?
    1. "Just how blind are you?"
    2. "Can you see enough to read those books?"
    3. "Tell me what you can see in this room."
    4. "Is your vision worse than 20/200 in either of your eyes?"

18. The nurse is working in a school health clinic, and a child comes in complaining of "something" in my eye." What should the nurse do first?
    1. Have the child wash hands.
    2. Refer the child to an ophthalmologist.
    3. Wash out the affected eye with tap water.
    4. Examine the eye for a foreign body.

19. A child assigned to the nurse's floor has dysfluencies. The nurse should recognize what symptoms?
    1. Stuttering.
    2. Substitution of one sound for another.
    3. Speaking in a monotone.
    4. Hypernasal speech.

20. Parents confide to the nurse that their child, who is 35 months old, does not talk and spends hours sitting on the floor watching the ceiling fan go around. They are concerned their child may have autism. The nurse should ask the parents which question?
    1. "Does your child have brothers or sisters?"
    2. "Does your child seek you out for comfort and love?"
    3. "Do you have trouble getting babysitters for your child?"
    4. "Does your child receive speech therapy?"

21. The nurse in the emergency department is caring for an 8-month-old who suffered a concussion from an automobile accident. The infant was in the car seat at the time. The nurse should assess the infant for which symptoms?
    1. Sweating, irritability, and pallor.
    2. Plethora and hyperthermia.
    3. Crying with fear.
    4. Negative Babinski reflex.

22. A 3-month-old is brought to the public clinic, and the parent tells the nurse that the baby is fussy, spits up constantly, and has a lot of gas, and that there is a family history of allergies. The nurse knows that these symptoms are related to which diagnosis?
    1. Failure to thrive.
    2. Sensitive to cow's milk.
    3. Phenylketonuria.
    4. Pancreatic insufficiency.

23. The nurse on the previous shift charted that a newborn demonstrated cutis marmorata. The nurse now caring for the baby should check which vital sign?
    1. Blood pressure.
    2. Respirations.
    3. Skin color.
    4. Temperature.

24. The nurse is caring for a newborn with Erb palsy and a phrenic nerve paralysis. The most effective way to promote respiratory effort is for the nurse to position the newborn in what way?
    1. Supine.
    2. On the affected side.
    3. On the unaffected side.
    4. Prone.

25. A 2-day-old baby is being readied for discharge but looks jaundiced. This is the mother's first baby. The nurse reviews the baby's birth records and notes that the baby has A+ blood type, and the mother has O+ blood type The nurse should check which blood test?
    1. Hepatitis B titer.
    2. Total bilirubin.
    3. Complete blood count.
    4. Sedimentation rate.

26. An infant at 12 hours of age has a positive Coombs test result and a bilirubin level of 18 mg/dL. The provider has ordered an exchange transfusion for the infant. As the transfusion is proceeding, the nurse should watch for which sign?
    1. Increasing jaundice.
    2. Lethargy.
    3. Temperature instability.
    4. Irritability.

27. A baby is brought into the clinic for follow-up review of phenylketonuria. The baby is 9 months old and weighs 22 lb. If the recommendation is to limit the phenylalanine in the diet to 25 mg/kg, this infant should have no more than _____/day.

28. The nurse working in the newborn nursery has to draw a heel-stick blood sample before an infant's discharge. What can the nurse do to decrease the pain the infant feels from this procedure? Select all that apply.
    1. Wrap the heel in a warm, damp cloth.
    2. Use EMLA before doing the stick.
    3. Swaddling the infant.
    4. Have the infant do non-nutritive sucking.
    5. Do the stick while the infant is asleep.

29. The nurse's unit is using the POPS pain scale for measuring pain in infants. The nurse knows this tool is which of the following?
    1. Pain Assessment Tool for infants 27 weeks to term gestation.
    2. The neonatal Postoperative Pain Measurement Scale for infants 32 to 60 weeks gestation.
    3. Premature Infant Pain Profile for infants 28 to 40 weeks gestation.
    4. Postoperative Pain Score for infants 1 to 7 months.

30. A child on the nurse's floor is having a polysomnogram. The parent wants to know what types of data are obtained from the sleep study. The nurse knows that which data can be provided? Select all that apply.
    1. Heart rate and respirations.
    2. Brain waves.
    3. Eye and body movements.
    4. Cyanosis or plethora.
    5. End-tidal carbon dioxide.

31. Parents tells the nurse that their 18-month-old is always curious about the environment and is learning new words every day. The nurse knows the baby is entering a phase of rapid _____ development.

32. Parents are concerned that their toddler refuses to sleep in the new toddler bed and wonder what to do. The nurse explains that the child is using "global organization." What does the nurse mean by this term?
    1. "The preoperational phase of developing cognitive thought starts around 3 years old."
    2. "The child is self-centered and does not want to learn."
    3. "The child sees changing to a toddler bed as changing the whole process of sleeping and going to bed."
    4. "The toddler may have a phobia to the bed."

33. Parents express concern about their 5-year-old who has started having more temper tantrums. The parents want to know if this is normal for this age. What should the nurse ask the parents about the tantrums? Select all that apply.
    1. "Does the child do anything right in front of you?"
    2. "Are the tantrums related to one specific aspect of life?"
    3. "Are the tantrums causing any harm to self or others?"
    4. "Have you consulted the Internet for any suggestions?"
    5. "How do you handle your child during a tantrum?"

34. Parents are told they must start taking their toddler to the dentist. They are concerned their child is too young and that the dentist will be too harsh with the child. The nurse suggests the parents do which of the following before the dental visit?
    1. Tell the child it will not hurt.
    2. Warn that they will have the dentist give a needle in case of bad behavior.
    3. Tell the child they will go along to the dentist so that they can model comfortable, safe behavior.
    4. Offer the child a treat for good behavior.

35. A 17-month-old is brought into the clinic, and the nurse notes the toddler has tooth decay on the maxillary upper incisors. The toddler is holding a bottle of juice, and the parent says the child cannot seem to be weaned from the bottle. The nurse could suggest which of the following tactics to assist the parent in weaning the toddler? Select all that apply.
    1. Hide the bottle, and tell the toddler that it is not needed anymore.
    2. Put only tap water in the bottle.
    3. Give the bottle only at night.
    4. Give the toddler a pacifier and take the bottle away.
    5. Do not give any bottles before bed.

36. Parents are frustrated with toilet training their 2-year-old. Both parents work full-time and claim they do not have time to spend on toilet training. What suggestions can the nurse give the parents to decrease their frustration?
    1. "You will have to invest some time if the child is to be toilet trained."
    2. "A child needs to be both physically and psychologically ready to learn the skills needed to be continent."
    3. "Do you think your child is stubborn?"
    4. "Have the child sit on the toilet until the child voids."

37. Parents are interested in switching their child from a booster seat to a regular seat belt. The child is 7 years old and weighs 51 lb. What can the nurse tell the parents about switching the child to a seat belt? Select all that apply.
    1. The safest place to ride in the car is in the front seat.
    2. The child needs to weigh 60 lb and be 8 years old to qualify legally for a seat belt.
    3. The seat belt should be worn low on the hips.
    4. Use a shoulder belt only if it does not cross the child's neck.
    5. Tether straps are optional.

38. The nurse goes to the kindergarten classroom to evaluate a rash. A 5-year-old has patches of vesicles on the chest and face rather than on the arms and legs. The child says it is very itchy. The teacher tells the nurse the child had a runny nose a couple of days ago. The nurse suspects that the rash is caused by which virus?
    1. Fifth disease (erythema infectiosum)
    2. Roseola (exanthema subitum)
    3. Scarlet fever (group A-B hemolytic streptococcus)
    4. Chickenpox (varicella zoster)

39. The clinic is doing a lead screening program for children in a low-income Hispanic community. The nurse working in the program wants to tell the parents the reasons to have their children screened for lead poisoning. Select all the following reasons that apply.
    1. Young children absorb 10% of the lead to which they are exposed.
    2. Homes built between 1900 and 1950 may contain lead-based paint.
    3. The blood level of lead should be below 12.8 mcg/dL.
    4. Lead can affect any part of the body, but the brain and kidneys are at greatest risk.
    5. Foods such as fruit, candy, and antacids contain lead.

40. A 9-year-old boy is brought to the clinic for a physical. The child's weight is 95 lb (95th percentile), and the height is 4 feet, 4 inches (50th percentile). Systolic blood pressure is 118 mm Hg, and diastolic blood pressure is 75 mm Hg. Reading the blood pressure graph in the following figure, the boy is in the _____ percentile for systolic and in the _____ percentile for diastolic readings for his age.

Blood Pressure Levels for Boys by Age and Height Percentile

Age (year)	HP Percentile	Systolic BP (mmHg) ← Percentile of Height →							Diastolic BP (mmHg) ← Percentile of Height →						
		5th	10th	25th	50th	75th	80th	95th	5th	10th	25th	50th	75th	80th	95th
1	50th	60	61	63	65	87	88	89	34	35	36	37	35	39	39
	90th	94	95	97	99	100	102	103	40	50	51	52	53	53	54
	95th	98	99	101	103	104	106	106	54	54	55	54	57	58	58
	99th	105	106	108	110	112	113	114	61	62	63	64	65	66	66
2	50th	84	85	87	88	88	92	92	39	40	41	42	43	44	44
	90th	97	89	100	102	102	106	106	54	55	56	57	58	58	59
	95th	101	102	104	105	105	109	110	59	59	60	61	62	63	63
	99th	109	110	111	113	113	117	117	66	67	63	69	70	71	71
3	50th	86	87	89	91	91	94	95	44	44	45	48	47	46	48
	90th	100	101	103	105	105	108	109	59	59	60	61	62	63	63
	95th	104	105	107	109	109	112	113	63	63	64	65	66	67	67
	99th	111	112	114	116	116	110	120	71	71	72	73	74	76	76
4	50th	88	89	91	93	93	96	97	47	48	49	50	51	51	52
	90th	107	103	105	107	107	110	111	62	63	64	65	66	66	67
	95th	106	107	109	111	111	114	115	66	67	68	69	70	71	71
	99th	113	114	116	118	118	121	122	74	76	76	77	78	78	79
5	50th	90	91	93	95	85	98	98	50	51	5 2	53	54	55	55
	90th	104	105	106	108	108	111	112	65	66	67	68	69	60	70
	95th	106	109	110	112	112	115	116	69	70	71	72	73	74	74
	99th	115	116	118	120	120	123	123	77	78	79	80	81	81	82
6	50th	91	92	94	95	98	99	100	53	53	54	55	56	57	57
	90th	105	106	109	110	110	113	113	66	68	69	70	71	72	72
	95th	109	110	112	114	114	117	117	72	72	73	74	75	76	76
	99th	116	117	119	121	121	125	125	80	80	81	82	83	84	84
7	50th	93	94	95	97	97	100	101	55	55	66	57	58	69	59
	90th	106	107	109	111	111	114	115	70	70	71	72	73	74	74
	95th	110	111	113	115	115	118	119	74	74	75	76	77	78	78
	99th	117	118	120	122	122	125	126	82	82	83	84	85	86	86
8	50th	94	95	97	99	99	102	102	56	57	63	60	60	60	61
	90th	107	109	110	112	112	115	116	71	72	72	73	74	76	76
	95th	111	117	114	116	116	119	120	76	76	77	78	79	79	80
	99th	119	120	122	123	123	127	127	83	84	83	86	87	87	88
9	50th	95	96	88	100	100	103	104	57	58	60	60	61	61	62
	90th	109	110	112	114	114	117	118	72	73	74	75	76	76	77
	95th	113	114	116	116	116	121	121	76	77	78	79	80	81	81
	99th	120	121	123	125	125	128	129	81	85	88	87	88	88	89
10	50th	97	98	100	102	102	105	106	50	59	60	61	61	62	63
	90th	111	112	114	115	115	119	119	73	73	74	75	76	77	78
	95th	115	116	117	119	119	122	123	77	78	79	80	81	81	82
	99th	122	123	125	127	127	130	130	85	86	86	88	88	89	90

41. The nurse is working in a school health clinic, and a teen mentions that her older sister just had a baby born with an open spine (myelomeningocele). The teen is wondering if there is anything she can do to prevent this from happening to her baby when she decides to have children. The best response the nurse can offer this teen is to do what about her daily diet?
1. Take a multivitamin with folic acid daily.
2. Eat more fruits and vegetables daily.
3. Have breakfast every morning.
4. There is nothing that can be done to decrease the risk.

42. A 16-year-old comes into the clinic for a physical examination. The teen weighs 180 lb and is 5 feet, 5 inches tall. According to the following figure, the basal metabolic index is _____.

Body Mass Index Table

	Normal						Overweight					Obese										Extreme Obese														
BMI	19	20	21	22	23	24	25	26	27	28	29	30	31	32	33	34	35	36	37	38	39	40	41	42	43	44	45	46	47	48	49	50	51	52	53	54
Height (inches)														Body Weight (pounds)																						
58	91	96	100	106	110	115	112	124	129	134	138	143	145	153	155	162	167	172	177	181	186	191	196	201	205	210	215	220	224	229	234	239	244	248	253	258
59	94	99	104	109	114	119	124	128	133	138	143	148	153	158	163	168	173	178	183	188	193	196	203	208	212	217	222	227	232	237	242	247	252	257	262	267
60	97	102	107	112	118	123	128	133	138	143	148	153	155	163	168	174	179	184	189	194	199	204	209	215	220	225	230	235	240	245	250	255	261	266	271	276
61	100	106	111	116	122	127	132	137	143	148	153	158	164	169	174	180	185	190	195	201	206	211	217	222	227	232	238	243	248	254	259	264	269	275	280	286
62	104	109	115	120	129	131	136	142	147	153	158	164	169	175	180	186	191	196	202	207	213	218	224	229	235	240	246	251	256	262	267	273	278	284	289	295
63	107	113	118	124	130	135	141	148	152	158	163	169	175	180	186	191	197	203	205	214	220	225	231	237	242	248	254	259	266	270	278	282	287	293	299	304
64	110	116	122	128	134	140	145	151	157	163	169	174	180	186	192	197	204	209	215	221	227	232	238	244	250	256	262	267	273	279	285	291	296	302	308	314
65	114	120	126	132	136	144	150	156	162	168	174	180	186	192	198	204	210	216	222	228	234	240	246	252	258	264	270	276	282	288	294	300	306	312	318	324
66	118	124	130	136	142	148	155	161	167	173	179	186	192	198	204	210	216	223	229	235	241	247	253	260	266	272	278	284	291	297	303	309	315	322	328	334
67	121	127	134	140	146	153	159	166	172	178	185	191	198	204	211	217	223	230	236	242	249	255	261	268	274	280	287	293	299	306	312	319	325	331	338	344
68	125	131	138	144	151	158	164	171	177	184	190	197	203	210	216	223	230	236	243	249	256	252	269	276	282	289	295	302	308	315	322	328	335	341	348	354
69	128	135	142	147	155	162	169	176	182	189	196	203	209	216	223	230	236	243	250	257	263	270	277	284	291	297	304	311	318	324	331	338	345	351	358	365
70	132	139	146	153	160	167	174	181	188	195	202	209	216	222	229	236	243	250	257	264	271	278	285	292	299	306	313	320	327	334	341	348	355	362	369	376
71	138	143	150	157	165	172	179	186	193	200	208	215	222	229	236	243	250	257	266	272	279	286	293	301	308	315	322	329	338	343	351	358	366	372	379	386
72	140	147	154	162	169	177	184	191	199	206	213	221	228	235	242	250	258	265	272	279	287	294	302	309	316	324	331	338	346	353	361	368	375	383	390	397
73	144	151	159	166	174	182	189	197	204	212	219	227	235	242	250	257	265	272	280	288	295	302	310	318	325	333	340	348	355	363	371	378	386	393	401	408
74	148	155	163	171	179	186	194	202	210	218	225	233	241	249	256	264	272	280	287	295	303	311	319	326	331	342	350	358	365	373	381	389	396	404	412	420
75	152	160	168	176	184	192	200	208	216	224	232	240	248	256	264	272	279	287	295	303	311	319	327	335	343	351	359	367	375	383	391	399	407	415	423	431
76	155	164	172	180	189	197	205	213	221	230	238	246	254	263	271	279	287	295	304	312	320	328	336	344	353	361	369	377	386	394	402	410	418	426	435	443

43. A 12-year-old girl with a thoracic myelomeningocele has had numerous urinary tract infections and has difficulty doing her clean intermittent self-catheterization. She and her parents are seeking an alternative way to empty her bladder. The surgeon has offered to do a Mitrofanoff procedure. The nurse knows that the surgeon will use the _____ to create a continent conduit between the bladder and the abdominal wall.

44. The parent of a school-aged child who is a paraplegic and uses a wheelchair states that the child is allergic to latex. The nurse knows that the most important intervention for this child is which of the following?
1. Giving antihistamines and steroids after procedures.
2. Prevention of contact with latex products.
3. Doing a radioallergosorbent test before each procedure.
4. Using only latex-free gloves when doing procedures.

45. A 5-month-old with a lumbar myelomeningocele is admitted to the unit with an Arnold-Chiari malformation. The nurse knows this infant has which diagnosis?
1. Hydrocephalus.
2. Anencephaly.
3. Tethering of the spinal cord.
4. Perinatal hemorrhage.

46. A 4-week-old infant has a hip dysplasia and is wearing a Pavlik harness. The nurse notices what when the infant's diapers are changed?
1. Diaper dermatitis.
2. Talipes equinovarus.
3. Leg shortening and limited abduction.
4. Pain.

47. Which of the following is the primary goal for a newborn with a cleft of the soft palate?
    1. Prevent ear infections.
    2. Help the mother bond with the baby.
    3. Repair the cleft palate.
    4. Establish feeding and sucking.

48. When an infant is born with a herniation of the abdominal wall with intestine present and the peritoneal sac absent, it is called a _____.

49. What are the two organizations in the United States that make and govern the recommendations for immunization policies and procedures?
    1. National Advisory Committee on Immunization and American Medical Association.
    2. U.S. Public Health Service Centers for Disease Control and American Academy of Pediatrics.
    3. National Immunization Program and Pediatric Infectious Disease Association.
    4. National Institutes of Health and Minister of National Health and Welfare.

50. A nurse is working in a well-child clinic administering immunizations to preschoolers. The nurse should do which procedure to minimize local reactions to the biological drugs?
    1. Apply EMLA cream 1 hour before.
    2. Change the needle on the syringe after drawing up the biological drug.
    3. Inject into the vastus lateralis or ventrogluteal muscle.
    4. Use distraction such as telling the child to hold the breath.

51. The nurse is assisting with a sports physical session at a local grade school. A fixed splitting of the S_2 sound is heard in an otherwise healthy child. The nurse knows that this is a diagnostic sign of which cardiac defect?
    1. Mitral regurgitation.
    2. Atrial septal defect.
    3. Functional murmur.
    4. Pericardial friction rub.

52. During a 15-month well-child examination, the physician hears an innocent murmur. The nurse knows which of the following about such a murmur? Select all that apply.
    1. It is short in duration.
    2. It is an S_2 murmur.
    3. It is loudest in the pulmonic area.
    4. It is fixed and can be heard in many positions.
    5. It is grade III or less.

53. A child is giggling and laughing, and the nurse gently places one hand on the child's front and back of their chest. The sounds can be felt through the skin. This finding is called vocal _____.

54. A child returns from surgery, having had tonsils and adenoids removed. When the parents are getting ready for discharge, the nurse instructs them to do what to care for their child. Select all that apply.
    1. Some secretions may be blood-tinged for a few days.
    2. Run a cool mist vaporizer in the bedroom.
    3. Pain relief should be provided every 4 hours.
    4. The child can resume a normal diet.
    5. The child should blow the nose and cough every 4 hours.

55. A 2-year-old is brought to the emergency department for fever and ear pain. The parents note the child has had many ear infections and that polyethylene tubes have been recommended, but the parents cannot afford surgery. The child is diagnosed with bilateral otitis media. The toddler is carrying a baby bottle full of juice, and a parent is carrying a pack of cigarettes. What one preventive measure could be taught the parents to decrease the incidence of ear infections?
    1. Wean the toddler from the bottle.
    2. Give the toddler a decongestant before bedtime.
    3. Encourage the parent to smoke outside the house.
    4. Have the child's hearing checked.

56. An 18-month-old, who attends day care, has been having a barking, hoarse-sounding cough that comes in spasms with very noisy respirations for the last 2 nights. The parent is concerned that the child has picked up an infection at day care. The day-care staff indicates the child does not cough during the day, has no fever, and is eating and drinking well. The nurse knows that this description is most likely which condition?
    1. Laryngotracheobronchitis.
    2. Bacterial tracheitis.
    3. Asthma.
    4. Acute spasmodic laryngitis.

57. An 11-month-old was born at 28 weeks' gestation and required 2 weeks of ventilation. The baby is currently well and is being seen in the clinic. The physician recommends that the baby receive preventive therapy for respiratory syncytial virus for the next 5 months. The nurse knows that the physician will order which medication?
    1. RespiGam.
    2. Ribavirin.
    3. Palivizumab (Synagis).
    4. Pneumococcal vaccine.

58. Three preschool children and their Middle East–born parents come to a homeless shelter. The family has been homeless for 3 months. The children appear somewhat unkempt but nourished. One of the children has several enlarged cervical lymph nodes and is running a low-grade fever. Which chronic infectious illness should be suspected in the child?
    1. Chlamydial pneumonia.
    2. Tuberculosis.
    3. Pertussis (whooping cough).
    4. Asthma.

59. A teacher has a pupil with head lice (pediculosis capitis). The nurse should see what to diagnose the infestation? Select all that apply.
    1. Crawling insects.
    2. White flakes in the hair.
    3. Nits attached close to scalp.
    4. Inflammatory papules.
    5. Dark brown hair.

60. A 7-year-old child in a classroom is disruptive with loud talking, short attention span, difficulty organizing work, unable to finish assigned class work, and moodiness. Which of the following is the most likely diagnosis for this child?
    1. Enuresis.
    2. Sexual abuse.
    3. Learning disability.
    4. Attention deficit/hyperactivity disorder.

61. A child is diagnosed with schizophrenia. The child is taking haloperidol (Haldol), and the family has been instructed to watch for extrapyramidal side effects. The nurse knows that extrapyramidal side effects include which symptoms in a child?
    1. Abnormal movements and twitches.
    2. Inappropriate behaviors.
    3. Excessive aggressiveness.
    4. Thoughts of suicide.

62. A sports physical is being performed on a 12-year-old male. He is evaluated as a Tanner stage II. The nurse sees which of the following physical characteristics?
    1. Enlarging penis.
    2. Height spurt.
    3. Gynecomastia.
    4. Deepening voice.

63. A 15-year-old girl who is an avid basketball player comes to the clinic for menstrual irregularities. She skips meals and has lost some weight. She mentions that she has menstrual periods every 2 weeks. The nurse knows that women who have menstrual periods less often than every 21 days are _____.

64. The high-school nurse is setting up a smoking prevention campaign for the students. Which of the following is the nurse's best approach?
    1. Discuss health consequences of smoking.
    2. Use scare tactics and point out the negative effects of smoking.
    3. Offer alternatives to smoking such as chewing gum and doing activities that distract.
    4. Have the adolescents talk with their parents about smoking.

65. A child with moderate asthma is wheezing and coughing. Before the physician sees the child, the nurse should perform which test?
    1. Skin testing for allergens.
    2. P_{CO_2} levels.
    3. Metered dose inhaler.
    4. Peak flowmeter.

66. The physician orders montelukast (Singulair) for a 10-year-old who has moderate, persistent asthma. The nurse should instruct the child and parents about which characteristic of the medication? Select all that apply.
    1. This is an add-on medication to the child's regular medications.
    2. The child is too young to be taking this medication.
    3. It is not to be used to treat acute episodes.
    4. The parents will need to give up smoking.
    5. The child will require chest physiotherapy in conjunction with the medication.

67. The nurse is caring for a child dying from leukemia. The parents want to know how comfortable the nurse is in giving doses of pain medication that are larger than customary to their child. The nurse knows that the parents are asking about which ethical principle of care?
    1. Double effect.
    2. Cultural influences.
    3. Honesty.
    4. Withholding pain medication.

68. The parents of a 19-year-old ask the nurse what they should do in terms of long-term care placement for their severely disabled child. Which of the following is the nurse's best response?
    1. "How much care do you want?"
    2. "Do you have other children who could take your child into their home?"
    3. "Do you have a detailed plan of care?"
    4. "Are you working with an agency or social worker about this matter?"

69. Parents of a 2-year-old with Down syndrome are told the child should be screened for atlantoaxial instability. The nurse tells the parents that which of the following are symptoms of this instability?
    1. Mental retardation.
    2. Neck pain and torticollis.
    3. Vision and hearing loss.
    4. Delayed secondary sexual development.

70. Early signs and symptoms of hydrocephalus in infants include which of the following?
    1. Confusion, headache, diplopia.
    2. Rapid head growth, poor feeding, confusion.
    3. Papilledema, irritability, headache.
    4. Full fontanels, poor feeding, rapid head growth.

71. A newborn with suspected hydrocephalus is transferred to the intensive care unit for further evaluation and treatment. The baby's nurse knows which of the following?
    1. To use sedation as needed to keep the baby from crying or being fussy.
    2. To keep the crib in a flat and neutral position.
    3. To expect the infant to sleep more than a baby without hydrocephalus.
    4. To not use any scalp veins for intravenous infusions.

72. Which of the following is immediate postoperative care for an infant diagnosed with hydrocephalus who had a shunt placed?
    1. Wet-to-dry dressing changes at both the shunt insertion site and the abdominal incision site.
    2. Inform the parents they will have to measure the child's head at least once a day.
    3. Position the infant's head off the shunt site for the first 2 postoperative days.
    4. Complete vital signs and neurological checks every 4 hours.

73. In preparing the patient and family for hospital discharge, which of the following signs and symptoms of shunt malfunction and infection should the nurse include in the teaching plan? Select all that apply.
    1. Emesis, lethargy.
    2. A change in neurological behavior.
    3. Fever, irritability.
    4. Diarrhea or constipation.
    5. Redness along the shunt system.

74. The parents of an infant with hydrocephalus ask about future activities in which their child can participate in school and as an adolescent. The nurse should tell the parents which of the following?
    1. A helmet should be worn during any activity that could lead to head injury.
    2. Only non-contact sports should be pursued, such as swimming or tennis.
    3. Because of the risk of shunt system infection, swimming is not a sports option.
    4. The child should wear a life alert bracelet; then there is no need to be aware of the shunt system.

75. While assisting with a lumbar puncture procedure on an infant or small child, the nurse should do which of the following?
    1. Have the patient in a clean diaper to avoid contamination of the site.
    2. Monitor the patient's cardiorespiratory status at all times.
    3. Position the patient in the prone position with the head to the left.
    4. Start an intravenous line to facilitate use of conscious sedation.

76. A 10-month-old has fallen out of the high chair and is brought to the emergency department. Put the following components of the nurse's assessment into the correct order.
    1. Airway____
    2. Bleeding____
    3. Appetite____
    4. Breathing____
    5. Circulation____
    6. Level of consciousness____

77. Guillain-Barré is a progressive motor weakness secondary to an autoimmune response from a viral illness or immunizations. Guillain-Barré shows which of the following symptoms? Select all that apply.
    1. Always fatal after 18 to 24 months.
    2. Progresses cephalocaudally.
    3. Complications are associated with immobility.
    4. Respiratory support is a nursing priority.
    5. Tube feedings or total parental nutrition may become necessary.

78. An adolescent Hispanic is complaining of knees swelling and hurting, hands and feet being cold all the time, frequent headaches, and a red rash on the cheeks and nose. The nurse suspects which of the following?
    1. Multiple sclerosis.
    2. Normal adolescent concerns.
    3. Myasthenia gravis.
    4. Systemic lupus erythematosus.

79. As a component of discharge teaching, the nurse knows that treatment regimen for a 15-year-old with systemic lupus erythematosus includes which of the following? Select all that apply.
    1. High-protein diet.
    2. Low salt intake.
    3. Exposure to the sun.
    4. Killed-virus vaccines.
    5. Systemic corticosteroids.
    6. Antimalarials.

80. A 12-year-old cut a hand while climbing a barb-wired fence. What should the nurse discuss with the parents regarding need for tetanus vaccine? Select all that apply.
    1. No tetanus vaccine is necessary; it is too soon.
    2. Tetanus is a potentially fatal disease.
    3. Puncture wounds are less susceptible to tetanus.
    4. There will be mild soreness at the injection site.
    5. Tdap should be administered.
    6. Td should be administered.

81. A parent calls the nurse for dosing information for Pepto-Bismol and aspirin for children who are 8 and 9 years old and are ill. The nurse states which of the following? Select all that apply.
    1. 1 tbs of Pepto-Bismol after every diarrhea stool.
    2. 81-mg baby aspirin every 4 hours.
    3. No medications are necessary.
    4. Pepto-Bismol contains aspirin.
    5. Diet as tolerated.
    6. Reye syndrome is associated with aspirin use.

82. In children with meningitis, there is the potential for many complications occurring from damage to the nervous system. Which of the following is/are the most common, nonlethal complication(s)?
    1. Cranial nerve deficits.
    2. Epilepsy.
    3. Bleeding intracranially.
    4. Cerebral palsy.

83. A child is admitted to the nurse's unit with a suspected diagnosis of meningitis. The nurse should tell the parent which of the following?
    1. Antibiotics are not initiated until the cerebrospinal fluid cultures are definitive for specificity to prevent resistance.
    2. Antibiotics are useless against viral infections, so they are not used for meningitis.
    3. Antibiotics should be started before the cerebrospinal fluid cultures are definitive because culture results may take up to 3 days.
    4. Antibiotic initiation is based on the age, signs, and symptoms of the patient, not on the causative agent.

84. A child arrives at the pediatric emergency department, having had a generalized seizure at home and a recent sore throat and mild fever. During the nurse's assessment, the child begins to have generalized tonic-clonic seizure activity. The drug of choice and method of administration the nurse expects the physician to order are which of the following?
    1. Lorezapam and diazepam, combined in an intravenous solution of D_5W.
    2. Lorezapam given intravenously or diazepam given directly into a vein.
    3. Phenobarbital administered in an intravenous solution of D_5W, 0.45 normal saline.
    4. Phenytoin in a dextrose solution given intravenously over 1 hour.

85. Parents of a child with generalized seizures ask the nurse for information to give their child's teachers. Which of the following should be included?
    1. A soft-padded spoon should be kept nearby to put between the child's teeth at the onset of a seizure.
    2. Roll the child onto the abdomen, with the head to the left, so any contents can flow from the mouth.
    3. If a seizure lasts longer than 10 minutes, the parents or an ambulance should be called.
    4. As the child grows, medication dosages may need to be adjusted to control seizure activity.

86. Which of the following best describes the type of seizure displayed in the figure?

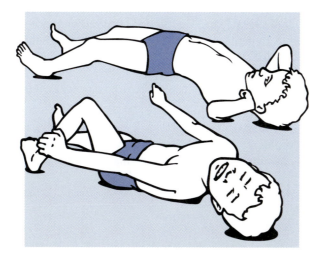

 1. Tonic-clonic.
 2. Absence.
 3. Atonic.
 4. Akinetic.
 5. Myoclonic.
 6. Infantile spasm.

87. Which of the following best describes the type of seizure displayed in the figure?

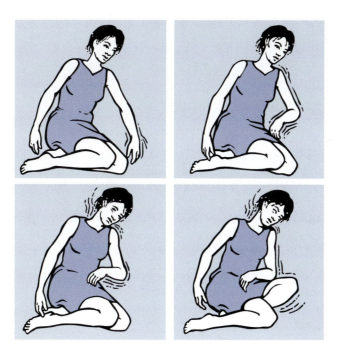

 1. Infantile spasm.
 2. Febrile seizure.
 3. Simple partial seizure with motor signs.
 4. Simple partial seizure with sensory signs.
 5. Atonic partial seizure.
 6. Absence seizure.

88. A 14-year-old sustained a grade III concussion while playing football. Which of the following statements made by the parents indicates that further patient education is needed?
    1. "Our child will not be able to play football until recovery is complete."
    2. "Our child needs to get back to school quickly, as there are midterms next week."
    3. "Our child's headaches may continue for the next 6 months; we should call the physician if the headaches get worse."
    4. "If our child suffers another concussion before recovery is complete, brain injury will be compounded."

89. The nurse is doing discharge teaching for a 3-month-old with a new shunt that was placed for hydrocephalus. Which of the following are signs and symptoms of hydrocephalus that the parents may see if the shunt malfunctions? Select all that apply.
    1. Vomiting.
    2. Irritability.
    3. Poor feeding.
    4. Headache.
    5. Sunken fontanel.
    6. Seizures.
    7. Inability to wake up infant.
    8. Hyperactivity.

90. When introducing solid foods into an infant's diet, it is important to introduce one food at a time in order to rule out _____.

91. The injection site of choice for a 6-month-old receiving immunizations is the _____.

92. Infants should ride in a _____ car seat until they weigh 9 kg and are approximately 1 year old.

93. According to Piaget, the school-age child is in the _____ stage of cognitive development.

94. According to Freud, the most significant achievement of toddlers is _____.

95. Seizures that originate in one hemisphere are called _____.

96. The term _____ is commonly defined as stiffness of the neck.

97. Which of the following applies to brain tumors? Select all that apply.
    1. Brain tumors are the most common malignancy in the United States.
    2. Although an exact cause is unknown, an association has been linked to paints and radiation.
    3. All children with brain tumors present with very similar manifestations.
    4. Brain tumors in children usually occur below the cerebellum.
    5. Symptoms of brain tumors always appear rapidly.

98. Which of the following applies to cerebral palsy? Select all that apply.
    1. It is the most common chronic disorder of childhood.
    2. Hyperbilirubinemia increases the risk of cerebral palsy.
    3. It is a progressive chronic disorder.
    4. Most children do not experience any learning disabilities.
    5. There is a familial tendency seen in children with cerebral palsy.

99. Which of the following applies to encephalitis? Select all that apply.
    1. Usually caused by a bacterial infection.
    2. A chronic disease.
    3. Most commonly seen after a varicella infection in the newborn population.
    4. Newborns diagnosed with encephalitis often have extensive neurological problems.
    5. Can be seen with meningitis.

100. Which approach gives the most support to parents grieving over a terminally ill newborn?
1. State "You are both still young and will be able to have more children."
2. Avoid the parents; let them ask you questions.
3. Offer rationalizations for the child's terminal illness.
4. State "You are still feeling all the pain of your child's illness."

1. 1. Newborns may not void spontaneously in the first 12 hours of life, but they void within the first 24 hours of life.
   2. Most, but not all, babies lose approximately 10% of their body weight in the first 3 to 4 days of life.
   3. **All infants, whether breastfed or bottle-fed, should regain their birth weight by 10 days of life.**
   4. Many babies do not initially awaken spontaneously for nursing; initially, the mother may need to offer the baby the breast every 2 to 3 hours.

   TEST-TAKING HINT: Infants gain weight once they are nursing.

2. 7.5.
   Change 3400 g to kg, and then multiply by 2.2 lb/kg. Divide 3400 g by 1000 g/kg = 3.4 kg. Multiply 3.4 kg by 2.2 lb/kg = 7.5 lb.

   TEST-TAKING HINT: The test taker must know the correct formulas and equivalencies to use.

3. 1. Hypotonia is of concern because a floppy, limp infant may have suffered a birth insult or has a genetic condition such as Down syndrome.
   2. Babies have a symmetric appearance and do not develop hand preference (asymmetry) until 18 to 24 months.
   3. Opisthotonic posture is an arched back and marked head lag, indicating a baby who is neurologically injured.
   4. **A full-term, healthy newborn initially has a flexion posture because it has been curled up in the uterus.**

   TEST-TAKING HINT: The nurse should expect to see an infant who has tone and strength, although not in its fully developed state.

4. 1. The Landau reflex occurs when the infant is suspended prone; the infant will raise the head and extend the trunk upward.
   2. Clonus is elicited by a brisk dorsiflexion of the foot that elicits oscillating movements of the ankles and knees.
   3. **A fencing posture describes an asymmetric tonic neck reflex and should disappear by 3 to 4 months of age.**
   4. The Moro reflex is another name for the startle reflex.

   TEST-TAKING HINT: The asymmetric tonic neck reflex is a specific posture that is assumed by the newborn when the head is turned or moved quickly.

5. 1. All states do newborn screening.
   2. **All states currently do screening for phenylketonuria and hypothyroidism.**
   3. Babies have to be nursing or feeding for 24 hours before the test is valid. If the baby goes home before the 24 hours, the newborn screen is repeated the next day.
   4. The baby will also be screened before discharge.

   TEST-TAKING HINT: The parents want to know what the test is looking for and not how or when the test is performed.

6. 1, 2, 4, 5.
   1. **Learn as much as possible about the child.**
   2. **Expect to have some conflict with cultural differences and age.**
   3. Children who are adopted when they are older than 2 years of age know their biological families and have feelings about their adoption. It is best to discuss this openly with the child.
   4. **Setting clear behavioral expectations for the child will aid in the assimilation to the family.**
   5. **It is always good to retain some part of their original name, such as a middle name, to maintain the link with their previous family and culture.**

   TEST-TAKING HINT: When children are older, they have memory of the previous family, and this will need to be incorporated into the rearing of the child.

7. 2, 3, 5.
   1. Young children who are experiencing a divorce have very poor self-esteem and blame themselves for the separation.
   2. **They exhibit loss of appetite and poor sleep patterns.**
   3. **Preschool and early school–aged children feel the parent who is leaving the family is abandoning them. They also develop increased anxiety.**
   4. Older school aged–children may become dictatorial and aggressive and show a decline in school performance.
   5. **The 5-year-old can verbalize feelings about divorce and the changes that are going to take place within the family.**

   TEST-TAKING HINT: This child is a young, school-aged child and is in the Piaget stage of ego formation.

8. **2, 3, 6.**
   1. Larger day cares do not necessarily have qualified staff and age-appropriate activities for the child or infant.
   2. **In choosing a day care, it is important for parents to see that the health and safety requirements of the law are maintained.**
   3. **Each child gets the attention that is required for maintaining a healthy, happy child. Caretakers should be loving and supportive of the children and parents.**
   4. Activities should be age-appropriate for the child.
   5. Child-care ratios should be small, as well as class size, and staff should not feel they have more work to do than they can manage.
   6. **Child-care ratios should be small, as well as class size, and staff should not feel they have more work to do than they can manage.**

   TEST-TAKING HINT: The infant is only 6 months old.

9. **1, C; 2, E; 3, F; 4, A; 5, D; 6, B.**

   TEST-TAKING HINT: First, match the word with the definition you know, then look for matches that are less familiar.

10. 1. Cleft lip and palate occur in many syndromes such as trisomy 13 and VATER association, but they are not associated with Turner syndrome.
    2. A weak, high-pitched cry is seen in babies with cri du chat.
    3. **A low-set posterior hairline, webbing of the neck, and lymphedema of the hands and feet are characteristic of Turner syndrome.**
    4. Small genitalia and long, thin arms and legs are seen with Klinefelter syndrome; this is seen only in males.

    TEST-TAKING HINT: Turner syndrome is a sex chromosome anomaly that is missing one complete X chromosome. It is the only known monosomy defect that produces a viable fetus.

11. 1. The triple marker screen, amniocentesis, and chorionic villus sampling require either a venipuncture or uterine puncture.
    2. **The ultrasound is appropriate for a noninvasive procedure. It would detect multiple gestations and structural abnormalities, but it would not detect biochemical abnormalities.**

3. The triple marker screen, amniocentesis, and chorionic villus sampling require either a venipuncture or uterine puncture.
4. The triple marker screen, amniocentesis, and chorionic villus sampling require either a venipuncture or uterine puncture.

TEST-TAKING HINT: The only test that does not require a blood sample is the ultrasound. Biochemical testing, however, should be encouraged because it will provide valuable information about the pregnancy.

12. 1. **In a probability equation, chance has no memory, and each pregnancy is an independent event.**
    2. The probability of having a child with cystic fibrosis is 1 chance in 4, whether the first or the fourth baby.
    3. The probability of having a child with cystic fibrosis is 1 chance in 4, whether the first or the fourth baby.
    4. The probability of having a child with cystic fibrosis is 1 chance in 4, whether the first or the fourth baby.

    TEST-TAKING HINT: Probability is a risk assessment term and denotes that a risk is present for the family.

13. 1. It is appropriate to develop a pedigree once the provider has discussed this issue with the patient.
    2. It is appropriate to take a family history once the provider has discussed this issue with the patient.
    3. **Working as a team with the provider and sharing this information enables the provider to make appropriate decisions.**
    4. It is appropriate to make a referral for genetic counseling once the provider has discussed this issue with the patient.

    TEST-TAKING HINT: The young woman is questioning whether mental retardation can be inherited. The provider will need to discuss what her understanding of that concept means to her.

14. 1. Some Jewish sects believe in numerous dietary kosher laws that they must follow.
    2. Muslims believe that Allah cures but sometimes works through humans to get treatment.
    3. Catholics encourage anointing of the sick.
    4. **Jehovah's Witnesses eat nothing that has come in contact with blood. They are opposed to transfusions, and many**

are opposed to albumin, globulin, and factor replacement. Generally, they are not opposed to non-blood plasma expanders.

TEST-TAKING HINT: The child's complete blood count is low, and the child will require blood or a blood volume expander.

15. 1, C; 2, B; 3, E; 4, D; 5, A.

TEST-TAKING HINT: Select the beliefs that are familiar within a specific culture to determine the country of origin, then consider cultural values to determine the ones you are less sure about.

16. 1. People tend to "do other things" while talking. The family does not hear well, so this will be inappropriate.
    2. **When communicating with parents who are hearing-impaired, maintain good eye contact, and allow them to read lips.**
    3. It is best to talk in short but concrete ideas, and for teaching complex material, drawings and charts should be used. Enunciate clearly, and talk slowly.
    4. The visit requires that the family be able to understand what is being said by the provider. A trained hearing dog is not part of this priority.

TEST-TAKING HINT: The parents are deaf. Scheduling an interpreter for the hearing-impaired will benefit the family in hearing the entire message. In helping the family benefit from the visit, also utilize the senses of sight, touch, and smell to communicate.

17. 1. The term "legally blind" means a person with central visual acuity of 20/200 or less in the better eye using corrective lens.
    2. This statement asks the teenager to tell if there is enough vision to read books, which may not be the case.
    3. **Having the teenager explain what can be seen will assist in learning the teen's visual capabilities. Asking the teenager to explain initiates rapport and builds trust.**
    4. This statement asks the teenager to tell you if there is enough vision to read books, which may not be the case.

TEST-TAKING HINT: This is a teenager with a chronic disability; therapeutic communication is always appropriate to use in interactions.

18. 1. Although washing the child's hands needs to occur, this is not the first priority.

2. Many eye injuries require immediate care with follow-up by an ophthalmologist.
3. Irrigating the eye, unless there is a chemical injury, may further irritate the eye problem. With chemical injuries, time is of the essence in diluting the chemical. This injury is stated to be a foreign body.
4. **Examine the eye, and check for a foreign body before attempting to treat the injury or determining the plan of action.**

TEST-TAKING HINT: The first step in the nursing process is to assess the problem.

19. 1. **Dysfluency is speech with abnormal rhythms, such as repetitions in sounds or words. A stutter is described as tense repetitions of sounds or complete blockages of sounds.**
    2. Children who substitute or omit consonants have articulation errors.
    3. A child who speaks in a monotone has a voice disorder. Hypernasal speech is prominent in children with palatal weakness and cleft palate repair.
    4. Hypernasal speech is prominent in children with cleft repairs of the hard and soft palate.

TEST-TAKING HINT: The definition of fluent speech is understandable speech.

20. 1. It is important to discuss the findings that the parents have presented and not peripheral information that may or may not be necessary to their concern.
    2. **Children with autistic-like features lack many social skills, such as seeking reciprocity and comfort from parents and maintaining eye contact when someone is speaking with them. They have an inability to develop peer relationships.**
    3. It is important to discuss the findings that the parents have presented and not peripheral information that may or may not be necessary to their concern.
    4. It is important to discuss the findings that the parents have presented and not peripheral information that may or may not be necessary to their concern.

TEST-TAKING HINT: Autism is a complex developmental disorder that presents with behavioral and intellectual deficits. Language acquisition is an indicator of cognitive development.

21. 1. Post-concussion syndrome is a common finding in children who have suffered a head injury. Symptoms in the infant include pallor, sweating, irritability, and sleepiness. The symptoms begin within minutes to hours.
2. Plethora and hyperthermia may indicate a number of problems, such as being overdressed, crying, and stress.
3. Crying with fear in an 8-month-old is an expected behavior at this time.
4. Babies have a positive Babinski reflex until they are 2 years old; after that, it should be a negative finding.

TEST-TAKING HINT: Post-concussion syndrome is common in children younger than 1 year who have suffered a head injury.

22. 1. Babies who have failure to thrive can tolerate a cows' milk formula, but they need to have a diet modifier to increase calories, such as polycose powder or medium-chain triglycerides oil.
2. **Babies taking Neocate formula have sensitivity to cows' milk proteins as well as soy and hydrolyzed proteins. The parent is describing symptoms of a cows' milk allergy and mentions there are many family members with allergies.**
3. Phenylketonuria is an inborn error of metabolism, and the infants are placed on a low phenylalanine formula, such as LoFenalac.
4. Portagen formula is used to nourish babies with pancreatic insufficiency or intestinal resections.

TEST-TAKING HINT: Consider the symptoms and the history of allergies in other family members.

23. 1. This is an important vital sign to assess, but it is not specific to cutis marmorata.
2. This is an important vital sign to assess, but it is not specific to cutis marmorata.
3. This is an important vital sign to assess, but it is not specific to cutis marmorata.
4. **Cutis marmorata is transient mottling of the body when the infant is exposed to cold. It is important to check the baby's temperature. Cutis marmorata is a change in the color of the skin.**

TEST-TAKING HINT: This question involves a newborn.

24. 1. Placing the baby supine will compromise the function of the good lung.

2. To optimize the baby's breathing, position the baby with the affected side down. In this way, the good lung can expand fully. Babies are primarily thoracic breathers, so it is important to maximize use of the good lung. The baby also has an Erb/brachial palsy, which further limits the function on the affected side.
3. Placing the baby on the unaffected side will decrease the ability to expand the good lung maximally and increase the work of breathing.
4. Placing the baby prone compromises the function of the good lung.

TEST-TAKING HINT: A phrenic nerve paralysis results in diaphragmatic paralysis and paradoxical chest movements.

25. 1. The baby would not have a hepatitis B titer unless the mother was hepatitis B–positive.
2. **This baby has an ABO blood incompatability, with the mother being O+ and the baby being A+. The total bilirubin is a value that combines the unconjugated and the conjugated bilirubin levels. The newborn would have an increase in the unconjugated bilirubin (lipid-soluble) as a result of the presence of antibodies to the mother's blood type.**
3. The complete blood count does not necessarily explain the jaundice.
4. The sedimentation rate indicates inflammation somewhere in the body.

TEST-TAKING HINT: The baby is 2 days old; the mother's blood is O+; and the baby's blood is A+. Mothers with O+ blood type have the antibodies to types A and B, regardless of whether they have had other children.

26. 1. The baby is already becoming increasingly jaundiced and, if the bilirubin level is not controlled, runs the risk of kernicterus.
2. Lethargy is symptomatic of a number of risks that a newborn might encounter, such as sepsis, dehydration, and hypothermia.
3. **The signs of a blood exchange transfusion reaction are focused on an unstable temperature. If the newborn becomes too cool, the infant could develop respiratory distress or bradycardia. If the baby's temperature becomes too high, there would be a dramatic change in blood pressure, with either hypertension or hypotension causing vascular**

collapse. If the baby becomes hyperthermic, the donor red blood cells
could also be damaged, further
increasing the jaundice.
4. Irritability would be symptomatic of a
number of risks that a newborn might
encounter, such as sepsis, dehydration,
hypothermia.

**TEST-TAKING HINT: The question is asking
for signs of a transfusion reaction in a
newborn.**

27. **250 mg.**
Convert the weight of 22 lb to kilograms.
There are 2.2 kg per pound of body weight, so
divide 22 lb by 2.2. The baby weighs 10 kg. By
multiplying 10 kg by 25 mg/kg recommendation per day, the total intake of phenylalanine
per day for this infant is 250 mg.

**TEST-TAKING HINT: The test taker must
know the correct formulas and equivalencies to use.**

28. **1, 3, 4.**
   1. **Wrapping the foot in a warm wash-
cloth increases the vasodilation and
makes obtaining the sample easier.**
   2. Using EMLA cream on the heel before
the stick has not been shown to decrease
the pain response of the infant.
   3. **Swaddling appears very effective in
decreasing neonatal pain.**
   4. **Non-nutritive sucking appears very effective in decreasing neonatal pain.**
   5. The baby will feel the pain whether asleep
or awake.

**TEST-TAKING HINT: The question is asking
for nursing measures that will help decrease the pain with a heel stick.**

29. 1. The Pain Assessment Tool would not
likely be used on an inpatient unit other
than a neonatal intensive care unit.
   2. The Neonatal Infant Pain Scale would not
likely be used on an inpatient unit other
than a neonatal intensive care unit.
   3. The Premature Infant Pain Profile would
not likely be used on an inpatient unit
other than a neonatal intensive care unit.
   4. **The acronym POPS stands for
Post-Operative Pain Score.**

**TEST-TAKING HINT: The acronym indicates
the name of the correct test.**

30. **1, 2, 3, 5.**
   1. A polysomnogram can record the heart
rate and respirations.
   2. A polysomnogram can record the brain
waves.

3. A polysomnogram can record the eye
movements and body movements.
4. Unless the child is being videotaped while
asleep, the polysomnogram is not able to
pick up cyanosis or plethora.
5. **A polysomnogram can record the
end-tidal carbon dioxide.**

**TEST-TAKING HINT: A polysomnogram is a
complex diagnostic tool that records electrical and muscle movements.**

31. **Cognitive.**
Piaget's late phase of sensorimotor development occurs between 12 and 24 months and
is a time when cognitive development occurs
rapidly. Reasoning skills are still very primi-
tive. The main cognitive skill of early childhood is language acquisition.

**TEST-TAKING HINT: Language acquisition is
the main cognitive achievement of early
childhood.**

32. 1. Preoperational thought starts around
2 years of age and continues until late
in the third year.
   2. Toddlers are self-centered, but they are
curious and want to learn. They love to
explore their environment and try new
things.
   3. **Toddlers think in very broad terms; it
is difficult for them to see that changing the bed will not change the entire
process of sleeping. Global organization is when change in one part of the
whole changes the entire whole.**
   4. The toddler is globally afraid of changes
but is not phobic about the bed.

**TEST-TAKING HINT: Preoperational thought
implies that the child does not think in
logical patterns. Global organization is
changing one part and affecting the entire
thing.**

33. **1, 2, 3, 5.**
   1. **Many children who have difficulty
with temper tantrums are described
by the family as "bad" or "difficult" in
all aspects of their life. This description often carries over into all the
activities and conversations that the
family has with the child and degrades
the positive aspects of the child's
personality.**
   2. **Tantrums are frequently associated
with only one aspect of a child's life,
and this should be identified quickly so
that changes can be instituted in the
approach to the problem.**

3. **Tantrums that result in harm to the child or to others should be dealt with quickly; professional help may be needed.**
4. The Internet is a frequent source of conflicting information, but families frequently seek help from it. Not all the information on the Internet is appropriate or correct.
5. **Discipline and inappropriate behavior management techniques may worsen the temper tantrums.**

TEST-TAKING HINT: Consider the child's age and what are appropriate and inappropriate behaviors for this age.

34. 1. It would be more appropriate for the parents to tell the child what "might" happen at the visit rather than say the visit will not hurt. Often, children perceive simple activities such as looking in the mouth or touching the skin as invasive and hurtful.
2. Telling the child that there are consequences for having fear of something new is inappropriate.
3. **Modeling appropriate behavior for the child by having the child go with a parent creates a positive preparation for attending the dentist.**
4. Bribing a child to "be good" sets up a negative approach to teaching a child. The child will then want a treat for every visit to the dentist.

TEST-TAKING HINT: The parents may be projecting their fear of the dentist onto the child.

35. **1, 2, 5.**
1. **Hiding the bottle and offering a cup is a good way to start to wean a toddler.**
2. **Putting only drinking water in the bottle is a good way to start to wean a toddler.**
3. Nighttime bottles should be discontinued as soon as the child is able to drink fluids from the cup. Nighttime bottles allow the milk or formula to coat the teeth all night long, encouraging tooth decay.
4. Starting to use a pacifier with a toddler who should be weaned from the bottle by 11 to 12 months of age is inappropriate.
5. **Nighttime bottles should be discontinued as soon as the child is able to drink fluids from the cup. Nighttime bottles allow the milk or formula to coat the teeth all night long, encouraging tooth decay.**

TEST-TAKING HINT: Weaning should occur before the first birthday unless medically

indicated. The bottle should be less appealing and less available to the child once the child is able to drink from a cup.

36. 1. The parents have indicated that neither one has the motivation or time to do the toilet training.
2. **The child is 2 years old and may not be physically, emotionally, or psychologically ready to toilet train.**
3. A toddler will say "no" to most questions; that does not make the child stubborn.
4. Having the child sit on the toilet for more than 2 or 3 minutes is inappropriate.

TEST-TAKING HINT: Most children initiate toilet training at 18 to 24 months on their own.

37. **2, 3, 4.**
1. The safest place for a child to ride in a car is in the middle of the back seat.
2. **Legally, a child must weigh 60 lb and be 8 years old to ride in a seat belt without a booster.**
3. **The seat belt, whether in a booster or on a seat, should be worn low on the hips and not across the abdomen.**
4. **The shoulder strap, for safety purposes, should be across the chest and not across the face or neck.**
5. Tether straps help to secure the seat belt in position when using a car seat or booster seat and should not be optional.

TEST-TAKING HINT: The child's age and weight determine the seat belt/booster seat requirements.

38. 1. Fifth disease is caused by the parvovirus, and the rash is initially described as "slapped cheek," with this impression lasting 3 to 4 days.
2. Roseola is caused by herpesvirus type 6 and is usually seen in children from 6 months to 3 years of age.
3. Scarlet fever is a bacterial disease and has a rash that feels like sandpaper.
4. **The most likely diagnosis for this child is chickenpox, which is caused by the varicella zoster virus. This is commonly seen in young children and is highly contagious to others in the classroom and at home. It initially presents with a high fever for 3 to 4 days.**

TEST-TAKING HINT: The pruritic nature of the rash and the distribution primarily on the trunk in clusters and patches give clues as to its cause.

39. 2, 4.
1. Young children absorb most of the lead that enters their body.
2. **Homes built between 1900 and 1950 most likely contain lead-based paints.**
3. The acceptable blood level is 2.3 mcg or less.
4. **Lead can affect any part of the body, but the brain, nervous system, kidneys, and blood are likely to be most affected.**
5. In Hispanic and Arabic cultures, some painted jars in which candy is stored are painted with lead paints. Some medicinals, such as Azarcon, Greta, Paylooh, Surma, and Lozeena, are sources of lead.

TEST-TAKING HINT: Low-income families are often at risk for lead exposure. Often, families who have immigrated from other countries are unaware of risks such as lead toxicity in the community.

40. 95th/90th.
The blood pressure table for boys 1 to 17 years is based on height for age. The vertical column represents the percentiles for a specific age. The horizontal columns represent the percentiles of blood pressure for a specific height. Locating the blood pressure percentile shows the systolic pressure to be in the 95th percentile and the diastolic pressure to be in the 90th percentile.

TEST-TAKING HINT: Find the 50th percentile vertical line for systolic pressure, and follow it to age 9. Find the 50th percentile on the vertical line for diastolic pressure, and follow it to age 9.

41. 1. The American Academy of Pediatrics recommends a daily intake of 0.4 mg of folic acid daily for all women of childbearing age.
2. Although eating fruits and vegetables is part of a healthy lifestyle, the young woman will not gain any additional folic acid in her diet through those foods.
3. Although eating fruits and vegetables and eating breakfast is part of a healthy lifestyle, the young woman will not gain any additional folic acid in her diet through those foods.
4. The addition of folic acid at 0.4 mg daily to the diet will decrease the risk of having a baby with a neural tube defect by 50% to 70%.

TEST-TAKING HINT: The teen is looking for a suggestion for preventing neural tube defects.

42. 30.
Change the height to inches. Locate the height of 65 inches on the vertical axis. Locate the weight of 180 lb on the horizontal axis on the same line as the height. Look up at the basal metabolic index line at the top, and it indicates the BMI is 30. This classifies as obese.

TEST-TAKING HINT: Weight for a person's height is the determinate of a BMI.

43. appendix.
The appendix is used to create the stoma between the bladder and the abdominal wall. The abdominal stoma allows the young woman to perform the clean intermittent catheterization comfortably with less dexterity required.

TEST-TAKING HINT: The family is looking for an alternate way to do clean intermittent catheterizations. The appendix is not a necessary piece of bowel, so it can be utilized easily for this procedure.

44. 1. Giving antihistamines and steroids before and after procedures will help to decrease the response to the exposure.
2. **The most important intervention for any person with latex allergy or sensitivity is to prevent contact with latex products.**
3. Once the radioallergosorbent test confirms that a person is allergic to latex, the test does not need to be repeated.
4. Using latex-free gloves is one way to decrease exposure to latex.

TEST-TAKING HINT: This is a known allergy in a child at risk for latex sensitivity or allergy.

45. 1. Arnold-Chiari malformation is a herniation of the brainstem into the cervical spinal canal through the foramen magnum.
2. Anencephaly is absence of the brain.
3. Tethering of the spinal cord occurs when the tissue surrounding the cord adheres to the underlying bony or tissue structure of the spinal canal.
4. Perinatal hemorrhage is one cause of hydrocephalus but is not a brain malformation.

TEST-TAKING HINT: Type 2 Arnold-Chiari malformation is frequently seen in infants and children with myelomeningocele.

46. 1. Diaper dermatitis should be assessed with the diaper change, but it is not specific to the risks of wearing a Pavlik harness.

2. Talipes equinovarus is congenital clubfeet and does not occur as a result of the harness.

3. An infant wearing a Pavlik harness is at risk of leg shortening on the affected side and limited abduction. The straps on the harness may need adjustment and lengthening frequently.

4. Pain of any kind warrants further assessment.

TEST-TAKING HINT: The child has hip dysplasia and is wearing a corrective (therapeutic) device, the Pavlik harness. It is important to check for problems or complications that are caused by the harness.

47. 1. Infants with clefts of the palate are at greater risk for ear infections once they are eating and sucking on a breast or bottle.

2. It is important to help the mother bond with the baby, but nursing or sucking on the bottle helps to create positive feelings between the baby and the mother.

3. The cleft palate is not repaired until the baby is closer to 9 to 11 months of age when speech begins.

4. The primary goal of any newborn with a cleft palate is to establish feeding and sucking.

TEST-TAKING HINT: Getting started with feeding and nursing is difficult for the newborn with a cleft palate.

48. **gastroschisis.**
   A herniation of the abdominal wall without a peritoneal sac and intestines penetrating outside the abdominal cavity is a gastroschisis.

   TEST-TAKING HINT: The stem of the word, "gastroc," is stomach, and "schisis" is a split. This is different from an omphalocele, which has the peritoneal sac present and intact.

49. 1. The National Advisory Committee on Immunizations is a subgroup of the U.S. Public Health Service. The American Medical Association makes recommendations on adult care.

2. The two organizations in the United States that govern the recommendations on immunization practices are the Advisory Committee on Immunization Practices (ACIP) of the U.S. Public Health Service and the Committee on Infectious Diseases of the American Academy of Pediatrics.

3. The National Immunization Program is a part of the U. S. Public Health Service. Pediatric Infectious Disease Committee makes recommendations on treatment of known infectious diseases in children.

4. Canada has its own advisory committee called the National Advisory Committee on Immunization under the Minister of the National Health and Welfare Department.

TEST-TAKING HINT: The United States Public Health Service is the umbrella organization for all national health issues. The American Academy of Pediatrics has been instrumental in combating infectious diseases in the United States and publishes the Red Book on recommendations for preventing and managing infectious diseases in children.

50. 1. EMLA cream does not decrease local reactions.

2. EMLA cream does not decrease local reactions, and changing the needle has not been shown to decrease local reactions.

3. The vastus lateralis and the ventrogluteal muscles are recommended sites for a child of any age. The deltoid muscle can be used in children over 18 months of age.

4. Using distraction will minimize pain but not minimize local reactions.

TEST-TAKING HINT: The question is asking for a procedure that the nurse can perform to minimize local reactions.

51. 1. Mitral regurgitation is best heard between S_2 and the beginning of S_1. It is accentuated by exercise.

2. The S_2 sound is caused by the closure of the pulmonic and aortic valves. A fixed splitting of the S_2 sound is indicative of an atrial septal defect.

3. A functional murmur does not denote a cardiac defect but may indicate anemia or some other physiological abnormality.

4. The pericardial friction rub is a high-pitched grating sound that is indicative of pericarditis.

TEST-TAKING HINT: The S_1 sounds are caused by closure of the tricuspid and mitral valves. The question involves an S_2 sound and is indicative of closure of the semilunar valves.

52. **1, 3, 5.**
   1. An innocent murmur does not have an anatomic or physiological abnormality;

it is a sound of short duration, grade III or less, and is best heard in the pulmonic area of the chest (second intercostal space close to the sternum).

2. An S_2 murmur is considered pathological until proved otherwise.

3. **An innocent murmur does not have an anatomic or physiological abnormality; it is a sound of short duration, grade III or less, and is best heard in the pulmonic area of the chest (second intercostal space close to the sternum).**

4. Murmurs that are innocent or functional vary in their intensity and the position in which they can be heard. Pathological murmurs are fixed and radiate throughout the chest.

5. **An innocent murmur does not have an anatomic or physiological abnormality; it is a sound of short duration, grade III or less, and is heard best in the pulmonic area of the chest (second intercostal space close to the sternum).**

TEST-TAKING HINT: This is an otherwise healthy child. The Erb point (second and third intercostal space, midclavicular) is a frequent site to locate innocent murmurs.

53. fremitus.
The conduction of voice sounds through the chest and respiratory tract is called vocal fremitus. The decrease in fremitus indicates obstruction in the airways, as would occur with asthma or pneumothorax. The increase in fremitus occurs with pneumonia.

TEST-TAKING HINT: Fremitus is the conduction of voice sounds through the respiratory tract.

54. 1, 2, 3.
1. **The nurse should alert the parents to the fact that the child may have some blood-tinged secretions for a few days afterwards.**
2. **Using a cool mist vaporizer helps to decrease the viscosity of the secretions. Pain relief every 4 hours is indicated.**
3. **Using a cool mist vaporizer helps to decrease the viscosity of the secretions. Pain relief every 4 hours is indicated.**
4. The child should not be eating foods that are rough or fibrous but rather stay on a soft or liquid diet for a few days to allow healing.
5. Blowing the nose and coughing are contraindicated because this may loosen the clot that has formed over the surgical site.

TEST-TAKING HINT: The care and comfort measures are those that enable the parents to relieve pain and have decreased stress and worry about the surgery.

55. 1. **Weaning the toddler off the bottle is the best tactic.**
2. Giving the toddler a decongestant before bedtime is not recommended because the primary problem is obstruction of the eustachian tube due to intrinsic or extrinsic causes. Decongestants thicken and make passage of fluid out of the middle ear more difficult.
3. Smoking outside the house is frequently recommended as a way to prevent exposure of second-hand smoke to children, but the smoke still clings to the parents' clothing and hands and continues to be a source.
4. Following treatment for otitis media, it is important to have the child's hearing checked because drainage from the middle ear may persist beyond the days of treatment. It will not prevent recurrence of the otitis media.

TEST-TAKING HINT: The question is asking for a major preventive measure for otitis media.

56. 1. Laryngotracheobronchitis is seen in infants and young school-aged children and is viral in origin with accompanying symptoms of brassy cough, low-grade fever, hoarseness, but otherwise well appearance.
2. Bacterial tracheitis is caused by staphylococcus with a croupy cough, purulent secretions, high fever, and a need for antibiotics.
3. Asthma is a chronic inflammatory disease of the airways. In susceptible children, inflammation causes cough, wheezing, and chest tightness.
4. **This is the history of a child with acute spasmodic laryngitis. Symptoms of inflammation are absent or mild. Some children are thought to be predisposed to this with allergy or psychogenic factors as an underlying cause.**

TEST-TAKING HINT: The child is well during the day and asymptomatic for fever or loss of appetite.

57. 1. RespiGam is also a prophylactic for respiratory syncytial virus, but it is primarily an immunoglobulin G that provides neutralizing antibodies against subtypes A and B of the virus. It must be given intravenously

monthly, which is more difficult in terms of administration.

2. Ribavirin is an antiviral agent and is given in a hospital for treatment of respiratory syncytial virus.

3. **The American Academy of Pediatrics recommends that infants born before 32 weeks gestation and younger than 2 years who have chronic lung disease should receive palivizumab (Synagis) monthly as a prophylactic to prevent respiratory syncytial virus during the winter months.**

4. The pneumococcal vaccine could be given during these 5 months but would not protect the infant from respiratory syncytial virus.

TEST-TAKING HINT: The infant is premature, and the winter season is starting.

58. 1. Chlamydial pneumonia is a sexually transmitted disease that would not be expected unless sexual abuse had occurred.

2. **The chronic infectious illness for which this child is at risk is tuberculosis. The disease may present as asymptomatic or include fever, enlarged lymph nodes, anorexia, weight loss, night sweats, and, occasionally, hemoptysis. It is recommended that Mantoux skin tests be performed annually for at-risk populations such as the homeless, first-generation immigrants, and residents of correctional facilities.**

3. Pertussis is an acute respiratory tract infection that lasts approximately 4 to 6 weeks.

4. Asthma is not contagious.

TEST-TAKING HINT: Tuberculosis is on the rise in homeless and immigrant populations, and the child is in both categories.

59. 1, 3, 4.

1. **The lice can be seen crawling about on the scalp.**

2. The nits can be described as "looking like dandruff," but it could also be dandruff or seborrhea that is seen.

3. **Nits can be seen, especially behind the ears and the nape of the neck and close to the hair shaft.**

4. **Often there are scratch marks and inflammatory papules as a result of the itching and scratching of the scalp.**

5. Head lice can be found in short and long hair and even in coarse curly hair.

TEST-TAKING HINT: Pediculosis capitis is common in classrooms. Because of the

frequency, many schools require the nurse to see the louse walking on the scalp before exclusion from the classroom is permitted. Nits can be confused with dandruff, hair spray, and lint.

60. 1. Enuresis is bed-wetting, which can have an array of causes.

2. It is important to rule out sexual abuse before deciding on the attention deficit/hyperactivity disorder diagnosis. It is also important to have a medical provider do a complete physical examination and have both the teacher and the family complete behavioral checklists before making that diagnosis.

3. It is important to rule out a learning disability before deciding on the attention deficit/hyperactivity disorder diagnosis. It is also important to have a medical provider do a complete physical examination and have both the teacher and the family complete behavioral checklists before making that diagnosis.

4. **The most likely diagnosis is attention deficit/hyperactivity disorder because the child has the classic symptoms.**

TEST-TAKING HINT: Classic symptoms of attention deficit/hyperactivity disorder are impulsiveness (talking loud), inattentiveness (difficulty organizing work), hyperactive-impulsive behavior (moodiness and unable to finish assigned class work).

61. 1. **Extrapyramidal symptoms are motor neuron responses that go from the brain to the spinal cord and present as tics, jerkiness, incoordination, and loss of involuntary muscle control.**

2. The medication is given to control the inappropriate behaviors, such as aggressiveness. If the symptoms started with the medication, it would be important to report this to the provider.

3. The medication is given to control inappropriate behaviors, such as aggressiveness. If the symptoms started with the medication, it would be important to report this to the provider.

4. Thoughts of depression would warrant further evaluation of the appropriate medication for treatment.

TEST-TAKING HINT: Pyramidal tracts control voluntary muscle movements, such as balance and walking. Extrapyramidal tracts are those that control involuntary motor movements, such as tics, twitches, and spasms.

62. 1. **A Tanner stage II male (early puberty) shows signs of an enlarging penis and loosening of scrotal skin. Puberty occurs from 9½ to 14 years for typical growing boys.**
    2. Height spurts occur toward the end of mid-puberty.
    3. Mid-puberty shows signs of breast enlargement (gynecomastia) due to elevated estrogen levels. This is temporary.
    4. A deepening of the voice occurs with changes in the larynx toward the end of puberty.

    TEST-TAKING HINT: This is a Tanner stage II male.

63. **anovular.**
    Young women who have periods more frequently than every 21 days, after ruling out sexually transmitted diseases, are anovulatory. These young women have adequate estrogen levels but inadequate progesterone levels. Unopposed estrogen can place a young woman at risk for endometrial carcinoma.

    TEST-TAKING HINT: The young woman is an athlete and has also lost weight.

64. 1. Using examples of short-term consequences, such as stained teeth, unpleasant odor, and stains on fingers, will emphasize the teens' most immediate needs of being accepted by their peers. These unpleasant effects may appear attractive.
    2. Teens feel they are "invincible" and safe from harm.
    3. **It is always best to focus on prevention of smoking, and take a positive approach to how a teen might resist smoking. Peer support groups work well in redefining the teens' peer groups and gives them tactics to use against smoking.**
    4. Talking with parents is not always an option for a teen.

    TEST-TAKING HINT: Teens are interested in becoming adults and are increasingly concerned about how their peer group sees them.

65. 1. Skin testing is done by an allergist to help determine triggers for the asthma.
    2. Taking PCO_2 levels would be helpful but would require the provider to order a blood gas.
    3. A metered dose inhaler is the device that is used to administer the medications.
    4. **The Expert Panel recommends that peak flow monitoring be used in** children with asthma to determine the severity of an exacerbation and to guide therapeutic decision making.

    TEST-TAKING HINT: The child has moderate asthma. The peak flowmeter is recommended for all children with moderate-to-severe asthma as a simple tool for offices and for patient home use.

66. **1, 3.**
    1. **Leukotriene modifiers such as montelukast are given orally and are indicated for add-on to low-dose inhaled corticosteroids in moderate persistent asthma.**
    2. The leuketriene modifiers are appropriate for children as young as 2 years old.
    3. **The leukotriene modifiers are not to be used for acute asthma attacks.**
    4. Although the parents should give up smoking and for the sake of their child's asthma, it is not affected by the medication.
    5. Chest physiotherapy is beneficial for children who are motivated and can help with respiratory distress. It is not affected by the use of montelukast.

    TEST-TAKING HINT: The child has moderate persistent asthma and is currently taking low-dose medications.

67. 1. **The ethical principle of double effect states that an action has good intentions and that a bad intention is permissible if the action itself is good or neutral, the good effect must not be produced by the bad effect, and there is a compelling reason to allow the bad effect to occur if the good effect is the primary reason for the action. The child may require doses of pain relievers higher than is considered safe in order to relieve the pain. If the child dies during this treatment, the overwhelming reason for the excess medication was to make the child comfortable and decrease the intense pain.**
    2. There is no principle of cultural influences. There is only acknowledgment of cultural differences in the dying process, honesty in dealing with the child and the family, and using pain medication to relieve pain as indicated by the circumstances.
    3. There is no principle of honesty. There is only acknowledgment of cultural differences in the dying process, honesty in dealing with the child and the family, and using pain medication to relieve pain as indicated by the circumstances.

4. There is no principle of withholding pain medication. There is only acknowledgment of cultural differences in the dying process, honesty in dealing with the child and the family, and using pain medication to relieve pain as indicated by the circumstances.

TEST-TAKING HINT: The child is terminally ill and in great pain.

68. 1. The parents obviously want their son cared for in the best and safest manner possible.
2. The parents may not have other relatives who are capable or willing to take care of the child.
3. **It is always best to ask the parents what plan of care has already been instituted.**
4. Many social service agencies have counselors who can assist parents with developing a specific plan and asking the right questions. Before offering this service it is important to ask if they already have a plan of care.

TEST-TAKING HINT: The parents are asking the nurse about a very personal decision. This is a very emotional issue and should be dealt with accordingly.

69. 1. All children with Down syndrome have mental retardation.
2. **Atlantoaxial instability is ligamentous laxity of the atlantoaxial joint. The symptoms of neck pain, torticollis, and loss of bowel and bladder control indicate that instability is already present. The purpose of the x-rays is to prevent symptoms by limiting activities if instability is present.**
3. Children with Down syndrome may have vision and hearing loss and should be screened before 2 years of age for both.
4. Children with Down syndrome attain puberty at the same age as nondisabled children.

TEST-TAKING HINT: Children with Down syndrome have hypotonia, and the more active they become, the more they are at risk for displacement of the atlantoaxial joint.

70. 1. These are signs of increased intracranial pressure in an older child.
2. Confusion is not easily assessed in an infant.
3. These are signs of increased intracranial pressure in an older child.
4. **Previously undiagnosed, one of the first signs of hydrocephalus is a bulging**

fontanel, followed by irritability, poor feeding, and overall rapid head growth.

TEST-TAKING HINT: The test taker should recognize that examination of fontanel and head circumference is a mainstay of the infant examination.

71. 1. No products that interfere with levels of consciousness are used so as not to confuse assessment.
2. The head of the crib is slightly elevated to help decrease intracranial pressure.
3. Infants with hydrocephalus are often irritable and do not sleep well.
4. **These may interfere with surgery and shunt placement.**

TEST-TAKING HINT: Answer 4 should be known by a nurse about any patient who is having surgery on the head.

72. 1. Dressings should be dry and free of drainage.
2. Once a shunt is determined to be functioning properly, head measurements are done at office visits.
3. **Position the head on the side opposite the surgical site to prevent pressure on the shunt and valve. This provides better visibility to watch for signs of bleeding or infection.**
4. Vital signs and neurological checks will be performed much more frequently, usually every 1 to 2 hours initially.

TEST-TAKING HINT: Knowing postoperative care, the test taker can eliminate answers 1 and 4.

73. 1, 2, 3, 5.
1. **Emesis and lethargy can be signs of increased intracranial pressure and may indicate an infectious process.**
2. **A change in behavior can be a sign of increased intracranial pressure and can be a sign of shunt malfunction.**
3. **Fever and irritability can be an indication of a possible shunt infection.**
4. Although diarrhea may be a sign of illness, it is usually not a shunt complication, nor is constipation.
5. **Redness along the shunt system can be an indication of a possible infectious process.**

TEST-TAKING HINT: The test taker should be able to identify signs of increase intracranial pressure and signs of infection.

74. 1. **The risk of shunt breakage or obstruction is extremely low.**
2. There is no reason why athletics need be restricted. Recent studies have shown little evidence of shunt injury or malfunction with sport participation.
3. The shunt is a sterile, closed system, without any external opening so there is no risk of infection from swimming.
4. Even with the alert bracelet, close contacts should be aware to provide care, if necessary.

TEST-TAKING HINT: The test taker may assume a child with a shunt may be at higher risk of injury.

75. 1. Diapers are kept rolled down and out of the way during a lumbar puncture.
2. **Airway, breathing, and circulation are always the priority during procedures.**
3. Positioning the patient should facilitate the opening of the vertebral spaces, either by a lateral or sitting-type position.
4. Conscious sedation is not utilized during a lumbar puncture.

TEST-TAKING HINT: Cardiorespiratory status is always the priority in any procedure.

76. 1, 4, 5, 6, 2, 3.
1. **Always first priority to assess.**
4. **Second aspect of ABC priority.**
5. **Third aspect of ABC priority.**
6. **Important after stabilization of the "ABC."**
2. **Important but not first priority.**
3. **Least important.**

TEST-TAKING HINT: The test taker should always assess ABCs first.

77. 3, 4, 5.
1. Progressive but full recovery is possible, taking months to years.
2. Neuromuscular progression is from feet to head.
3. **Due to the progressive paralysis, immobility is a major concern.**
4. **The respiratory tract muscles may become compromised with the progression.**
5. **Adequate calorie intake is essential to prevent catabolism.**

TEST-TAKING HINT: The test taker should be able to eliminate answer 1 because in nursing there are few absolutes. Just knowing that some sort of immobility is involved should lead the test taker to answers 3, 4, and 5.

78. 1. Multiple sclerosis appears initially as a neurological disorder.
2. The offered signs and symptoms are not normal in any age group.
3. Myasthenia gravis is a neuromuscular disorder.
4. **Butterfly rash, arthritic symptoms, Raynaud phenomenon (cold hands and feet), and headaches when all are seen together, are indicative of systemic lupus erythematosus.**

TEST-TAKING HINT: The test taker should know symptoms of all the involved diseases to determine which one it is.

79. 2, 4, 5, 6.
1. Low protein to keep BUN within normal range.
2. **Low salt to help control blood pressure.**
3. Worsens butterfly rash.
4. **More susceptible to infections and a lowered immune response.**
5. **First line therapy.**
6. **Indicated treatment.**

TEST-TAKING HINT: Butterfly rash should be recognized as a sign of lupus erythematosus and that it will worsen with sun exposure.

80. 2, 5.
1. Required tetanus boosters are given at 5 years of age. If a "dirty" wound occurs before 10 years after the last dose, a booster is necessary.
2. **Tetanus is a potentially fatal disease.**
3. Puncture wounds are more susceptible to tetanus, especially in rural areas.
4. This is a possible side effect of tetanus vaccine.
5. **Due to the increase in incidence of pertussis in adolescents and adults, this is the vaccine of choice.**
6. No longer the vaccine of choice, tetanus/diphtheria/pertussis is the vaccine used to help control the growing incidence of pertussis.

TEST-TAKING HINT: Pertussis outbreaks are occurring as immunity wanes, so there is a need to use tetanus/diphtheria/pertussis for boosters.

81. 3, 4, 5, 6.
1. Pepto-Bismol contains bismuth subsalicylate, an aspirin component, and is contraindicated in children.
2. Aspirin is contraindicated in children with viral symptoms due to the association with Reye syndrome.

3. **Allow the body to rid itself of harmful agents. This is first-line advice.**
4. **Pepto-Bismol contains bismuth subsalicylate, an aspirin component.**
5. **This is first-line advice if there is no vomiting.**
6. **Reye syndrome is associated with aspirin use and viral illness in children.**

TEST-TAKING HINT: Many people are unaware of the aspirin in Pepto-Bismol and the link to Reye syndrome.

82. 1. **If infection extends into the area of the cranial nerves, increased pressure may cause sensory deficits.**
2. Although this is a possible complication, it is not the most common.
3. Although there is often purpura and petechiae with meningitis, there is no intracranial bleeding.
4. This condition is usually an injury incurred during the neonatal period.

TEST-TAKING HINT: The test taker should know about complications in children with bacterial meningitis. With meningitis there is an increase in intracranial pressure which can put pressure on the cranial nerves.

83. 1. A delay in administering antibiotics can be fatal.
2. Cerebrospinal fluid cultures may require up to 3 days to determine the causative agent.
3. **Immediate antibiotic therapy is necessary to prevent death and avoid disabilities.**
4. Antibiotic choice is based on the most likely causative agent for that particular age group. If the culture indicates a resistant organism, the antibiotic can be changed.

TEST-TAKING HINT: The test taker may be tempted to choose answer 2 if the urgency of early treatment is not understood.

84. 1. Although these are the correct drugs, they are not administered simultaneously.
2. **These continue to be the drugs of choice for in-hospital management of tonic-clonic activity. These are the recommended methods of administration; diazepam compromises intravenous tubing.**
3. Phenobarbital is not the drug of choice for in-hospital management of tonic-clonic activity.
4. Intravenous phenytoin is given by slow intravenous push. Dextrose causes phenytoin to precipitate.

TEST-TAKING HINT: The test taker needs to know emergency care of a child having tonic-clonic seizures.

85. 1. Trying to insert something into a seizing person's mouth can lead to injury.
2. Anyone having a seizure should be rolled onto the side.
3. If a child has seizure activity at school, the parent should be notified as soon as possible.
4. **Growth spurts occur, and medications will need to be adjusted. Teachers should be made aware and notify a parent or guardian if they notice even mild seizure activity.**

TEST-TAKING HINT: Answer 3 can be eliminated because the test taker should recognize the need for full communication between school and home. Also, seizure activity lasting more than 5 minutes requires medical attention.

86. 1. Tonic-clonic seizures consist of sustained, generalized stiffening of the muscles in symmetric, rhythmic contractions and relaxations of major muscle groups. Level of consciousness is impaired.
2. **Absence seizures are characterized by a blank stare and no muscle activity.**
3. Atonic seizures are characterized by an abrupt loss of tone.
4. Akinetic seizure is another term for atonic seizure.
5. Myoclonic seizures are characterized by sudden contractures of a muscle or muscle group.
6. Infantile spasms occur during the first year of life.

TEST-TAKING HINT: Answer 6 can be eliminated by the age of the child depicted.

87. 1. Infantile seizures occur during the first year of life.
2. Febrile seizures occur in young children, usually before 4 years.
3. **There is no change in the level of consciousness; motor symptoms are evident.**
4. No sensory involvement is depicted.
5. Atonic seizures are characterized by an abrupt loss of tone.
6. Absence seizures are characterized by a blank stare with no muscle activity.

TEST-TAKING HINT: Answers 1 and 2 can be eliminated by the age of the patient depicted.

88. 1. This statement indicates that the parents understand the potential severe consequences of receiving a second concussion while recovering from the first one. Football is a contact sport in which there is an increased risk of concussion. The child should not participate in contact sports until cleared by the physician.
  2. **Short-term memory loss is a frequent side effect of concussions. Until effects of the concussion have subsided and the child is cleared by a physician, the child should not take school tests that often rely on short-term memory.**
  3. Headaches can occur for up to 6 months after the initial impact. Headaches that continue to worsen, however, could be indicative of the development of other injuries.
  4. This statement indicates that the parents understand the potential severe consequences of receiving a second concussion while recovering from the first one.

TEST-TAKING HINT: Because answers 1 and 4 have the same rationale, the choice is further limited to either answer 2 or 3.

89. 1, 2, 3, 6, 7.
  1. **As the shunt malfunctions and cerebrospinal fluid builds up, the child will exhibit symptoms of increased intracranial pressure. Vomiting is one of the possible signs of increased intracranial pressure.**
  2. **As the shunt malfunctions and cerebrospinal fluid builds up, the child will exhibit symptoms of increased intracranial pressure. Irritability and change in neurological status are two of the possible signs of increased intracranial pressure.**
  3. **As the shunt malfunctions and cerebrospinal fluid builds up, the child will exhibit symptoms of increased intracranial pressure. Poor feeding is one of the possible signs of increased intracranial pressure.**
  4. As the shunt malfunctions and cerebrospinal fluid builds up, the child will exhibit symptoms of increased intracranial pressure. Headache is very difficult to assess in an infant.
  5. A sunken fontanel is a sign of dehydration. With increased intracranial pressure, the brain is edematous and expands in size. This would result in an enlarged rather than a sunken fontanel.
  6. **As the shunt malfunctions and cerebrospinal fluid builds up, the child will exhibit symptoms of increased intracranial pressure. Seizure is one possible sign of increased intracranial pressure.**
  7. **As the shunt malfunctions and cerebrospinal fluid builds up, the child will exhibit symptoms of increased intracranial pressure. A declining neurological status evidenced by the inability to wake a child up is one of the possible signs of increased intracranial pressure.**
  8. A declining neurological status is a sign of increased intracranial pressure. Hyperactivity is not a sign of a declining neurological status.

TEST-TAKING HINT: The test taker needs to knows signs of increased intracranial pressure.

90. Allergies.
Infants should be introduced to solid foods after 6 months of age. Iron-fortified infant cereals are recommended first, followed by the introduction of vegetables, then fruits. New foods should be introduced about every 3 to 5 days so the caregiver has the opportunity to identify any food allergies the baby may have.

TEST-TAKING HINT: The question requires knowledge of the nutritional needs of an infant as well as the safety concerns that involve children of this age.

91. Vastus lateralis.
The vastus lateralis muscle can be used for immunizations of children of all ages. It is a particularly good choice for infants because it is the most developed muscle for this age group. This area is also appealing because it has few major nerves and blood vessels.

TEST-TAKING HINT: The test taker must have knowledge of intramuscular injection sites and acceptable volumes for children of varying ages.

92. Rear-facing.
An infant should always ride in a rear-facing car seat until older than 1 year and over 9 kg.

TEST-TAKING HINT: The question requires knowledge of infant safety.

93. Concrete operations.
During the concrete operations stage of cognitive development, the school-age child is able to take into account another person's point of view. School-age children are also able to classify, sort, and organize facts in order to use them for problem solving.

TEST-TAKING HINT: The question requires knowledge of Piaget's stages of cognitive development.

94. Toilet training.
Freud believed that during the anal-urethral stage of psychosexual development, a child must achieve toilet training. Freud believed that children may have long-lasting difficulties if they do not master toilet training.

TEST-TAKING HINT: The question requires knowledge of Freud's stages of development.

95. Partial or focal seizures.
Seizures originating in both hemispheres are called generalized seizures.

TEST-TAKING HINT: The question requires knowledge of names of different seizure types.

96. Nuchal rigidity.
Nuchal rigidity is assessed when a child has a fever or appears septic.

TEST-TAKING HINT: The test taker needs to know how a health-care provider commonly assesses for meningitis.

97. 2, 4.
1. Brain tumors are the most common solid tumor. Leukemia is the most common malignancy in the United States.
2. **Although an exact cause is unknown, an association has been linked to paints and radiation.**
3. The manifestations can vary depending on where the tumor is located.
4. **Brain tumors in children usually occur below the cerebellum. Brain tumors in adults usually occur above the cerebellum.**
5. Symptoms of brain tumors can appear rapidly or slowly, depending on whether the tumor is fast- or slow-growing.

TEST-TAKING HINT: The test taker can eliminate answer 1 because brain tumors are not the most common malignancy in the United States.

98. 1, 2.
1. **Cerebral palsy is the most common chronic disorder of childhood.**
2. **There is an increased risk of cerebral palsy in infants with hyperbilirubinemia.**
3. Cerebral palsy is a nonprogressive chronic disorder.
4. Approximately 75% of children with cerebral palsy experience learning disabilities.

5. There is no familial tendency seen in children with cerebral palsy.

TEST-TAKING HINT: The test taker needs to have a good knowledge of cerebral palsy.

99. 4, 5.
1. Although it can be caused by a variety of organisms, encephalitis is usually a viral infection.
2. Encephalitis is an acute disease.
3. Encephalitis is most commonly seen after a herpes infection in the newborn population. It is often seen after a varicella infection in older children.
4. **Newborns diagnosed with encephalitis often have extensive neurological problems.**
5. **Encephalitis can be seen with meningitis.**

TEST-TAKING HINT: The test taker should be led to answers 4 and 5 by knowing that encephalitis is usually viral in origin.

100. 1. State "You are both still young and will be able to have more children."
2. Avoid the parents; let them ask you questions.
3. Offer rationalizations for the child's terminal illness.
4. **State "You are still feeling all the pain of your child's illness."**
Support to grieving families varies with the needs of the family. General guidelines in support of grieving families are to deal openly with their feelings and accept the family's grief response. Avoid judgmental or rationalizing statements. Focus on their feelings. Provide referral to self-help groups or professional help if appropriate.

TEST-TAKING HINT: The test taker should understand that answers 1, 2, and 3 are incorrect. General guidelines in support of grieving families are to deal openly with their feelings of grief, pain, guilt, anger, or loss. Stay with the family either sitting quietly or talking, if they indicate a need to talk. Avoid offering rationalizations for the child's terminal illness.

Glossary

Absence seizure — Temporary loss of consciousness.

Acute renal failure — Acute failure of the kidney to perform its essential functions. May be due to trauma; any condition that impairs flow of blood to the kidneys; toxins such as mercury, tetrachloride, or ethylene glycol; bacterial toxins; glomerulonephritis; acute obstruction of the urinary tract.

Adrenal gland — Triangular gland covering superior surface of each kidney; composed of outer cortex and inner medulla.

Advocacy — Promotion of rights of individuals or groups, including self-determination, autonomy, respect, equality, dignity.

Airway — Passageway for air to and from lungs; device used to prevent or correct obstructed respiratory passages.

Akinetic seizure (drop attack) — Sudden, momentary loss of muscle tone.

Albuminemia — Level of albumin in the blood.

Alcohol poisoning — Consuming and absorbing too much alcohol.

Anemia — Reduction in number of circulating red blood cells; exists when hemoglobin content less than that required to provide oxygen demands of body.

Anencephaly — Congenital absence of brain and spinal cord.

Anorectal malformation — Congenital deformity of anus and rectum.

Anterior fontanel — Unossified space or soft spot at junction of coronal, frontal, and sagittal sutures.

Anticholinergic — Agent that blocks parasympathetic nerve impulses; effects include dry mouth and blurred vision.

Anticipatory guidance — Information concerning normal expectations of age group or disease entity in order to provide support for coping and problems before they arise.

Antipyretic — Fever-reducing agent, such as acetaminophen.

Apgar score — System of scoring infant's physical condition 1 minute and 5 minutes after birth; includes heart rate, respiration, muscle tone, response to stimuli and color; each rated 0, 1, or 2; maximum total score 10.

Aplastic anemia — Caused by deficient red cell production due to disorders of bone marrow.

Appendectomy — Surgical procedure to remove appendix.

Appendix — Worm-shaped process projecting from the blind end of the cecum.

Aspirated — Drawing in or out as by suction; foreign bodies may be aspirated into the nose, throat, or lungs on inspiration; withdrawing of fluid from a cavity by suction.

Assent — Process by which children (younger than 18 years) give consent for medical treatment.

Assessment — Obtaining a careful and complete history from the patient; physical examination to determine how a disease process has altered physical and mental status.

Atonic seizure — Generalized seizure with sudden loss of muscle tone; may be sudden drop of the head.

Atrophy — Wasting or decrease in size of muscles.

Auscultate — Listening for sounds within the body.

Autonomy — Functioning independently.

Autosomal-dominant — Trait or characteristic expressed in offspring, even though trait is carried on only one of the homologous chromosomes.

Azotorrhea — Excessive loss of nitrogenous products through urine and feces.

β-thalassemia (Cooley anemia) — Resulting from inheritance of a recessive trait responsible for interference with rate of hemoglobin synthesis.

Bacterial endocarditis — Bacterial infection of muscle that lines heart; usually confined to external lining of valve.

Bacterial meningitis — Bacterial inflammation of lining of brain and spinal column.

Benzoyl peroxide — Keratolytic agent.

Bile — Secretion of liver; passes from bile duct of liver into common bile duct and into duodenum as needed.

Biliary atresia — Closure or absence of some or all of major bile ducts.

Bladder exstrophy — Congenital eversion of urinary bladder; abdominal wall fails to close, and inside of bladder may be seen to protrude through abdominal wall.

Bowel obstruction — Blockage of lumen of intestine.

Brachycephaly — Coronal suture fuses prematurely and results in a wide head.

Bradycardia — Slow heart rate.

Bronchiectasis — Chronic dilatation of a bronchus or bronchi with a secondary infection that usually involves the lower portion of the lung.

Bronchoscopy — Examination of bronchi through a bronchoscope.

Brudzinski sign — Test for meningeal inflammation; child lies supine with neck flexed; positive result occurs if resistance to flexion occurs.

Carbon monoxide poisoning — Poisoning can occur from small amounts of carbon monoxide inhaled over a long time or from large amounts inhaled in a short time.

Cardiac demand — Amount of blood needed for normal filling pressures to meet metabolic demands.

Celiac disease — Intestinal malabsorption syndrome; characterized by diarrhea, malnutrition, bleeding tendency, and hypocalcemia.

Central nervous system prophylaxis — Chemotherapeutic drugs administered intrathecally to prevent cancer in central nervous system.

Cerebellum — Portion of brain connected to brainstem and involved in synergic control of skeletal muscles; plays a role in coordination of voluntary muscular movements.

Cerebral palsy — Nonprogressive paralysis resulting from developmental defects in brain or trauma at birth.

Cerebrospinal fluid — Water cushion protecting brain and spinal cord from physical impact.

Cervical spine precautions — Stabilization of cervical spine to prevent injury.

Chelation therapy — Removal of metallic ions held by chemical bonds from blood and soft tissues, bone, and brain.

Child abuse — Emotional, physical, or sexual abuse of a child.

Child-proofing measures — Removal of objects identified as being harmful to a child.

Cholestyramine — Resin used to treat itching associated with jaundice.

Chronic renal failure — Failure of kidneys to perform their essential functions for a long time; may be due to trauma, toxins, obstruction, or infection.

Chronically ill child — Living with a long-term illness.

Circulation — Movement in a regular or circular course.

Cleft lip — Congenital cleft or separation of upper lip.

Cleft palate — Congenital fissure in roof of mouth, forming a communicating passageway between mouth and nasal cavities.

Coma — Abnormal deep stupor occurring in illness, as a result of illness or due to an injury.

Compartment syndrome — Condition in which a structure, such as a nerve or tendon, is constricted in a space.

Concussion — Common result of a blow to the head; usually causes unconsciousness.

Confidentiality — Right to privacy of the medical record and other health information.

Confusion — Not being aware of or oriented to time, place, or person.

Congenital — Present at birth.

Congenital aganglionic megacolon (Hirschsprung disease) — Due to failure of development of myenteric plexus of retrosigmoid area of the large intestine; colon above inactive area dilates, and there is chronic constipation.

Congenital heart disease — Any pathological condition of the heart that is diagnosed at birth.

Congenital heart failure — Heart failure diagnosed at birth.

Congenital hypothyroidism — Due to deficiency of thyroid secretion, resulting in lowered basal metabolism; diagnosed at birth.

Consciousness — State of awareness; implies an orientation to time, place, and person.

Constipation — Difficult defecation; infrequent defecation, with passage of unduly hard and dry fecal material.

Contact precautions — Used to prevent exposure to a contagious disease.

Contracture — Shortening of muscle or scar tissue, resulting in deformity.

Craniosynostosis — Premature closure of skull sutures.

Croup — Childhood disease characterized by barking cough, laryngeal spasm.

Cryptorchidism — Failure of testicle to descent into the scrotum.

Cushing triad — Bradycardia; irregular respirations and hypertension.

Cystic fibrosis — Inherited disease of exocrine glands affecting pancreas, respiratory system, and apocrine glands.

Decerebrate posturing — Extremities stiff and extended, head retracted.

Decorticate posturing — Posture of patient with lesion at or above upper brainstem; patient rigid with arms flexed, fists clenched, and legs extended.

Defects with decreased pulmonary flow — Obstruction of pulmonary blood flow with another defect, such as atrial septal defect.

Defects with increased pulmonary flow — Increased blood volume on right side of heart; increases pulmonary blood flow; e.g., ventricular septal defect.

Dehydration — Condition resulting from excessive loss of body fluid.

Delegation — Assigning or sharing activities with other individuals who have appropriate authority to accomplish task.

Delirium — State of mental confusion and excitement characterized by disorientation to time, place.

Detachment — Becoming separate.

Diabetes insipidus — Polyuria and polydipsia; caused by inadequate secretion of vasopressin (antidiuretic hormone).

Dialysate — Fluid used to remove or deliver compounds or electrolytes that the failing kidney cannot excrete or retain in the proper concentration.

Diarrhea — Frequent passage of unformed watery bowel movements.

Disequilibrium syndrome — Neurological signs and symptoms caused by cerebral edema in patients undergoing dialysis.

Droplet (airborne) precaution — Type of standard precaution; patient may have a serious illness transmitted by airborne droplet, such as varicella and tuberculosis.

Dysphagia — Inability or difficulty in swallowing.

Dystrophy — Disorder in which muscles weaken and atrophy.

Edema — Local or generalized condition in which body tissues contain excessive amount of tissue fluid.

Encephalitis — Inflammation of brain.

Encopresis — Associated with constipation and fecal retention.

Enema — Solution introduced into rectum and colon to stimulate bowel activity to cause emptying of lower intestine.

Enterocolitis — Inflammation of intestines and colon.

Enuresis — Involuntary discharge of urine after the age by which bladder control should have been established.

Epidural hematoma — Blood located over or upon dura.

Epiglottitis — Inflammation of epiglottis, which is a thin leaf-shaped structure located immediately posterior to root of tongue.

Epilepsy — Recurrent seizure pattern.

Epinephrine 1:1000 subcutaneous injection — Drug used as cardiac stimulant and vasoconstrictor and to relax bronchioles.

Epispadias — Congenital opening of urethra on dorsum of penis.

Erythema infectiosum (fifth disease) — Viral illness with rash on face (slapped-cheek appearance), arms, and legs.

Esophageal atresia — Esophagus ends in a blind pouch instead of stomach.

Esophagus — Muscular canal extending from pharynx to stomach.

Ethical principles — Principles relating to moral actions and value systems: autonomy, beneficence, nonmaleficence, veracity, justice, fidelity.

Eustachian tube — Auditory tube extending from middle ear to pharynx.

Exanthema subitum (roseola) — Viral illness in young children; has a rose-pink macular rash.

Factor VIII deficiency (hemophilia A) — Bleeding disorder resulting from congenital absence of factor VIII (antihemophilic factor).

Fiber — Components of food that are resistant to chemical digestion; includes portions of food made up of cellulose, hemicelluloses, and pectin.

Fistula — Abnormal tube-like passage from a normal cavity or tube to a free surface or to another cavity; can be congenital or can result from abscesses, injuries, or inflammatory processes.

Fluid maintenance — Volume needed to replace fluid losses from insensible, evaporative, and fluid lost through urine and feces.

Followership — Assertive use of personal behaviors that contribute to health-care team achievement in collaboration with leaders and managers.

Fundus — Larger part; base or body of a hollow organ; portion of an organ most remote from its opening.

Galactosemia — Inborn error of metabolism; inherited as autosomal recessive trait.

Gastroenteritis — Inflammation of stomach and intestinal tract.

Gastroesophageal reflux — Persistent reflux of acid contents of stomach into lower esophageal area.

Gastrostomy tube — Surgical insertion of a tube primarily to supply nutrition.

Genetic counseling — Application of what is known about human genetics in providing advice to those concerned about possibility of their offspring being free of hereditary abnormality.

Glomerulonephritis — Form of nephritis in which lesions involve primarily the glomeruli; may be acute, subacute, or chronic; frequently follows infection of upper respiratory tract due to particular strains of streptococci.

Gluten — Protein found in wheat, rye, and barley.

GoLYTELY — Trade name for polyethylene glycol electrolyte; gastrointestinal lavage solution.

Gonadotropin — Gonad-stimulating hormone.

Grief reaction — Emotional reaction following loss of a love object.

Growth hormone — Hormone liberated by anterior pituitary; important in regulating growth.

Gynecomastia — Development of abnormally large mammary gland in the male.

Heimlich maneuver — Technique for removing a foreign body from trachea or pharynx.

Hemarthrosis — Bloody effusion into cavity of a joint.

Hematuria — Hematin in urine.

Hemiplegia — Paralysis of half the body.

Hemodialysis — Method for providing function of the kidneys by circulating blood through tubes of semipermeable membranes.

Hemolytic uremic syndrome — Acute condition consisting of microangiopathic hemolytic anemia, thrombocytopenia, and acute nephropathy; etiology unknown.

Hemophilia — X-linked hereditary blood disorder characterized by greatly prolonged coagulation time; blood fails to clot, and abnormal bleeding occurs.

Hepatitis — Inflammation of liver; may be caused by a variety of agents, including viral infections, bacterial invasion, and physical or chemical agents.

Hepatitis B — Hepatitis caused by hepatitis B virus.

Hepatitis B surface antigen — Antigen to hepatitis B virus.

Hepatitis B immune globulin — Standard solution consisting of globulins derived from blood plasma of human donors who have high titers of antibodies against hepatitis B.

Hepatitis B vaccine — Vaccine prepared directly from human blood; used to vaccinate persons at high risk of coming in contact with carriers of hepatitis B or with blood or fluids from such individuals.

Hirschsprung disease — Megacolon due to failure of development of myenteric plexus of rectosigmoid area of large intestine.

Hodgkin disease — Disease of unknown etiology producing enlargement of lymphoid tissue, spleen, and liver with invasion of other tissues.

Hydrocephalus — Increased accumulation of cerebrospinal fluid within brain ventricles.

Hydronephrosis — Collection of urine in the renal pelvis due to obstructed outflow.

Hyperthyroidism — Disease caused by excessive levels of thyroid hormone.

Hypospadias — Abnormal congenital opening of urethra on undersurface of penis.

Hypothyroidism — Clinical consequences of inadequate levels of thyroid hormone.

Hypotonia — Decreased muscle tone.

Immunosuppressive — Acting to suppress body's natural immune response to an antigen.

Imperforate anus — Anus without an opening.

Informed consent — Consent for medical treatment based on legal capacity, voluntary action, and comprehension.

Inguinal hernia — Hernia in inguinal area.

Intestinal villi — Multiple minute projections of intestinal mucosa into lumen of small intestines.

Intracranial pressure — Pressure of cerebrospinal fluid in subarachnoid space between skull and brain.

Intradermal — Within substance of the skin.

Intrathecal chemotherapy — Chemotherapeutic administered into spinal column.

Intussusception — Inner segment of intestine pushed into another segment.

Jaundice — Condition causing yellowness of skin, whites of eyes, mucous membranes, and body fluids due to deposition of bile pigment resulting from excess bilirubin in the blood.

Jejunal biopsy — Biopsy of portion of jejunum.

Kasai procedure — Used to treat biliary atresia; small intestine used to create a bile duct; rest of intestine attached to side of small intestine.

Kawasaki disease — Mucocutaneous lymph-node syndrome.

Kernig sign — Symptom of meningitis; evidenced by reflex contraction and pain in hamstring muscles when attempting to extend leg after flexing the thigh upon the body.

Ketogenic diet — Diet that produces acetone or ketone bodies or mild acidosis.

Lead poisoning — Usually chronic; caused by ingestion or inhalation of large amount of lead, causing damage to central and peripheral nervous systems, the blood-forming organs, and gastrointestinal tract.

Leadership — Use of personal traits and power to influence others toward a shared vision or goal.

Leukemia — Acute or chronic disease characterized by unrestrained growth of leukocytes and their precursors in tissues; classified according to dominant cell type and severity of disease.

Low-phenylalanine diet — Diet having decreased amounts of essential amino acids; used in treatment of phenylketonuria.

Malabsorption — Inadequate absorption of nutrients from intestinal tract, especially small bowel.

Malaise — Discomfort, uneasiness, or indisposition; often indicative of infection.

Malignancy — Neoplasm or tumor that is cancerous.

Malpractice — Failure of a health-care professional to act in a reasonable and prudent manner.

Management — Process of providing structure and direction to accomplish prescribed organizational goals.

Maple syrup urine disease — Inherited metabolic disease involving defective amino acid metabolism; named because of characteristic odor of the urine and sweat.

Meningitis — Inflammation of spinal cord or brain.

Meningocele — Congenital hernia in which meninges protrude through opening of skull or spinal column.

Mentor — Experienced professionals who provide guidance to new members of a profession.

Miscarriages — Termination of pregnancy at any time before fetus has attained extrauterine viability.

Mucositis — Inflammation of mucous membrane.

Munchausen syndrome by proxy — One person fabricates an illness and induces it in another.

Myelomeningocele — Spina bifida, with portion of cord and membranes protruding.

Myxedema — Clinical and metabolic manifestations of hypothyroidism.

Nasal decongestant — Agent that reduces nasal swelling.

Near-drowning — Asphyxiation due to immersion in liquid.

Necrotizing enterocolitis — Severe disease of newborn, especially those prematurely born; inflammation of intestines and colon.

Nephrotic syndrome — End result of a variety of diseases that damage capillary wall of arteries of glomerulus; leads to loss of large amount of protein in urine that, in turn, results in hypoalbuminemia and edema.

Neuroblastoma — Malignant hemorrhagic tumor composed principally of cells resembling neuroblasts that give rise to cells of sympathetic system.

Neurogenic bladder — Dysfunction from lesions of central nervous system or nerves supplying the bladder.

Neurogenic shock — Sudden loss of autonomic nervous system signals to smooth muscle in vessel walls.

Neurological checks — Assessment of the neurological system, including vital signs, level of consciousness, muscle activity and strength, and pupillary response.

Neutropenia — Abnormally small number of neutrophil cells in blood.

Newborn assessment — History and physical examination of a newborn.

Nissen fundoplication — Surgical reduction of size of opening into fundus of stomach and suturing the removed end of the esophagus.

Non-Hodgkin lymphoma — Cancer that starts in lymph glands.

Normal growth and development — Expected growth (height, weight, head size) and achieving expected developmental milestones.

Nuchal rigidity — Stiff neck.

Nurse practice act — Law or statute in each state that outlines the scope of nursing practice in that state.

Nursing intervention — All aspects of nursing care for patients; requires full knowledge of assessment and planning stages.

Obstructive defects — Blockage of a structure that prevents it from functioning properly.

Obtunded — Too dull or blunt as sensitivity to pain.

Occult blood — Blood in such minute quantity that it can be recognized only by microscopic examination or by chemical means.

Opaque — Impenetrable by visible light rays or by other forms of radiant energy such as x-rays.

Osmotic pressure — Pressure that develops when two solutions of different concentrations are separated by semipermeable membrane.

Osteosarcoma — Malignant tumor of bone.

Otitis media — Inflammation of middle ear.

100% Oxygen via nonrebreather mask — Used in medical emergencies to deliver oxygen to patients who can breathe on their own.

Palpate — To examine by touch or feel.

Pancreas — Gland located behind stomach; both an exocrine and endocrine gland.

Pancytopenia — Reduction in all cellular elements of blood.

Patient-controlled analgesia — Drug administration method that permits patient to control rate of drug delivery to control pain.

Pediatric trauma — Physical injury or wound in a child caused by external force or violence.

Peristalsis — Progressive wave-like movement that occurs involuntarily in hollow tubes of the body, especially alimentary canal.

Peritoneal dialysis — Removal of toxic substances from body by perfusing specific warm sterile chemical solutions through peritoneal cavity.

Peritonitis — Inflammation of peritoneum.

Pharyngitis — Inflammation of pharynx.

Phimosis — Stenosis or narrowness of preputial orifice so that foreskin cannot be pushed back over glans penis.

Pituitary gland ("master gland") — Endocrine gland that secretes hormones, which include growth and reproductive hormones.

Pneumothorax — Collection of air or gas in pleural cavity.

Poisoning — State produced by introduction of poison into the body.

Polycythemia — Excess of red blood cells.

Polycythemia vera — Chronic, life-shortening, myeloproliferative disorder involving all bone-marrow elements.

Polyhydramnios — Excess of amniotic fluid in the bag of waters in pregnancy.

Posturing — Attitude or position of body.

Prioritization — Organization of work to emphasize accomplishing tasks that take precedence over others.

Proteinuria — Protein; usually albumin in the urine.

Purpura — Condition characterized by hemorrhages into the skin, mucous membranes, internal organs, and other tissues.

Pyloric stenosis — Narrowing of pyloric orifice.

Reed-Sternberg cells — Giant connective tissue cells with one or two large nuclei that are characteristic of Hodgkin disease.

Renal diet — Used in treatment of chronic renal failure; protein restricted to meet recommended dietary guidelines for age; phosphorus may be restricted; minerals such as potassium may be restricted.

Respiratory precautions — Part of universal precautions for infection prevention and control; to prevent transmission of respiratory infections; may involve use of mask or isolation for patient.

Reticulocyte — A red blood cell containing network of granules or filaments representing an immature stage in development.

Reye syndrome — Syndrome characterized by acute encephalopathy and fatty infiltration of liver and possibly pancreas, heart, kidney, spleen, and lymph nodes.

Rheumatic fever — Systematic, febrile disease that is inflammatory and nonsuppurative in nature and variable in severity, duration, and sequelae; frequently from severe heart or kidney disease.

Risk management — Process of identifying, analyzing, and treating potential hazards in a given health-care setting.

Rotavirus — Group of viruses that are a major cause of epidemic acute gastroenteritis and sporadic acute enteritis in infants and small children.

Rovsing sign — Palpation or percussion of another part of abdomen that causes tenderness in right lower quadrant.

Scope of practice — Actions and duties allowable in nursing practice, as defined by each state's nurse practice act.

Seizure — Sudden attack of pain, disease, or certain symptoms.

Serial neurological assessments — Neurological assessments taken at frequent intervals.

Sexual abuse — Misuse of or excessive or improper use of sex with an underage child.

Shaken baby syndrome — Closed-head injury caused by baby being shaken.

Short-bowel syndrome — Inadequate absorption of ingested nutrients due to a surgical procedure in which considerable length of intestinal tract has been removed or bypassed.

Sickle cell anemia — Hereditary chronic form of anemia in which abnormal sickle or crescent-shaped erythrocytes are present; due to presence of abnormal type of hemoglobin (hemoglobin S) in red blood cells.

Spasticity — Increase in muscle tone.

Special needs child — Child who has special health-care needs, such as a child with chronic illness, is developmentally delayed, or has a congenital disability.

Spina bifida occulta — Failure of vertebrae to close without hernia protrusion.

Spinal cord injury — Usually the result of trauma causing some type of physical disability.

Splenic sequestration — Pooling of quantities of blood in spleen causing a decrease in circulating blood volume; found in children with sickle cell disease and beta thalassemia.

Sputum — Substance expelled by coughing or clearing the throat.

Steatorrhea — Fatty stools seen in pancreatic diseases.

Stoma — Artificially created opening between two passages or body cavities or between a cavity or passage and the body's surface.

Stool — Waste matter discharged from bowels.

Stridor — Harsh sound during respiration; high-pitched and resembling blowing of the wind due to obstruction of air passages.

Subdural hematoma — Hematoma located beneath dura; usually result of head injuries.

Subglottic — Beneath glottis.

Sudden infant death syndrome — Completely unexpected and unexplained death of an apparently well, or virtually well, infant.

Supine — Lying on the back.

Sympathomimetic — Adrenergic.

Tachycardia — Abnormally rapid heartbeat.

Tachypnea — Abnormally rapid respiratory rate.

Tay-Sachs disease — Autosomal-recessive trait inherited disease characterized by neurological deterioration.

Terminally ill child — Child suffering from disease that will cause death.

Testicular torsion — Twisting of testicle.

Therapeutic open communication — Foundation of clinical nursing practice; promotion of development of another person by building trust.

Thrombocytopenea — Abnormal decrease in number of blood platelets.

Tonsillectomy — Surgical procedure to remove tonsils.

Total parenteral nutrition — Provides vital nutrients intravenously in those who cannot eat enough nutrients for growth.

Tracheoesophageal fistula — See **Esophageal atresia.**

Tracheostomy — Incising skin over trachea and making a surgical wound in the trachea in order to permit an airway during tracheal obstruction.

Trendelenburg position — Patient's head in low and body and legs are on elevated and inclined plane.

Tuberculosis — Infectious disease caused by the tubercle bacillus *Mycobacterium tuberculosis*; characterized pathologically by inflammatory infiltrations, formation of tubercles, caseation, necrosis, abscesses, fibrosis, and calcification primarily in the respiratory system.

Type I diabetes mellitus — Chronic metabolic disorder marked by hyperglycemia; presents as acute illness with dehydration and often ketoacidosis.

Type II diabetes mellitus — Chronic metabolic disorder often asymptomatic in early years.

Umbilical hernia — Protrusion of hernia sac containing intestine at inguinal opening.

Urinary tract infection — Infection of urinary tract with microorganisms.

Vaccine information statement — Statement of information about a vaccine.

Varicella (chickenpox) — Acute, highly contagious viral disease; characterized by an eruption that makes its appearance in successive crops and passes through stages of macules, papules, vesicles, and crusts.

Vaso-occlusive crises — Most common type of crisis in children with sickle cell disease; may have local or generalized pain due to ischemia.

Vastus lateralis — One of three muscles of thigh.

Ventricle — A small cavity; either of two lower chambers of the heart; one of the cavities of brain.

Ventriculoperitoneal shunt — Catheter diverting cerebrospinal fluid, usually from lateral ventricle to peritoneum.

Vesicant — Agent used to produce blisters.

Vesicoureteral reflux — Urine flowing back from bladder to a ureter.

Vomiting — Ejection through mouth of gastric contents.

Von Willebrand disease — Congenital bleeding disorder.

Wheezing — Production of whistling sounds during difficult breathing, such as in asthma.

Wilms tumor — Rapidly developing tumor of kidney; usually occurs in children.

Yankauer suction — A device with both proximal and distal ends; proximal end with an elongated suction tip; distal end connects to a suction source.

Index